PHARMACOLOGY - RESEARCH, SAFETY TESTING AND REGULATION

MEDICINAL PLANTS AND SUSTAINABLE DEVELOPMENT

PHARMACOLOGY - RESEARCH, SAFETY TESTING AND REGULATION

Additional books in this series can be found on Nova's website
under the Series tab.

Additional E-books in this series can be found on Nova's website
under the E-books tab.

BOTANICAL RESEARCH AND PRACTICES

Additional books in this series can be found on Nova's website
under the Series tab.

Additional E-books in this series can be found on Nova's website
under the E-books tab.

MEDICINAL PLANTS AND SUSTAINABLE DEVELOPMENT

CHANDRA PRAKASH KALA
EDITOR

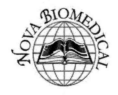

Nova Science Publishers, Inc.
New York

Library of Congress Cataloging-in-Publication Data
Medicinal plants and sustainable development / editor, Chandra Prakash Kala.
      p. ; cm.
  Includes bibliographical references and index.
  ISBN 978-1-61761-942-7 (hardcover)
  1. Medicinal plants. 2. Sustainable development. I. Kala, C. P.
  [DNLM: 1. Plants, Medicinal. 2. Conservation of Natural Resources. 3.
Ethnobotany--methods. QV 766]
  SB293.M433 2010
  633.8'8--dc22
                          2010034037

Published by Nova Science Publishers, Inc. † New York

Contents

Introduction

Medicinal Plants and Sustainable Development

Chandra Prakash Kala

Today, the world witnesses a global resurgence of interests in the plant based drugs and cosmetics. The revival of traditional health care systems, which is mainly plants-based, has several ramifications including the challenging tasks of meeting the health care needs of ever increasing human population. The decline in medicinal plants is unpresidented as majority of raw material for preparing herbal medicine is sourced from the wild and commercial operations have not adopted sustainable harvesting practices. People across the world use medicinal plants in several health care practices, and loss of this valuable resource have direct bearings on these traditional health care systems.

Realizing the criticalities of ongoing issues associated with the medicinal plants, countries across the world have started finding out the solutions for various existing problems. Studies are going on to explore the possibilities of domesticating wild medicinal plants through rural and modern biotechnologies. Besides, various medicinal plants related issues, such as, bio-prospecting and bio-piracy, identifying sustainable harvesting practices, safety and standardization of herbal drugs, strengthening legislation and policy on medicinal plants, developing market infrastructure, supply chain management, etc., are being dealt with the national to international levels.

There are studies available on the above mentioned issues, and information is being shared in bits and pieces, which may not serve the purpose of multidisciplinary medicinal plants sector. Here in this context, the present book 'Medicinal Plants and Sustainable Development' deals with multidisciplinary approach and contains information on different aspects of medicinal plants, which can be used as guiding tools. The book contains 18 chapters written by eminent scientists and academicians from different countries. There are case studies on the species to community level, and also documentation of medicinal plants as used by different ethnic groups. This book aims to provide academic and practitioners' insights into medicinal plants related issues from science and technology interventions to historical use patterns and indigenous knowledge systems.

The chapters in this book fall into four categories. The first five chapters describe medicinal plants conservation and cultivation strategies, of which two chapters focus on the conservation of threatened medicinal plants through cultivation. The second category of chapters deals with current trends and interventions of science and technology for medicinal plants. This section contains 6 chapters ranging from seed technology to mycorrhizal inoculation, in-vitro cytotoxicity, morphological markers, and diversity of phytoplasma with respect to the medicinal plants. The third section includes information on traditional use patterns and indigenous knowledge on medicinal plants. This section also discusses the diversity in medicinal plants and interactions of humans and animals with medicinal plants for curing various kinds of diseases. The fourth and final category of chapters of this book highlights issues associated with medicinal plants and sustainable development. This section of the book includes issues related to the community based enterprises, local health care promotion and empowering women and their roles in the medicinal plants sector.

The first chapter, by Růžičková et al., gives an overview on the technology of growing, breeding, physiology and the quality of caraway (*Carum carvi*) that occurs in several countries. The article also describes the policy issues and interventions made by the Czech Republic for production of high quality caraway by establishing an association of caraway growers – Czech Caraway. In second chapter, Gomez-Flores and Tamez-Guerra review sustainable agricultural practices and emphasize the need of reinforcement of medicinal plants farming by using sustainability practices. The authors of chapter 3, Dixit and Silori report medicinal plant species growing in hot desert conditions and their conservation through prioritization on the basis of 'purpose-part used' combinations of species.

Chapter 4, by Rawat and Vishvakarma examines cultivation practices and status of *Saussurea costus* and *Inula racemosa* - the endangered medicinal plants, in four different agro-ecosystems of the Himalayan cold desert between 2600 m to 3200 m elevations. The authors also suggest reviving cultivation of selected medicinal plants by providing scientific agro-techniques, creating value addition centers at local level, strengthening existing market and granting permits for cultivation and export. The authors of chapter 5, Butola et al. report on simple, low cost propagation protocol and post harvesting technology for *Heracleum candicans*- a threatened medicinal plant. The authors consider the *ex-situ* cultivation of threatened medicinal plant species as the most viable option not only for sustained supply of homogenous quality raw materials but also for conservation of existing populations in the wild.

The applications of science and technology have proven the significance and advantages for developing the medicinal plants sector. The second section of this book looks at the various scientific and technological applications in designing protocols for meeting the medicinal plants requirements of ever increasing human populations. The sixth chapter by Zubaida et al. explores seed science and technology of some important medicinal plants, especially of Solanaceae family. The authors discuss their findings in detail by using different treatments viz; distilled water, pre-chilling, NaNO3, CaNO3, hot water treatment, and 100ppm GA3. In the seventh chapter of this book, screening of some important medicinal plants, such as, *Capparis erythrocarpos, Cussonia arborea, Dracaena steudneri, Lannea schimperi, Pseudospondias microcarpa, Rauvolfia vomitoria, Sapium ellipticum* and *Zehneria scabra* for cytotoxicity is discussed by Kisangau et al. by using brine shrimp and CellTiter-Blue cell viability assays.

Chapter 8 by Bhoon looks for mycorrhizal inoculation of the high valued medicinal plants of the sub-tropical region. The author investigates the effects of mycorrhizal inoculation on the quality and bioactive phyto-constituent of 12 important medicinal plants, such as, *Centella asiatica*, *Bacopa monnieri*, *Silybum marianum*, *Asparagus racemosus*, *Andrograhis paniculata*, *Ocimum sanctum*, *Clitoria ternatea*, *Acalypha indica*, *Phyllanthus amarus*, *Lepidium sativum* and *Adhatoda vasica*. The medicinal plants selected by Bhoon are used in the Ayurvedic Pharmacies and also traded internationally. Chaturvedi et al. in chapter 9 stress that of many diseases, phytoplasma diseases are the major constraints in profitable cultivation and production of medicinal plants, which lowers the quantum and quality of medicinal plants. The authors discuss in detail the occurrence, symptomatology, molecular characterization, transmission, taxonomy, genetic diversity and management approaches on medicinal phytoplasmas. In chapter 10, Bhatt and Bisht discuss characterization and development of morphological markers of two endangered medicinal plant species - *Swertia chirayita* and *S. angustifolia*. The chapter 11 in this book, by Shrestha and Dall'Acqua, deals with the phytochemical analysis of *Aconitum naviculare*, an endemic medicinal plant of the Himalaya.

The knowledge of medicinal plants, historically, was available with a few specialized herbal healers in rural communities; thus much of their use was observed as being primarily of local interest. This indigenous and traditional knowledge over a period of time have drawn immense commercial interests. The third section of this book reports on the significance of indigenous knowledge systems and medicinal plants. The authors of chapter 12, Jayanti et al. consider that humans have learnt the use of medicinal plants by observing animals. In Western Ghats - one of the two biodiversity hotspots of India, their study concludes that the highest number of medicinal plants occur in the dry forests, followed by the wet-evergreen patches, and the moist deciduous forests.

In Chapter 13, Ayyanar and Ignacimuthu report indigenous uses and diversity of endemic medicinal plants in a protected area of Western Ghats– the Kalakad Mundanthurai Tiger Reserve of India. The authors stress the need of immediate conservation of medicinal plants in the Western Ghats realizing that the majority of medicinal plants in this biodiversity hotspot are declining rapidly due to anthropogenic pressures. In chapter 14, Phondani et al. describe the indigenous uses of medicinal plants growing in the middle Himalayan region and used by traditional herbal practitioners for preparing medicinal formulations. Chapter 15, the last chapter in this section, looks into the traditional herbal formulations prepared by herbal practitioners for curing the urogenital disorders.

One school of thought believes that the sustainability of the medicinal plants cannot be achieved merely by promulgating a ban on their export or by fencing areas rich in medicinal plants. People's participation is required to meet the desired objectives. The last section of this book includes 3 chapters dealing with sustainable development of medicinal plants. Apart from *in-situ* and *ex-situ* conservation, Torri et al., in chapter 16, consider role of women as important factor in the medicinal plants sector. Here the authors point out that in numerous societies, it is mainly women who are wild plant gatherers and managers, home gardeners and plant domesticators, herbalists and healers. This chapter further reviews the key role that women entrepreneurs can play in reinforcing local health care and empowering poor rural indigenous and tribal women. Chapter 17 by Kala reviews various traditional and ongoing management and conservation practices with respect to the medicinal plants and their long term sustainability. In the final chapter of this book, chapter 18, Kandari et al. explore sustainable development strategies through domestication of important medicinal plants by using simple and cost effective technology such as, polyhouse and shade netting.

The objective of developing this book was to incorporate different viewpoints of the scholars working in different set up but with a focus on developing the medicinal plants sector. The authors hope that this book provides answers to many critical questions and also helps academicians, policy makers, scientists and different stakeholders of the medicinal plants for designing the future course of action.

A. Medicinal Plants Conservation and Cultivation Strategies

In: Medicinal Plants and Sustainable Development
Editor: Chandra Prakash Kala

ISBN 978-1-61761-942-7
© 2011 Nova Science Publishers, Inc.

Chapter 1

The System of Caraway (*Carum carvi* L.) Production in the Czech Republic

Gabriela Růžičková[1], Antonín Vaculík[2],
Prokop Šmirous[2] and Blanka Kocourková[1]*

[1]Department of Crop Science, Breeding and Plant Medicine, Faculty of Agronomy,
Mendel University, Zemědělská 1, 613 00 Brno, the Czech Republic
[2]AGRITEC, Research, Breeding and Services, Ltd.,
Zemědělská 16, 787 01 Šumperk, the Czech Republic

Abstract

This chapter gives an overview on 10 years of work of Czech scientists on the technology of growing, breeding, physiology and quality of caraway (*Carum carvi* L.). This crop belongs to *Apiaceae* (*Umbelliferae*) family and it is the most cultivated spice and medicinal plant in the Czech Republic with mainly carminative and antibacterial properties. Its growing area varies between 1600 – 2000 hectares from year to year. Caraway fruits contain the essential oil with high ratio of D-carvone. The growers of this crop have established their own association – Czech Caraway in 1996. The association has obtained the Protected Designation of Origin (PDO) of the "Czech Caraway" on 20th May 2008 by the Commission Regulation (ES) No. 433/2008. This act has confirmed high level of Czech caraway production as very important trading factor.

Keywords: caraway, *Carum carvi* L., Czech Caraway, Český kmín, D-carvone.

* Department of Crop Science, Breeding and Plant Medicine, Faculty of Agronomy, Mendel University, Zemědělská 1, 613 00 Brno, Czech Republic. E-mail: gabriela.ruzickova@mendelu.cz, phone: +420 545 133 361, fax: +420 545 133 302

Introduction

Caraway (*Carum carvi* L.) is a volatile oil spice crop with a long tradition of farming in Czech lands. Probable region of its origin is Asia Minor and Central Asia, from where caraway spread on the Continent. The seeds of caraway were found during the archaeological works in lacustrian dwellings from 3rd Century B. C. It was a favourite spice of ancient Egyptians, Romans and Greeks (Mičánková, 1991). Primarily, the caraway was collected from natural localities. Caraway is known from Czech historical period and it is mentioned in Cosmas chronicle from 1073. In 19th century, together with the development of chemical industry, caraway was introduced into the cultivation as a raw material for the essential oil extraction. Consequently, large areas of caraway were brought under farming in Czech Republic. The seeds from The Netherlands were imported into Czech lands. The breeding of Czech varieties has started in 40-ties of 20th century with shattered types, and continued with new varieties in 60-ties. The first non-shattered variety was registered in 1978 and it stabilized the commodity as for the yield parameters. Although this crop is a small but very important commodity of Czech agriculture sector, it definitely needs the use of all knowledge from the research, breeding, growing and trading for the keeping and improving of its situation and stability among the minor commodities. The association Czech Caraway was established in the Czech Republic in 1996. The association has applied to European Commission for the Protected Designation of Origin (PDO) of the Czech caraway varieties in 2004. This Designation bases on climatic and soil conditions and traditions of production typical for the Czech lands. The Commission has registered PDO "Czech caraway" 20. 5. 2008 by the Commission Regulation (ES) No. 433/2008 into the Register of Protected Designations of Origin and Protected Geographical Indication. This act has confirmed high level of Czech caraway production, which is entangling not only for the growers and processors but also very important trading factor (Vaculík et al., 2008).

Biological Characteristics

Caraway (*Carum carvi* L.; $2n = 2x = 20$; *Apiaceae*) is cross-pollinated plant species. The plant is allogamous (60 – 70 % heterogamous) and mostly cultured as annual (winter type) or biennial (spring type) form (Smýkalová et al., 2009). The most cultivated form of caraway in the Czech Republic is a biennial crop- typical for the potato production regions. It does not demand warm climate, but needs a lot of sunlight, which implicates the creation of the vegetative organs and formation of the generative organs in second year.

Caraway is a long day crop. Low level of the light delays and decreases the yield of the achenes. Caraway is also demanding a lot of water, in both vegetative years. In the first year, the highest amount of water is needed in August when the root system and the leaf rosette are formed. In second year, caraway needs the moisture in the period of intensive growth, from the end of April till the end of May. Later precipitation does not balance the negative influence of the lack of winter moisture. Long term precipitation during the flowering prolongs this period, caraway matures non-uniformly and the quality of the production is decreased. Because the different weather course during the years, the yields of the achenes highly varies (Kocourková, 1996).

The development is slow in the beginning of the vegetation period. Caraway germinates at 6 – 8 °C, the optimum temperature for germination is around 12 – 24 °C. Caraway emerges 14 – 24 days at soil temperature 9 °C and air temperature 10 – 14 °C. The formation of the leaf rosette takes one month. In the first year, caraway forms the root of fusiform shape, transversely wrinkled, slightly branched and the leaf rosette with pedunculated leaves (Kocourková, 1996). Good developed plants are resistant to hard frosts (-30 °C). The generative organs are formed after the end of the juvenile phase which implicates complete pass of the vernalisation stage. Taking up of the juvenile phase depends on the nutritional state of the plants. The plants should have approximately 13 – 14 leaves and the root diameter minimal of 7 mm. The vernalisation starts when the soil temperature in 5 – 10 cm under the ground level decreases below 12 °C. The vernalisation could also run in spring, after warmer period, when weaker plants thicken and reach defined developed stage, in the case that a sufficient decrease of the temperature will come for required time. Caraway starts to vegetate in spring at 3 °C. Grooved stem, 30 – 120 cm height, branches and the number of the branches are influenced genetically and by the growth architecture. The stem is green; in the flowering stage has anthocyane colour. After long growth, in the beginning of flowering stage, caraway demands a sunshine period and the temperature between 16 – 22 °C. Too high temperature at fruits maturity causes the essential oil looses, lower temperature reduces the essential oil biosynthesis. After the flowering, the plant dies. Only the plants, which were not able to flower, continue to the next year.

Caraway occurs naturally on the sites with neutral soil reaction, high reserve of potassium and middle or higher reserve of nitrogen. The nutrition of caraway in the first year influences the state and production ability of the growth because the transition from the vegetative to generative phase needs relevant reserve of the nutrients in the roots. The size of the root influences the general formation of the plant, the height, the number of the branches, the number of the umbels and the weight of the achenes on the plant. The positive correlation of the essential oil content in the fruits and the seed germination on the root size was found (Vrzalová and Procházka, 1988). The soil reaction is really important for optimal growth of caraway. The application of calcium has a positive effect on acidic soils. Caraway grows and well develops on the sandy loam and clay loam soils with good water regime. The best soils are light, humid, and non-compacted soils in semiarid and semihumid regions. Caraway emergences uniformly and can form sufficient growth in summer period on these soils. In arid regions, if the irrigation is not possible, the problems with the establishing of the growths from later sowing terms can occur. The root and leave rosette formation in the period of growing (August - September) is delayed. In these areas, the yield stability is lower. Caraway has no use for shallow soils, sandy, drying, heavy or watered soils weeded by catch grass (*Agropyron repens*) (Vrzalová and Procházka, 1988).

Physiology

The breeding for non-shattering character was also studied from physiological point of view. The problem was very low germinability (20 – 70 %) although it was native of 90 – 98 % (Hradilík and Císařová, 1975a; Hradilík and Fišerová, 1980). The germinability of caraway is higher on the light than in the dark and increases dramatically by rinsing in the flow of distilled water, probably because of a depletion of inhibiting substance. Wild caraway does not germinate or germinates very little and is non-shattering due to high content of native abscisic acid (Hradilík and Císařová, 1975b). Abscisic acid is responsible for the dormancy of caraway and the content of this phytohormone is decreased during cold stratification dramatically with simultaneously increasing germinability of the achenes. The content of gas hydrocarbons in three varieties was evaluated. The production of ethylene in the plants is influenced by environmental stressors – light, temperature, water stress, herbicides, mechanical lesions and pathogen infections. The ethylene induces the maturity and the fruit fall, stimulates the biosynthesis of proteins, aromatic compounds and phytoalexins. Increased production of ethylene by the attacked plant can be expressed by the stimulation or inhibition of the processes leasing to the plant resistance. Abscisic acid (ABA) inhibits the seed germination and influences their dormancy. The amount of ABA is increased due to water or temperature stress dramatically, similarly as due to pathogenic attack. The problem of abscisic acid and ethylene relation to the shattering of caraway is not unambiguous although both regulators are in direct relation to this physiology reaction. The evaluation of the difference in production of ethylene, ethane and abscisic acid in the achenes or mature umbels between the individual varieties of caraway can be completed by the results from indolyl-3acetic acid content (IAA). IAA is important indicator of the dormancy depth, the content and composition of the essential oil, the non-shattering of the achenes and the resistance to the negative environmental factors and pathogens. On the bases of four years results it can be said that variety Rekord had the highest content of the essential oil, produced the highest amount of ethane and had the lowest germinability. Variety Prochan had the best germinability. The ABA content had ten times higher value in different years. These differences could be caused by the change of the climatic factors. The achenes with the lowest level of ABA produced the highest amount of ethylene and had the best germinability (Fišerová et al., 1999; Fišerová et al., 2008).

Forms and Varieties

Caraway is distinguished into two groups: caraway with the standard length of the growing season (Czech varieties, biennial form) and caraway with shortened length of the growing season (winter caraway and annual caraway) (Šmirous, 2005; Németh, 1998). Annual and biennial taxa differ in morphology, yield and also in chemical parameters. Biennial caraway contains about two times higher oil than annual caraway in a similar-sized seed (Zambori-Németh, 2005; Bouwmeester et al., 1998). According to Bouwmeester et al. (1995b), there was a positive relationship between seed weight and absolute amount of essential oil per seed for both annual and biennial caraway, whereas Zambori-Németh (2005) concluded that the content of essential oils and carvone did not show significant correlations with the morphological and production traits. The first foreign non-shattering variety was Bleija, which was created by the careful selection on the absence of divisive line in the peduncles of the buds, the flowers and the fruits.

The source for the selection was the offspring of two non-shattering plants found in barn the offspring of five non-shattering plants chosen from 2500 observed plants of traditional variety Volhouden. By the sequential selection, 12 stocks were created and they gave the base for the non-shattering variety Bleija, registered in the Netherlands in 1972 (Németh, 1998).

First Czech variety of intensive type was "Ekonom" (registered in 1964, shattering type). It was bred by František Procházka (1926 – 1989), who worked at breeding station Keřkov, division Česká Bělá. In 1978, the non-shattering variety "Rekord" was registered. The next variety "Prochan" was registered in 1989 and in 1996 was registered the variety "Kepron".

Table 1. Varieties of caraway in the Common catalogue of varieties of agricultural plant species — 28th complete edition (as 12. 12. 2009) from that three are of the Czech origin (Official Journal of the EU, 2009)

Variety	EU country of admission
Ass	*AT 20
Bleija	*NL x
Gintaras	*LT 34
Kepron	*SK 174
Kończewicki	*NL x, *PL 893
Maud	*HU 151223
Plewiski	*NL x
Prochan	*CZ 231, *NL x, *SK x
Rekord	*CZ x, *SK 104
Sylvia	*DK 14
Volhouden	*NL x

* - officially admitted a variety.

x - there are several persons considered as responsible for maintenance by the country admission number - it indicates persons considered as responsible for maintenance by the country admission.

There are 11 varieties of caraway registered in the Common Catalogue of Varieties of Agricultural Plant Species — 28th complete edition (as 12. 12. 2009) from that three are of the Czech origin (Official Journal of the EU, 2009) (Table 1). The varieties are not divided by the length of the vegetative period.

Table 2. Important parameters of Czech caraway varieties in the Czech Republic according to Central Institute for Supervising and Testing in Agriculture (www.ukzuz.cz, the results from 2000 – 2007)

	REKORD	PROCHAN[PO]
Year of registration	1978	1990
Yield of the achenes (%)	97*	101*
Days till maturity	199	199
Plants height (cm)	92	93
Weight of thousand seeds (g)	2.89	2.88
Essential oil content (%)	4.3	4.1
D-carvone content in the EO (%)	59.6	58.4

[PO] legal protection according to Czech law N. 408/2000 Sb.

*recalculation to the average yield of both varieties 2.02 t.ha^{-1} .

Rekord

This Czech biennial, non-shattering variety was registered in 1978. It was bred by the irradiation by 180 Gy of variety Ekonom in 1962. In following experiments, the full ripen non-shattering achenes were chosen. It is one of the middle early varieties. The height of the plants is middle, with erect growth. The leaves have rich green colour, middle fine parts. The umbels are white, rarely light pinkish.

The umbels are of middle size, situated in top part of the plant. It is suitable for the fruits production for food industry. The essential oil content in the fruits is high the carvone ratio in the oil is standard (over 50 %). It can be cultivated in all growing regions. There is a risk of lower yield of the achenes.

The health state is average with the hint of the higher sensitivity to the complex of root and stem pathogens (*Fusarium, Rhizoctonia* etc.) (Kadlec, 1996). The maintainers of this variety are Sativa Keřkov, a. s., SEMPRA PRAHA, a. s. and OSEVA PRO, s. r. o. Praha.

Table 3. Herbicides registered to caraway in the Czech Republic (Vaculík et al., 2008)

Active substance	Dose (concentration in %)	Term of application	Application comments
DICOTYLEDONOUS ANNUAL WEEDS			
Linuron	$1.5 - 2.5$ l.ha^{-1}	postemergently	application from 13 BBCH
Pendimethalin	$4.0 - 5.0$ l.ha^{-1}	preemergently, early postemergently	possible to the undersow in cereals, legumes and maize
DICOTYLEDONOUS WEEDS			
Fluroxypyr	$0.5 - 0.6$ l.ha^{-1}	postemergently	in occurrence of catch weed (*Galium aparine*), possible divided dose 2 x 0.3 l (from 14 BBCH)
MCPB	3.0 l.ha^{-1}	postemergently	in occurrence of common thistle (*Cirsium arvense*), max. till the beginning of the flowering, do not apply at the temperatures higher than 25 °C
MONOCOTYLEDONOUS, PERENNIAL WEEDS AND COUCH GRASS (*Agropyron repens*)			
Propaquizafop	$0.5 - 1.5$ l.ha^{-1}	postemergently	min. 2 leaves on weed grasses, do not apply in the phase of the stem with the buds
Haloxyfop-P-methyl	$0.5 - 1.25$ l.ha^{-1}	postemergently	min. 2 leaves on weed grasses, do not apply in the phase of the stem with the buds
Quizalofop-P-tefuryl	$1.0 - 2.5$ l.ha^{-1}	postemergently	min. 2 leaves on weed grasses, do not apply in the phase of the stem with the buds
Quizalofop-P-ethyl	$1.0 - 2.5$ l.ha^{-1}	postemergently	min. 2 leaves on weed grasses, do not apply in the phase of the stem with the buds

Prochan

Czech biennial variety, non-shattering, was registered in 1990. The original material, dutch variety Bleija, was irradiated by 30 Gy.

From the best strains, the population was created after the experiments during 1985 – 1989. It is middle early, with middle height and the average height is 96 cm. The umbels are middle to large and the leaves are green with fine parts.

The variety is well resistant to the frost killing and is resistant to lodging. The inflorescences are white with delayed flowering period from Rekord variety. The essential oil content is middle to high, with the standard content of carvone (over 50 %). This variety is suitable to all growing regions.

The advantage of this variety is high yield and certain resistance to the stem pathogens (Kadlec, 1996). The maintainers are Sativa Keřkov, a. s. and SEMPRA PRAHA, a.s.

Kepron

As at previous variety, the original material was Bleija, irradiated by 30 Gy and selected consequently. Also Kepron is biennial, non-shattering variety, used for food industry.

The essential oil content is middle high to high with the standard ratio of carvone (over 50 %). It can be cultivated in all production regions. The advantage is high yield, of 11 % higher in average than control variety Rekord and has no growing risks.

The maintainer of this variety is Sativa Keřkov, a. s., but the company has not prolonged the registration in the Czech Republic, so Kepron is not included in the State Catalogue of Registered Varieties yet.

Anyway, Kepron is still mentioned in Common Catalogue of the Varieties of Agricultural and Horticultural Crops of EU.

Currently, there is possible to buy the seeds of non registered varieties with shortened vegetative period. It is a winter form of caraway, recently called Alfa and spring form called as Sprinter. These varieties are favourite in the regions that are not suitable for biennial caraway.

The growing of these varieties does not correspond with the law about the turnover of the seed and seedlings. They have lower content of the essential oil and lower yield (Vaculík et al., 2008).

Breeding

The classical selection according to the morphological characters was one of the first methods of caraway breeding. In 60-ties of 20th century, the irradiation by the X-rays was used at the breeding of modern varieties, combined with the classical positive selection (Šmirous et al., 2004a and 2004b). In Germany, the breeding of annual caraway was focused on the development of genetic components for a synthetic variety (Pank, 2009).

The other method used for the experiments with annual caraway was a recurrent phenotypic selection. The results from 7 years of breeding activities showed that generally, the essential oil content and caryone ratio are influenced by time period (Smirous and Kocourkova, 2006). As for the genotypes, there were very high significant differences between them. Presently, there are selected genotypes considered as homozygous and homogenous available for further breeding (Smirous and Kocourkova, 2006; Šmirous, 2007; Šmirous et al., 2007).

Conventional caraway breeding is limited mainly by the available genetic variation of the caraway genepool. Thus, breeding barriers, such as low level of autogamy (cross-pollinated species), long vegetation period, narrow genetic variability and sensitivity to wilt diseases prevent the easy production of new healthy parental materials (clones). The process of developing new inbred parents generally takes a total of 7 – 10 years. Therefore, *in vitro* approach such as rapid method of inducing homozygosity and production of doubled haploid breeding lines could help to overcome these main obstacles limiting caraway breeding and speed up substantially the breeding process. The first report on androgenic doubled haploid production in caraway was reported by Smykalova et al. (2005, 2006, 2009). The in vitro androgenesis in annual (winter type) caraway representing third generation of forced (artificial) self-pollination has been studied with the aim to produce completely homozygous inbred lines.

Various induction conditions, such as temperature pretreatments, combination of growth regulators and carbon sources in a culture medium as well as the effect of genotype on in vitro androgenesis were examined. Cultured anthers produced embryogenic calli, and subsequently two types of regenerated plants were obtained, namely haploids of microspore origin, and diploids which may represent somatic regenerants (anther wall) or spontaneous doubled haploids. The ploidy status of regenerated plants was determined by flow cytometry. The colchicine treatment of haploid regenerants resulted in fertile doubled haploid plants.

Composition of the Achenes

Depending on planting conditions, caraway fruits contain 2 – 7 % of essential oil consisting of about 30 compounds. Carvone and limonene account for the main portion, about 95%. The ratio of these main monoterpenes leads to the main purpose of the essential oil. The other compounds of the essential oil are pinenes, thujone, camphene, fellanderene (Sedláková et al., 2001; Sedláková et al., 2003b).

In the field, for both annual and biennial caraway, formation of limonene started earlier than that of carvone, but both occurred during the early stages of seed development. The content of the two compounds reached a steady level several weeks before harvest, being higher in biennial than in annual caraway, apparently because carbon partition to essential oil formation in biennial caraway is more favourable than in annual caraway (Bouwmeester et al., 1998). Generally, D-limonene content negatively correlates with D-carvone, due to the fact that limonene is its precursor and decreases during the ripening (Baysal et al., 1999; Sedláková et al., 2003b; Bouwmeester et al., 1995a). The achenes content also lipids (13 – 21 %), nitrogen substances (25 – 36 %), fiber (13 – 19 %), non-nitrogen substance extractive (5 – 18 %), ash (5 – 7 %), wax (1.5 %) and water (9 – 13 %) (Bruneton, 1999). Sedláková et al. (2003a) studied the influence of the application of the growth regulators and fungicides on the essential oil content. It was concluded that the use of the growth regulators during caraway maturation and the use of fungicides affected positively the amount of essential oil in caraway.

The same team, Sedláková et al. (2003a), has investigated the application of Supercritical Fluid Extraction for the essential oil determination in small samples gathered during breeding as an alternative method. The results were used as a one of the criteria during breeding. Classical way of the essential oil determination does not allow this option. Table 6 shows the essential oil content in Czech varieties and different essential oil composition of some European caraway resources is mentioned in table 7.

Use of Caraway

Caraway is a traditional spice and medicinal plant with carminative and antibacterial properties. Seeds, seed cake and straw are valuable dietetic feeders for cattle, improving the synthesis of milk due to increasing taste and digestibility of nutrients, reduce meteorism and generally influenced the metabolism and health state positively. They are not suitable for milking cows because the essentials oil compounds can affect the type of milk smell after the consumption.

In feeding industry of pigs, caraway is used for improving of the atractivity of the feeders which have lower tolerance (Kameník, 1999).

Concerning the carvone, it has a several applications including as fragrance and flavor, potato spout inhibitor, antimicrobial agent, building block and biochemical environmental indicator (de Carvalho and da Fonseca, 2006).

Cizkova et al. (2000) studied the direct dependence of sprouting on residual carvone and its biodegradation products in tubers. S-carvone was converted into dihydrocarveol and dihydrocarvone especially in easily accessible tissues of sprouts, peels and half tubers. Sensory analyses confirmed that S-carvone treatment of stored tubers does not influence taste, odour or colour of cooked potatoes.

Vejrazka et al. (2008) confirmed good insecticidal effect of carvone against the grain weevil (*Sitophillus granarius*) and they detected the limit concentrations.

Technology of Growing

Crop Rotation of Caraway

The same fore crop and the same agrotechnology is recommended. Suitable fore crop are the cereals and root crops. Clover crops, ploughed meadows, the other grasslands and oil crops, rape seed respectively are not suitable. Caraway can be sown once after 6 years because of the transport of the pathogens and the pests. Also, it can be sown on the plots minimal 200 m from the current caraway growths or ploughed under growths. The growth of caraway is established by the sowing into the cover crop or as a pure crop. As the pure crop, caraway can be as the main crop or as subsequent crop after early harvested fore crops. For the cultivation of caraway in the cover crop, horse bean for green matter, sparsely sown cereals (spring wheat, spring barley, spring triticale), pea harvested in green maturity and also poppy are recommended. The use a poppy as cover crop is rare because of problematic weed control. The growing in maize is also tested. The cover crops are recommended in warmer regions (Kocourková, 1996).

Soil Preparation

After the harvest of the fore crop the stubble breaking is necessary with the stubble breaking care for the reducing of unwanted evaporation. After the stubble breaking, the application of total herbicide on the base of glyphosate in recommended in a suitable dose. After minimal of 18 days, the middle ploughing to depth 22 – 26 cm is performed with the application of the mineral fertilizers. If there is not possible to keep the time break between stubble breaking and ploughing, the stubble breaking can be eliminated and in the convetional technologies can be used deep ploughing from 30 to 35 cm in dependence on the depth of the topsoil profile. In the regions without water or wind erosion, the crude treatment of the plot together with the ploughing in autumn can be performed. It makes the spring preparation easy and saves the winter moisture (Králík, 2007).

Fertilization

Caraway is a plant having a high demand for the nutrition, for nitrogen mainly. The higher need of nitrogen in the first year of the vegetation is in the phase of intensive development of the leave rosette (July – August) and in second year in the phase of the formation of stems and branches. The highest uptake of potassium is in the phase of the prolongation growth and the flowering beginning. Phosphorus and calcium uptake is the highest in autumn in the first year and in the phase of the fruits formation. The amount of 30 – 40 t.ha^{-1} of biomass in the flowering period is needed to form the yield of the fruits of 1 – 2 t.ha^{-1}. For optimal development of the yield characters there is a premise that the soil is in the old power and the doses of the fertilizers will be: 120 – 180 kg.ha^{-1} of N, 140 kg.ha-1 of P_2O_5 (62 kg P) and 120 kg.ha^{-1} of K_2O (100 kg K). The fertilization can be provided before sowing, part of the phosphorus dose can be supplied in the superphosphate form in amount of 40 – 50 kg P_2O_5 (17.6 – 22.0 kg P) per hectare before the end of the vegetation in the autumn. The nitrogen is applied in the divided doses. The first 2/3 of planned dose is added in the year of the sowing. It is applied in the pure crop, before the sowing in the saltpeter form or the best form is ammonium sulphate form. The ammonium nitrate with urea added before the sowing has also been proven. At the undersowing of caraway, the nitrogen application should be provided after the harvest of the cover crop. The well-integrated growths in second year, with well-developed root neck (minimum of 5 mm in diameter) do not need additional nitrogen. Only the growths with the density lower than 100 plants per m^2 need to be fertilized. The saltpeter form of nitrogen prevails and the doses have to correspond with the actual assessment of the soil samples. Ammonium nitrate with urea could not be used in early spring because of burning of the plants damaged by the frost. The results from many experiments showed that the quality of the achenes (the essential oil content) can be increased by the application of some additional leave fertilizer with higher content of magnesium and sulphur.

Excessive amount of nitrogen has no positive effect on the higher yield or essential oil content (Králík et al., 2007).

The Growth Establishment

Sowing Term and Sowing Rate

Caraway is sown into 15 – 20 mm. The sowing rate results from the soil and climatic conditions during the emergence and from the way of cultivation. The rates range from 2.25 MGS.ha^{-1} (million of germinating seeds) to 3.37 MGS.ha^{-1} in worse soil conditions. These rates equate the doses 8 – 12 kg.ha^{-1} in dependence on biological value of the seeds and WTS (weight of thousand seeds). Currently, caraway is sown into 12.5 cm rows. The sowing of the pure crop has to be finished between 15. – 20.6. The results from the project showed that the highest yield was recorded at the growths established in April, the lowest in July. Caraway sown into the cover crop has to be sown at the same time or immediately after the sowing of the cover crop. Cover crops lying on the field longer than 20.7 cm need to have a decreased sowing rate. The sowing of caraway in warmer regions has to be performed as early as possible (till the end of April). Later term delays the flowering, maturity and harvest slightly but the yield is decreased significantly (Králík, 2007).

The Seed

The certified seed provides high purity and germinating ability. The higher category of reproductive material pays off in growing of caraway. The germinating ability should be min. of 70 %, the purity min. 97 %, the moisture max. 13 %.

Weed Regulation

Caraway is a crop with very small competitive ability against the majority of weed species and has slow development at the beginning. The timing of herbicides application is very important, especially at biennial caraway. There is a recommendation for regulating the perennial species (couch grass) and hardly regulated weeds (common thistle, sorrel) in a fore crop. The spectrum of the herbicides registered into caraway is narrow. The different sensitivity of cover crop and caraway to the herbicides plays the important role, as well as the coordination of the application term from the point of view of the efficiency and the sensitivity (Vaculík, 2006; 2007; 2008; Vaculík et al., 2008).

Plant Diseases

The health state of caraway is influenced by many factors: the weather conditions, physiological state of the plants after overwintering, the quality of soil preparation, the fertilization, the sowing term, the growth density etc. The spectrum of the fungi diseases of caraway is changed recently as the result of the changes in climatic conditions. High temperatures and low precipitation suit to termophile fungi as is *Ascochyta*, *Erisyphe*, cold and rainy weather is optimal for the development and spread of psychrophile species (*Mycocentrospora*). The growths with high density and highly weeded create the optimal microclimatis conditions for the development of pathogenic fungi. There is also the risk of the propagation and spread of them to the other growths. High concentration of rape can be also the risk of higher occurrence of *Sclerotinia sclerotiorum*. There is necessary to keep the crop rotation where caraway or other species from *Apiaceae* family can be on the same plot not earlier than after 5 – 6 years. As at the other crops, the certified seed is a guarantee that the seed growths were controlled for the occurrence of serious diseases. Among the pathogens cause the diseases of the roots and neck belong these species: *Rhizoctonia, Pythium, Fusarium, Cylindrocarpon, Phoma, Colletotrichum, Sclerotinia*. The stem diseases and leaves cause: *Mycocentrospora, Septoria, Ascochyta, Itersonilia, Erysiphe* and the flower diseases and achenes: *Erysiphe, Phomopsis*, bacteria. The easy regulated diseases are: *Mycocentrospora, Septoria, Erysiphe*. The diseases with complicated regulation are: *Phomopsis, Ascochyta, Itersonilia* and root and neck diseases.

The diseases can be spread by the seeds (*Mycocentrospora, Septoria, Ascochyta, Itersonilia*), by insect (*Phomopsis diachenii*, bakteriózy), by wind from the wild plants from *Apiaceae* family (*Erysiphe, Ascochyta phomoides*) and by soil (*Rhizoctonia, Pythium, Fusarium, Cylindrocarpon, Phoma, Mycocentrospora, Itersonilia, Colletotrichum, Sclerotinia*).

Table 4 shows the fungicides registered against the antracnose in the Czech Republic (Odstrčilová et al., 2002; Odstrčilová, 2006; Odstrčilová, 2007a and 2007b).

Table 4. Fungicides registered against the antracnosis in caraway in the Czech Republic (Vaculík et al., 2008)

Active substance	Mechanism of action	Dose (concentration %)	Protection period	Application comments
Copper oxichloride	contacted	3.5 – 4.0 kg.ha^{-1}	7	
Copper hydroxide	contacted	3.5 – 4.0 kg.ha^{-1}	7	
Copper hydroxide	contacted	3.5 – 4.0 kg.ha^{-1}	7	in the beginning of flowering
Copper oxichloride	contacted	3.5 – 4.0 kg.ha^{-1}	7	
Iprodione	contacted	3.0 l.ha^{-1}	-	in the beginning of creation of flower stem, 61 BBCH
Thiophanate-methyl	systemic	0.8 kg.ha^{-1}	-	1. application in the beginning of creation of flower stem, 2. application before flowering

Pest Control

One of the main pests attack caraway is *Aceria carvi* Nal. (1985) in the Czech Republic and can became a serious problem in major caraway-growing areas. So far, no effective method for its control is known.

A. carvi overwinters hidden within leaves of young caraway plants, the first symptoms are usually not visible before the start of flowering.

Though the initial density of the pest is low, the mite population multiplies during the season when the pest attacks plant tissues and causes development of galls on leaves and flowers.

Comparison of healthy plants and plants infested by *A. carvi* showed that infested plants had significantly more umbels but produced far fewer seeds, and the yield of caraway was thus substantially decreased (Zemek et al., 2005).

Table 5. Insecticides registered in the Czech Republic against Depressaria daucella and Cnephasia spp. (Vaculík et al., 2008

Active substance	Mechanism of action	Dose (concentration in v %)	Application comments
Pirimiphos–methyl	Contacted, feeding and breathing nervous poison, nonsystemic; quickly penetrates into tissues	1.5 l.ha^{-1}	After the first record of occurrence of caterpillars, entirely before flowering
B.thuringiensis ssp. *kurstaki*	Biological formulation	1.5 l.ha^{-1}	After the first record of occurrence of caterpillars; before flowering or after the beginning of flowering, in the period of 1. instar of caterpillars
B.thuringiensis ssp. *kurstaki*	Biological formulation	1 kg.ha^{-1}	After the first record of occurrence of caterpillars; before flowering or after the beginning of flowering, on the caterpillars
Deltamethrin	Contacted, feeding and nervous poison, nonsystemic	0.1 l.ha^{-1}	After the first record of occurrence of caterpillars; before flowering or after the beginning of flowering, seed growths
Deltamethrin	Contacted, feeding and nervous poison, nonsystemic	0.3 – 0.5 l.ha^{-1}	After the first record of occurrence of caterpillars; before flowering or after the beginning of flowering, seed growths
Deltamethrin	Contacted, feeding and nervous poison, nonsystemic	0.2 l.ha^{-1}	After the first record of occurrence of caterpillars; before flowering or after the beginning of flowering, seed growths
Deltamethrin	Contacted, feeding and nervous poison, nonsystemic	0.1 l.ha^{-1}	After the first record of occurrence of caterpillars; before flowering or after the beginning of flowering, seed growths
Lambda-cyhalothrin	Contacted, feeding and nervous poison, nonsystemic; irritates insect to moving	0.2 l.ha^{-1}	After the first record of occurrence of caterpillars; before flowering or after the beginning of flowering

The adults overwinter on the vegetative tops of caraway and then, they attack the whole plant in second year. They are spread passively by wind, actively by movement and probably by the seed.

The pest control is indirect – the selection of good seed, the establishment of new growths, the isolation. The direct control represents application acaricides, in the first year preventively and in spring after overwintering in second year.

There is one formulation registered against *A. carvi* in the Czech Republic – Pyridaben, in dose 0.375 kg.ha^{-1}. It is contacted and feeding nervous poison, nonsystemic, inserts into the tissues. It is applied in the first year after the harvest of surrounding growths (July – August) and in second year in spring after vegetation renovation (April) (Vaculík et al., 2009).

An interesting effect of Aceria attack on the abscisic acid and ethylene content in the fruits was recorded. This stressor increased the highest values of stimulating phytohormones also. These substances can disturb the dormancy and cause the highest germinability (Fišerová et al., 1999).

The other important pest of caraway is *Depressaria daucella* Denis et Schiffermüller (1775). The symptoms are appeared as the umbels spun into the balls, bitten flower peduncles and seeds (in May), later the holes covered by the arachnoid cap in the stems are present. *Depressaria* is spread from the host plants – *Carum carvi* L., *Foeniculum vulgare* var. *vulgare* Mill., *Petroselinum hortense* L., *Daucus carota* L., *Anethum graveolens* L. and the other species from *Apiaceae* family.

The caterpillars eat through into the stems and form chrysalis. The butterflies incubate in July and August and the adult (imago) overwinters. The natural enemies are the parasitoids from *Hymenoptera*.

Caraway is treated after the first record of housenek on generative organs, the limited occurrence is not given. There are some pyrethroid, organophosphate and also biological (*B. thuringiensis* ssp. *kurstaki*) formulations registered in the Czech Republic against this pest. The basic method is isolation of the growths from all of host crops harvested in that year.

The control represents the establishment of new growths as much as far from the host crops harvested in the same year.

The formulations registered against both pests are mentioned in the table 5 (Vaculík et al., 2008).

Harvest and Postharvest Treatment

The ripeness of caraway starts in the first decade of July in lowlands and in the end of July in foothills. The plants begin to be reddish brown and the fruits are light brown. The achenes from main umbels and two thirds of the umbels of the first branch are hard, easily divided into two mericarps with typical spicy flavour and they have uniform colour. The harvest is not delayed because of possible decrease of the quality by the rain.

Also, the early harvest is not recommended because the pectins in the fruit peduncles did not allow divide the individual mericarps. The growths are harvested directly by the harvest machines, which have to be adjusted to reduce the damage of the achenes. Caraway fruits could not be steamy.

The seeds with the moisture higher than 13 % loose their vitality and germinability. So, the seeds have to be dry to the value lower than this limit, the maximal drying temperature is 35 °C. Market caraway has to be protected from the direct light. The occurrence of the living pests is not allowed, the maximal limit is 10 acarids per 1 kg of fruits.

The other problem could be the absorbing the smells from the surrounding during the store. The achenes yield can reach 2 t.ha^{-1} when keep good agrotechnology (Králík, 2007; Vaculík et al., 2009).

Quality Control

The quality of caraway fruits used in pharmaceutical and food industry is given one of the main criteria – the essential oil content and D-carvone content, respectively. The amount of caraway processed in the pharmaceutical industry reaches 10 – 15 % of total caraway production (Sedláková et al., 2001). The minimal limit of the essential oil (30 ml.kg^{-1} of dried drug) and D-carvone content in the essential oils required by the Czech Pharmacopoeia is 50 % (2006). Also, according to European Pharmacopoeia (6th Ed) caraway fruits contain not less than 30 ml.kg^{-1} of essential oil in dried drug. The specification in the application for designation of origin (PDO) for Czech caraway requires also minimum of 50 % of D-carvone. The steam distillation at Clavenger apparatus and GC methods are required for the assessment by the several standards. Table 6 describes the essential oil content of Czech caraway varieties.

Table 6. Essential oil content and ration of carvone and limonen in 2008 in Czech varieties (Jarošová, 2009)

	Essential oil content (%)	Carvone in EO (%)	Limonene in EO (%)
KEPRON	4.54	53.93	46.08
PROCHAN	4.59	55.71	44.29
REKORD	4.48	58.04	41.95

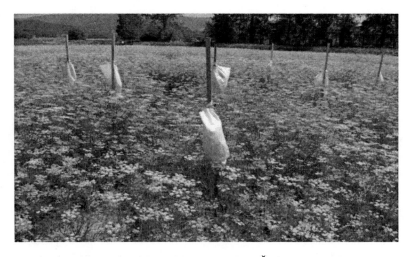

Biennial caraway in flowering stage with the isolators (author: Šmirous, P., 2009).

Table 7. Essential oil composition of various European caraway resources in % (Růžičková et al., 2009)

	RT (min)	Kepron	Prochan	Rekord	Czech annual	OP-CC-02	Raw Poland	Konzevicki (PL)	Italian
D-limonene	4.22	29.65	29.44	23.48	32.95	23.77	34.54	20.26	18.2
Fenchone	6.8	1.31	1.40	1.45	1.66	1.42	1.31	1.49	
S-linalool	8.71	3.75	4.12	4.52	4.33	4.09	3.89	4.56	
Trans-dihydrocarvone	9.46	0.37	0.04	0.07	0.13	0.06	0.11	0.20	14
D-Carvone	10.98	52.40	52.61	56.87	46.18	57.84	48.36	59.81	23.3
Dihydrocarveol	11.74	0.34	0.14	0.19	0.12	0.20	0.25	0.36	4.5
Anethol	11.92	7.39	8.41	9.11	9.20	8.53	7.98	8.87	3.3
Cadiene	15.38	0.13	0.15	0.16	0.16	0.15	0.14	0.17	0.5

Unfortunately, recent studies showed that there were no significant differences between Czech varieties in the essential oil content. These works studied the influence of use of various mills on the essential oil content, the influence of time of storage and the use of different extraction methods on the quality of caraway (Sedláková et al., 2003). Table 7 shows the differences in chemical composition between various genotypes (Růžičková et al., 2009).

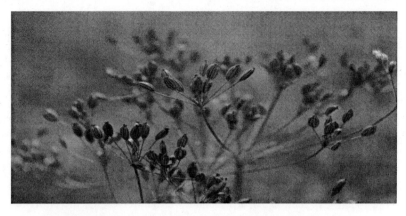

Biennial caraway in maturation phase (author: Šmirous, P., 2009).

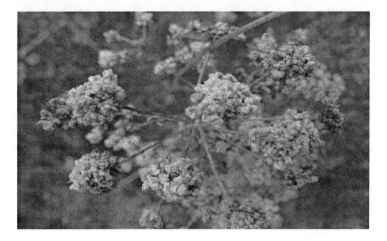

Biennial caraway, umbels attacked by *Aceria carvi* (author: Růžičková, G., 2008).

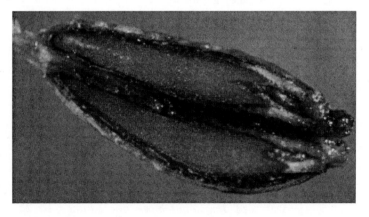

Biennial caraway, variety Kepron, longitudal section (author: Fišerová, H., 1998).

Conclusion

The most cultivated registered varieties of caraway (*Carum carvi* L.) - REKORD, KEPRON, PROCHAN, in the Czech Republic were compared with respect to the standard requirements for caraway yield and quality given by the variety REKORD as described by Central Institute for Supervising and Testing in Agriculture. The yield characters were not influenced by the varieties, even in the different growing localities. These characters were strongly affected by the weather course in the experimental years. As the new contribution for the growing practice can be considered the possibility of cultivation of caraway in cover crop (spring wheat with lowered sowing rate of wheat), and the fact that caraway can be grown in the less suitable localities, such as, in lower and warmer locations, the short term droughts may impose the negative effects.

On the basis of minimal morphological differences, it can be possible to distinguish the "winter" genotypes from the varieties with the standard length vegetative period, e.g. biennial varieties. The other important output resulted from the experiments is the "Application of the registration of the pesticide in extent use via minority uses" according to the Act No. 326/2004 Sb. on phytosanitary care and changes of some other related acts. Two herbicides for pre-emergent (linuron, 450 g, 2.0 l.ha^{-1}) and post-emergent (propyzamide, 50 %, 3.0 kg.ha^{-1}) application were suggested. Both preparations had high selectivity against the caraway plants. Beside this, linuron (450 g) in the suggested dose showed very good or excellent efficacy against weeds and in all observed years, the yield of the achenes was the highest from the pre-emergently treated variants.

Acknowledgments

The authors want to thank for the support to these two projects: Ministry of Agriculture of the Czech Republic, National Agency for Agriculture Research No. EP 7043: Biodiversity of caraway (*Carum carvi* L.) and possibilities of its use in the integrated plant production. Ministry of Agriculture of the Czech Republic, National Agency for Agriculture Research, project QF 4056: Use of current caraway varieties (*Carum carvi* L.) and new methods of its breeding for improvement of quantitative and qualitative parameters.

References

Baysal, T. and Starmans, D.A.J. (1999). Supercritical carbon dioxide extraction of carvone and limonene from caraway seed. *Journal of Supercritical Fluids*, 14: 225-234.

Bouwmeester, H.J., Davies, J.A.R. and Toxopeus, H. (1995a). Enantiomeric composition of carvone, imonene, and carveols in seeds of dill and annual and biennial caraway varieties. *Journal of Agricultural and Food Chemistry*,43(12): 3057-3064.

Bouwmeester, H.J., Davies, J.A.R., Smid, H.G. and Weltren, R.S.A. (1995b). Physiological limitations to carvone yield in caraway (*Carum carvi* L.). *Industrial Crops and Products*, 4 (1): 39-51.

Bouwmeester, H.J., Gerhenzon, J., Konigs, M.C.J.M. and Croteau, R. (1998). Biosynthesis of the monoterpenes limonene and carvone in the fruits of caraway – I. Demonstration of enzyme activities and their changes with development. *Plant Physiology,* 117 (3): 901-912.

Bruneton, J. (1999). *Pharmacognosy, Phytochemistry and Medicinal Plants.* INTERCEPT Ltd, Andover, U. K.

De Carvalho, C.R. and Da Fonseca, M.R. (2006). Carvone: Why and how should one bother to produce this terpene. *Food Chemistry*, 95 (3): 413-422.

Cizkova, H., Vacek, J., Voldrich, M., Sevcik, R. and Kratka, J. (2000). Caraway essential oil as potential inhibitor of potato sprouting. *Rostlinna Vyroba,* 46 (11): 501-507.

Czech Pharmacopoeia 2009 (2009). Grada Publishing, Prague, Czech Republic.

European Pharmacopoeia (2008). 6th Edition, Supplement 6.6, 01/2010.

Fišerová, H., Kocourková, B. and Klemš, M. (1999). Physiological characteristics of registered varieties of caraway (*Carum carvi* L.). In: *Book of Abstracts from the seminar for caraway growers.* B. Kocourková and M. Manhalterová (Eds), pp. 27-34. Mendel University of Agriculture and Forestry Brno, Czech Republic.

Fišerová, H., Vašatová, V., Klemš, M. and Kocourková, B. (2008). Influence of the year, the variety and the locality on dormancy of caraway aachenes (*Carum carvi* L.). In: *Book of Abstracts from the 5th Conference on Medicinal and Aromatic Plants of Southeast European Countries.* G. Růžičková (ed) pp. 100. Mendel University of Agriculture and Forestry Brno, Czech Republic.

Hradilík, J. and Císařová, H. (1975a). Study of dormancy of caraway achenes (*Carum carvi* L.). *Rostlinná výroba,* 21 (4): 351- 364.

Hradilík, J. and Císařová, H. (1975b). The role of abscisic acid (ABA) in achenes of dormant cumin. *Acta Univ. Agric.* XXIII. 4: 748-753.

Hradilík, J. and Fišerová, H. (1980). The role of abscisic acid in achenes of dormant caraway *Carum carvi* L.. Acta univ. agric. (Brno), *Fac. Agron.* XXVIII, 2: 39-64.

Iacobellis, N.S., Cantore, L.P., Capasso, F. and Senatore, F. (2005). Antibacterial activity of *Cuminum cyminum* L. and *Carum carvi* L. essential oils. *Journal of Agricultural and Food Chemistry*, 55: 57-61.

Jarošová, I. (2008). *The influence of fungicides application on the essential oil content in caraway* (*Carum carvi* L.). Bc. Thesis, Mendel University of Agriculture and Forestry Brno, Brno, Czech Republic.

Kadlec, T. (1996). Varietal spectrum of caraway. In: Book of Abstract from the seminar *"The perspectives of caraway production in Czech agriculture"*, pp. 16-17.

Kameník, J. (1999). Czech caraway – association. In: *Book of Abstracts from the seminar for caraway growers.* B. Kocourková and M. Manhalterová (Eds) pp. 5-7. Mendel University of Agriculture and Forestry Brno, Czech Republic.

Kocourková, B. (1996). Biology and agrotechnology of caraway. In: Book of Abstracts from the seminar *"The perspectives of caraway production in Czech agriculture"*, Brno, pp. 11-14.

Kocourková, B., Sedláková, J. and Holubová, V. (1999). Morphological and qualitative traits of registered varieties of caraway. In: *Book of Abstracts from the seminar for caraway growers.* Kocourková, B. and Manhalterová, M. (Eds) pp. 34. Mendel University of Agriculture and Forestry Brno, Czech Republic.

Králík, J. (2007). *Increasing of qualitative and quantitative parameters of caraway (Carum carvi* L.). Ph.D. Thesis, Mendel University of Agriculture and Forestry Brno, Czech Republic, 136 p.

Králík, J., Jůzl, M. and Kocourková, B. (2007). The influence of the environment on the yield and essential oil content of caraway (*Carum carvi* L.). *Acta Universitatis Agriculturae et Silviculturae Mendelianae Brunensis,* LV (5): 83-94.

Mičánková, M. and Lejnar, J. (1991). *Plants in therapy, kitchen and cosmetics (1991).* SEUT Prague, Czech republic, 176 p.

Németh, E. (1998). *Caraway. The genus Carum.* Harwood Academic Publishers, The Netherlands, 195 p.

Odstrcilova, L., Ondrej, M., Kocourkova, B. and Ruzickova, G. (2002). Monitoring of incidence and determination of fungi on caraway, fennel, coriander and anise, consideration of disease importance and possibility of chemical protection. *Plant Protection Science,* 38 (Special 2): 340-343.

Odstrčilová, L. (2006). Diversity of fungl pathogens incidence in the Czech traditional regions of caraway cultivation. In: *Book of Abstracts* from 8th Conference of the European Foundation for Plant Patology, Coppenhagen, Denmark, p. 31.

Odstrčilová, L. (2007a). *The diseases of caraway and the possibilities of their control.* Ph.D. Thesis, Mendel University of Agriculture and Forestry Brno, Czech Republic, 107 p.

Odstrčilová, L. (2007b). Changes in the occurence of mycoflora on caraway seeds after fungicide application. *Plant Protection Science,* 43 (4): 146-150.

Official Journal of the European Union. Council Regulation (EC) No. 433/2008, 'Český kmín',Accessibleon<http://www.fsai.ie/uploadedFiles/ Legislation/Legislation_Update/Reg433_2008.pdf >.

Official Journal of the European Union. 2009/C 302 A/01 Common catalogue of varieties of agricultural plant species — 28th complete edition.. Accessible on-line from: < http://eurlex.europa.eu/JOHtml.do?uri=OJ%3AC%3A2009%3A302A%3ASOM%3AEN %3AHTML>.

Pank, F. (2009). Conventional breeding of medicinal and aromatic plants – fundamentals and examples. In: *Book of Abstracts from 4th International Symposium Breeding Research on Medicinal and Aromatic Plants.* Baričevič, D. and Ratajc, P. (Eds) pp. 25. University of Ljubljana, Ljubljana, Slovenia.

Růžičková, G., Reinöhl, V., Svoboda, Z., Mikulíková, R. and Kocourková, B. (2009). Quality assessment of some European caraway resources (*Carum carvi* L.) (2009) In: Book of Abstracts from 40th International Symposium on Essential Oils. Bicchi, C. and Rubiolo, P. (Eds). pp. 96. University of Turin, Savigliano, Italy.

Sedlakova, J. Kocourkova, B. and Kuban, V. (2001). Determination of essential oils content and composition in caraway (*Carum carvi* L.). *Czech Journal of Food Sciences,* 19 (1): 31-36.

Sedláková, J., Kocourková, B., Lojková, L. and Kubáň, V. (2003a). Determination of essential oil content in caraway (*Carum carvi* L.) species by means of supercritical fluid extraction. *Plant, Soil and Environment,* 49 (6): 277-282.

Sedláková, J., Kocourková, B., Lojková, L. and Kubáň, V. (2003b). The essential oil content in caraway spices (*Carum carvi* L.). *Horticulture Science,* 30: 73-79.

Šmirous, P., Kocourková, B. and Sedláková, J. (2004a). Cultivation and breeding caraway in the Czech republic. In: Proceedings from the 8th International Congress Phytopharm, Mikkeli, Finland, pp. 529-532.

Šmirous, P., Kocourková, B., Fišerová, H. and Králík, J. (2004b). Breeding of caraway in Czech Republic. In: Proceedings from 3rd Conference on Medicinal and Aromatic Plants of Southeast European Countries, M. Habán and P. Otepka (Eds) pp. 68-69, Nitra, Slovak Republic.

Šmirous, P. (2005). *The influence of recurrent phenotypic selection to the chosen yield characters of caraway* (*Carum carvi,* L.). Ph.D. Thesis, Mendel University of Agriculture and Forestry in Brno, Czech Republic, 79 p.

Smirous, P. and Kocourkova, B. (2006). Selection of useful caraway (*Carum carvi,* L.) genotypes for following breeding process. *Acta Universitatis Agriculturae et Silviculturae Mendelianae Brunensis,* 54 (2): 117-130.

Šmirous, P. and Kocourková, B. (2006). Choosing of suitable genotype sof caraway (*Carum carvi,* L.) for its further breeding. *Acta Universitatis Agriculturae et Silviculturae Mendelianae Brunensis,* LIV, 2: 117-130.

Šmirous, P., Kocourková, B. and Růžičková, G. (2006). Methods used for caraway (*Carum carvi* L.) breeding in The Czech Republic. In: Proceedings from 4rd Conference on Medicinal and Aromatic Plants of Southeast European Countries, pp. 231-233. Alma Mater Publishing House, Iasi, Romania.

Šmirous, P., Růžičková, G., Kocourková, B. and Fojtová, J. (2007). Variability of qualitative parameters of winter form of carawy (*Carum carvi* L.). In: *Book of Scientific Papers and Abstracts from the 1st International Scientific Conference on Medicinal, Aromatic and Spice Plants.* Habán, M. and Otepka, P. (Eds) pp. 15-19. Slovak University of Agriculture, Nitra, Slovakia.

Smykalova, I., Smirous, P., Kubosiova, M., Gasmanova, N. *and* Griga M. (2005). Dihaploid production via anther culture in Czech breeding lines of caraway (*Carum carvi* L.). In: International Conference on Plant Embryology, Cracow, Poland. Kuta, E. (Ed.) XII. *Acta Biologica Cracoviensia. Series Botanica,* 47 (1): 52.

Smykalova, I., Horacek, J., Smykal, P., Soukup, A., Gasmanova, N., Kubosiova, M. and Griga, M. (2006). Detection of dihaploid status using isozyme analysis and fluorescent microscopy in caraway. In: The International Conference Haploids in Higher Plants III., Touraev, A., and Forster B. (Eds.) pp. 43. Vienna, Austria.

Smykalova, I., Smirous, P., Kubosiova, M., Gasmanova, N. and Griga, M. (2009). Doubled haploid production via anther culture in annual, winter type of caraway (*Carum carvi* L.). *Acta Physiologiae Plantarum,* 31 (1): 21-31.

Vaculík, A. (2006). Influence of herbicide protection on quantitative and qualitative characteristics of caraway (*Carum carvi* L.). In: *Book of Abstracts from 4rd Conference on Medicinal and Aromatic Plants of Southeast European Countries*, pp. 6. Iasi, Romania.

Vaculík, A. (2007). *The influence of herbicidal treatment on the yield and Essentials oil content of spice plants in the Czech Republic.* Doctoral Thesis, Mendel University of Agriculture and Forestry in Brno, Fac. of Agronomy, Brno.

Vaculík, A. (2008). The influence of preemergently applied herbicides on the yield and duality of caraway (*Carum carvi* L.). *Acta Universitatis Agriculturae et Silviculturae Mendelianae Brunensis,* MZLU Brno, LIV, 2: 255 - 266.

Vaculík, A., Kocourková, B., Šmirous, P., Odstrčilová, L., Růžičková, G. and Seidenglanz, M. (2008). *The methodology of growing of caraway. Certified methodology.* Mendel University of Agriculture and Forestry in Brno, Agritec, Research, Breeding and Services, Ltd, Czech Caraway association, Brno, Czech Republic, 29 p.

Vejrazka, K., Hrudova, E., Kocourkova, B. and Cerkal, R. (2008). Insecticidal effect of carvone against the wheat weevil (*Sitophiius granarius* L.). In: Proceedings of the 4th International Congress on Flour – Bread '07, pp. 261-265, Croatia.

Vrzalová, J. and Procházka, F. (1988). *The System of Caraway Growing.* Ministry of Agriculture and Nutrition of ČSR.

Zambori-Németh, E. (2005). Taxon evaluation methods for caraway (*Carum carvi* L.) role and significance of the studied plant properties. *Kertgazdasag – Horticulture*, Special Issue, pp. 209-220.

Zemek, R., Kurowska, M., Kamenikova, L., Rovenska, G.Z., Havel, J. and Reindl, F. (2005). Studies on phenology and harmfulness of *Aceria carvi* Nal. (Acari: Eriophyidae) on caraway, *Carum carvi* L., in the Czech Republic. *Journal of Pest Science,* 78 (2): 115-116.

In: Medicinal Plants and Sustainable Development
Editor: Chandra Prakash Kala

ISBN 978-1-61761-942-7
© 2011 Nova Science Publishers, Inc.

Chapter 2

Sustainable Agriculture for Medicinal Plants

Ricardo Gomez-Flores and *Patricia Tamez-Guerra*
Departamento de Microbiología e Inmunología, Laboratorio de Inmunología y Virología,
Facultad de Ciencias Biológicas, Universidad Autónoma de Nuevo León, San Nicolás de
los Garza, N. L., México

Abstract

Globally, demand of medicinal plants (MP) has been increasing from the past decade and still the main trading products come from wild harvesting. This practice has led to an increase of MP threatened species. In order to fulfill the MP demand without increasing the number of threatened species, countries that lead the MP treading market or have a high MP diversity must look after sustainable practices to continue the production and commercialization of MP. Sustainable cultivation of MP species will assure that the biological resource is preserved for future generations and that harvested practices are being performed within the limits of their capacity for self-reproduction and natural dissemination. In addition, sustainable practices must follow an environment impact study to conserve the environment as a whole, to allow genetic prevalence of flora and fauna. In order to implement and reinforce the cultivation of MP by using sustainability practices within developing countries, the scientific, academic, and economic support of global agencies, as well as international MP treading guidelines must be involved.

Keywords: ecosystem conservation, management programs, medicinal plants, sustainable agriculture, threatened species, wild harvest.

* LIV-DEMI. FCB-UANL. AP 46-F Cd. Universitaria, San Nicolás de los Garza N.L., México 66450. Tel.: (5281) 8329-4000 ext. 6453; Fax: (5281) 8352-4212; Email: rgomez60@hotmail.com

Introduction

Medicinal plants (MP) marketing has been increasing in the past decade, and their high demand has prompted trading from local to international level. Annual worldwide MP imports, referred as pharmaceutical plants, reported in 2008 a total of more than 5,500 million dollars, compared with 1,200 millions in 2003 (COMTRADE, 2009). Nevertheless, MP production is not currently depending on normal agricultural sources, but from large-scale wild collections (http://www.bgci.org/resources/news/0525/).

The increasing commercialization of wild-collected, largely unmonitored trading, and habitat loss of MP has led to endanger native MP (Brower, 2008). As a matter of fact, by 2008 it was estimated that 9,000 MP species were under threatened status (Hawkins, 2008). Based on this information, MP conservation and reproduction strategies are of high priority. Thus, reproduction of MP must follow a sustainable agriculture model, in order to reduce or prevent such status and improve the MP commercial use and nature conservation (Lange, 2006).

Sustainable development is expressed by the relationship between people and the ecosystem around it, when both are satisfactory growing or even improving (Prescott-Allen and Prescott-Allen, 1996). Nevertheless, what the term sustainable in agriculture implies is not that simple. Specialists have pointed out that the term sustainable should be used as:

1. Assure persistence, demonstrating capabilities to continue for a long period of time
2. Implement a reliance system, which includes strategies to overcome development difficulties, especially related to ecosystem
3. Assure that this practice will not reduce natural resources (mainly water availability) (Dürbeck, 1999; Farnsworth and Soejarto, 1991; Groombridge and Jenkins, 2002).

Medicinal Plants Global Demand

Demand for a large variety of wild species is increasing with human needs and commercial trade. Developing countries and their indigenous MP populations produce, use and commercialize most MP (Harnischfeger, 2000; FAO, 1995). As a result, MP are not only being used as traditional medicines but also as trade commodities, which meet the demand of often distant markets. Under this scope, China and India are the major MP producers and exporters, followed by Germany, which mainly use wild-collected MP for trading purposes (COMTRADE, 2009). With the increased realization that some wild species are being over-exploited, a number of agencies are recommending that wild species be brought into cultivation systems (Lambert *et al.* 1997; WHO, 2006; WHO, IUCN and WWF, 1993), which have conservation impacts among native flora and fauna; that is why MP cultivation needs to follow an ecological risk impact study before implementing it. For example, it must be ensured that MP cultivation is done in a land where no other species might be endangered and assured that harvesting of MP wild populations are properly harvested to avoid environmental degradation and even loss of genetic diversity, which may lead to loss of incentives to preserve wild populations (Lange, 1998, 2004). Thus, MP production from sustainable agriculture is vital to improve the management programs of MP cultivation and to ensure their conservation. To assure the sustainable agriculture of MP production, international organizations have promoted the conservation of biological diversity worldwide, looking for economical support to implement this practice in developing countries (Lange, 2002; Bodeker et al., 1997).

Why is the Sustainability Program Implementation Critical?

Worldwide, around 70-80% of human population relies on MP as primary healthcare source (Pei, 2001). Thus, as population increases, the MP demand also increases (Hamilton, 2004). The market for MP in India was estimated to increase 20% annually (Subrat, 2002), whereas the MP collected from just one province in China (Yunnan) raised 10 times in 10 years (Pei, 2002). In a survey carried out by the Rainforest Alliance, companies involved in trade and production of MP revealed what 60–90 % of the traded volume was cultivated, but most species were wild collected (Laird and Pierce, 2002). Uniyal et al. (2000) reported that out of 400 MP species used by the Indian industry, less than 20 were cultivated. Similarly, reports from last decade of MP species being cultivated revealed that in China, only 100–250 (out of 1000 used and treaded) are being cultivated (Govaerts, 2001). In Hungary, a country with a long tradition of MP cultivation, only 40 MP are produced by cultivation, whereas in Europe, only 130–140 MP species are cultivated (Bernáth, J. 1999; Shan-An and Sheng, 1997; Verlet and Leclercq, 1999). This data revealed the high incidence of wild MP harvesting around the world.

It is known that MP collecting methods are often crude and wasteful, resulting in loss of quality and reduction in price; wild harvesting has negatively impacted in the species distribution and population, and has permanently damaged MP, especially within perennial plants. Inadequate harvesting of perennial plants may delay its recovery or could even lead to plant death; same results can be observed after extracting the roots (Lange, 2002; 2004).

Sustainable practices must assure not only the environmental stability after cultivation, but also that the harvesting practice does not degrade the environment in other ways (Schippmann, 1997). Global implementation of MP sustainable agriculture will be hard to implement in extremely low income populations, besides the opposition of changing the MP wild collection traditional activity, and the lack of knowledge about sustainable agriculture practices, undefined land use rights, and legislative and guidance policies (Iqbal, 1993).

Nevertheless, sustainable cultivation of MP may reduce wild harvesting and this may result in improving the developing countries economy, the cultural identity and livelihood security, and may gradually reduce the MP threatened species (Schippmann, 1997; Pinheiro, 1997; Mander, 1998). Among the actions to take in order to improve the sustainable agriculture of MP are:

1. MP growth in areas where the plant species are found, to achieve conservation of natural habitats
2. MP *ex situ* conservation in countries of high demand, like China, assuring agriculture practice and growth areas to avoid endangering other native plant species, and

3. Bioprospecting to achieve enough production to meet demand, but looking forward the biological diversity (Bernáth, 1999; Cunningham, 1997; -2001)

MP Production Strategies

Sustainable agriculture practices can take place as enrichment planting, under natural conditions more than under agriculture regime. Some strategies for MP production following a sustainable program are:

1. Growing specific species at small-scale in home gardens (to be used as family remedies)
2. Growing specific species at small scale by herbalist (to cover locally demand)
3. Cultivation by local people, where endemic MPs are located (Agelet et al., 2000; CBD, 1992).

Unfortunately, there are several reasons why the MP cultivation will never fit in the market. One example is the ginseng, whose cultivation fits the demand-cost economy model; the largest consumer group of wild ginseng believes that wild root shapes symbolizes the vitality and potency of the root. Based on this assumption, the price of wild ginseng in the market is 5–10 times higher than ginseng roots produced under growing agriculture models (Nantel et al., 1996; Robbins, 1998). As a result, ginseng is produced mostly at small-scale because large cultivation systems do not meet the herbalist demand.

Another example is the metabolite content; it is a challenge to meet the expectations of metabolite amounts in a specific MP in the market. Scientific studies have shown that secondary metabolites production, which represent the active ingredients of MP, may be induced under stress and plant competition, and may not be produced under mono-culture conditions. In this regard, herbalists from Botswana stated that cultivated MP do not have the efficacy of wild collected MP (Cunningham, 1994). To prevent this, agriculture growing conditions that induce metabolites production must be found and implemented for MP international treading success (Uniyal et al., 2000). As a matter of fact, in recent years, most international herbalist companies prefer cultivated MP, because this material can be certified at biodynamic or organic level (Laird and Pierce, 2002).

Advantages of sustainable agriculture of MP include:

1. Speed and facilitation of the treading process and certification to achieve self-consumption and exportation.
2. Harvest volumes will become easier to guarantee and improve their distribution, marketing and exportation schedule.
3. Cultivation of selected hybrids or MP traits will assure the active ingredient amount per weight, to meet herbal market expectation.
4. Better control of post-harvest treatment (drying, milling, packing, etc.).
5. Quality control to fit market regulations and consumer preferences between MP production lots, and

6. Speed the organic or biodynamic certification (Kuipers, 1997; Leaman, 2002; Pierce et al., 2002).

Benefits of MP sustainable agriculture include native plant germoplasm conservation strategies for most wild-harvested species and their habitats, given their current and potential contributions to local economies and their greater value to harvesters over the long term. In order to gradually increase or implement MP sustainable agriculture practice, adequate information about distribution, genetic diversity, wild populations and relative species are needed, in addition to the annual sustained yield that can be harvested without damaging natural flora (Leaman et al., 1997; Prescott-Allen and Prescott-Allen, 1996; Roling and Wagemakers, 1998).

MP Sustainable Use: The Sri Lanka Experience

Sri Lanka maintains about 3,500 species of plants and 100 species of ferns of which about 1,500 have medicinal value; of these MP, about 190 were found only in Sri Lanka. This reason was a key to support the MP cultivation project using a sustainability model, it was named "The Sri Lanka Medicinal Plant Conservation and Sustainable Use Project" (GOSL, 2004). The basic idea behind sustainable harvesting is that a biological resource must be harvested within the limits of its capacity for self-renewal. Responding to these factors, The Government of Sri Lanka (GOSL), adopted the developmental objective of the project as to *globally and nationally conserve significant medicinal plants, their habitats, species and genomes and promote their sustainable use.*
Project objectives based in a general biodiversity project included:

1. Conservation and sustainable use of medicinal plants found in the wild (*in situ*),
2. Production of medicinal plants *ex situ* as a substitute for harvesting from the wild, as a source of income for the herbalist communities, and
3. Provide incentives to protect and use forest resources responsibly (FAO 1995; Harnischfeger, 2000; Moerman, 1996; Palevitch, 1991).

Since the project was launched, the main lesson has been that traditional medicine and indigenous knowledge in general, could be supported through a disciplined and strategic manner. The project has served as a learning exercise from other countries under the World Bank's Indigenous Knowledge Development Program. Sustainable use of biological resources would seem self-evidently desirable, but there are complexities in its practical definition and attainment:

1. Human understanding of how ecosystems function is weak.
2. The standing stock of a resource can alter for reasons unconnected with its use (e.g. related to ecological succession). Production of medicinal plants *ex situ* as a substitute for harvesting from the wild, as a source of income for the herbalist and communities, and different sections of society can place different values on

resources, which can have contradictory implications for sustainability (Mander, 1998; Hamilton, 2005).

Conclusion

The increasing commercialization of medicinal plants has led to endangering native species. One approach to overcome this issue is to implement sustainable agriculture practices, mainly in countries with strong culture, diversity, use, and trading of medicinal plants.

Pro-ecology international organizations must support and implement projects to look after the environmental conditions needed to achieve sustainable agriculture practices for medicinal plants. Evaluation would include biodiversity, germoplasm persistence, environmentally friendly and reliable cultivation/harvesting systems, strategies to overcome development difficulties (i. e. water supply, soil erosion), and assurance that cultivation or sustainable harvesting of perennial plants will not reduce natural resources (native flora and fauna). In addition, harvesting practice monitoring and management prescriptions must be scheduled, following procedures to ensure cultivation/ harvesting management programs.

References

Agelet, A., Bonet, M.A. and Valles, J. (2000). Homegardens and their role as a main source of medicinal plants in mountain regions of Catalonia (Iberian Peninsula), *Economic Botany,* 54: 295–309.

Baker, J. T. Borris, R. P., Carté, B., Cordell, G. A., Soejarto, D. D., Cragg, G. M., Gupta, M. P., Iwu, M. M., Madulid, D. R., and Tyler, V. E. (1995). Natural product drug discovery and development: new perspectives on international collaboration. *Journal of Natural Products*, 58 (9): 1325-1357

Bernáth, J. (1999). Biological and economical aspects of utilization and exploitation of wild growing medicinal plants in middle and south Europe. In: *Proceedings of the Second World Congress on Medicinal and Aromatic Plants for Human Welfare.* WOCMAP II. Biological resources, sustainable use, conservation and ethnobotany. ISHS (Acta Horticulturae 500). Caffini, N., Bernath, J., Craker, L., Jatisatienr, A. and Giberti, G. (eds.), pp. 31–41. Leuven, The Netherlands.

Bodeker, G., Bhat, K.K.S., Burley, J., and Vantomme, P. Eds. (1997). *Medicinal plants for forest conservation and health care.* Rome, FAO (Non-wood Forest Products 11).

Brower, V. (2008). Back to nature: extinction of medicinal plants threatens drug discovery. *J. Natl. Cancer Inst*, 100: 838-839.

CBD. (1992) Convention on Biological Diversity. www.biodiv.org.

COMTRADE. (2009). *COMTRADE database,* United Nation Statistics Division, New York. leading countries of import and export of MAP material classified as pharmaceutical plants (SITC.3: 292.4 = commodity group HS 121190, HS1996).

Cunningham, A.B. (1994). Management of medicinal plant resources. In: *Proceedings of the 13th Plenary Meeting of AETFAT, Zomba, Malawi*, Seyani, J.H. and Chikuni, A.C. (eds.) Vol. 1. pp. 173–189, Limbe, Cameroon, Montfort.

Cunningham, A.B. (1997). The "Top 50" listings and the Medicinal Plants Action Plan. *Medicinal Plant Conservation*, 3: 5-7.

Cunningham, A.B. (2001). *Applied ethnobotany*. Earthscan People, wild plant use and conservation. People and Plants Conservation Manuals, London.

Dürbeck, K. (1999). Green trade organizations. Striving for fair benefits from trade in non-wood forest products. *Unasylva* 198. Retrieved from FAO website, www.fao.org/docrep/x2450e/x2450e04.htm

FAO Food and Agriculture Organization of the United Nations. (1995). *Non-wood forest products for rural income and sustainable development*. Rome, Italy.

Farnsworth, N.R. and D.D. Soejarto. (1991). Global importance of medicinal plants. In: *Conservation of medicinal plants*. Akerele, O., Heywood, V. and Synge, H. (eds.) pp. 25–51. University Press. Cambridge, UK.

GOSL. (2004). *Implementation Completion and Results Report*. Sri Lanka - Conservation and Sustainable Use of Medicinal Plants Project. Ministry Health and Indigenous Medicine/ Provincial Councils. South Asia. Report No. 29629.

Govaerts, R. (2001). How many species of seed plants are there? *Taxon*, 50: 1085–1090.

Groombridge, B. and Jenkins, M.D. (2002). *World atlas of biodiversity. Earth's living resources in the 21st century*. University of California Press. Berkeley, CA. USA.

Hamilton, A.C. (2004). Medicinal plants, conservation and livelihoods. *Biodiversity and Conservation*, 13: 1477-1517.

Hamilton, A. C. (2005). *Resource assessment for sustainable harvesting of medicinal plants*. *S*ource to Shelf: Sustainable Supply Chain Management of Medicinal and Aromatic Plants, International Botanical Congress, Vienna, Italy. http://www.plantlife.org.uk/international/assets/med-plants/what-are-med-plants/resource-assesment.pdf.

Harnischfeger, G. (2000). Proposed guidelines for commercial collection of medicinal plant material. *Journal of Herbs, Spices and Medicinal Plants*, 7 (1): 43–50.

Hawkins, B. (2008). *Plants for life: Medicinal plant conservation and botanic gardens*. Botanic Gardens Conservation International, Richmond, U.K.

Iqbal, M. (1993). *International trade in non-wood forest products, An overview*. FAO. Rome, Italy.

Kuipers, S.E. (1997). Trade in medicinal plants. In: *Medicinal plants for forest conservation and health care*. Bodeker, G., Bhat, K.K.S., Burley J., and Vantomme, P. (eds.) FAO, pp. 45–59. Rome, Italy.

Laird, S.A. and. Pierce, A.R. (2002). Promoting sustainable and ethical botanicals. Strategies to improve commercial raw material sourcing. Results from the sustainable botanicals pilot project. Industry surveys, case studies and standards collection. New York, Rainforest Alliance (www.rainforest-alliance.org/news/archives/news/news44.html).

Lambert, J., Srivastava, J. and Vietmeyer, N. (1997). *Medicinal plants. Rescuing a global heritage*. World Bank. World Bank Technical Paper 355), Washington DC.

Lange, D. (1998). *Europe's medicinal and aromatic plants. Their use, trade and conservation*. TRAFFIC International. Cambridge, UK.

Lange, D. (2002). The role of east and southeast Europe in the medicinal and aromatic plants' trade. *Medicinal Plant Conservation,* 8: 14–18.

Lange, D. (2004). Medicinal and aromatic plants: trade, production, and management of botanical resources. *Acta Hort.* (ISHS), 629: 177-197. http://www.actahort.org/books/629/629_25.htm

Lange, D. (2006). International trade in medicinal and aromatic plants. In: *Medicinal and Aromatic Plants,* Bogers, R.J., Craker, L.E., and Lange D. (eds.) pp 155-170. Springer. The Netherlands.

Leaman, D.J., U. Schippmann and L. Glowka (1997). Environmental protection concerns of prospecting and producing plant-based drugs. In: *International symposium on herbal medicine. A holistic approach. Documents, proceedings and recommendations.* Wozniak, D.A., Yuen, S., Garrett, M., and Schuman, T.M. (eds.) International Institute Human Resources Development. Honolulu. pp. 352–378. San Diego, CA, USA.

Leaman, D. (2002). Medicinal plants. Briefing notes on the impacts of domestication /cultivation on conservation. Paper for the "Commercial captive propagation and wild species conservation" workshop, 7–9.12.2001, Jacksonville, FL, USA.

Mander, M. (1998). *Marketing of indigenous medicinal plants in South Africa - A Case Study in Kwazulu-Natal.* FAO. Rome, Italy.

Moerman, D.E. (1996). An analysis of the food plants and drug plants of native North America, *Journal of Ethnopharmacology,* 52: 1–22.

Nantel, P., Gagnon, D. and Nault, A. (1996). Population viability analysis of American ginseng and wild leek harvested in stochastic environments. *Conservation Biology*, 10: 608–621.

Palevitch, D. (1991). Agronomy applied to medicinal plant conservation. In: *Conservation of medicinal plants.* Akerele, O., Heywood, V. and Synge, H. (eds.), pp. 168–178, University Press. Cambridge, UK.

Pei, S. L. (2001). Ethnobotanical approaches of traditional medicine studies: Some experiences from Asia. *Pharmaceutical Biology*, 39: 74-79.

Pei, S. L. (2002). *Ethnobotany and modernisation of traditional Chinese medicine.* In: Workshop on wise practices and Experimental learning in the Conservation and Management of Himalayan Medicinal Plants. Katmandu, Nepal.

Pierce, A., Laird, S. and Malleson, R. (2002). *Annotated collection of guidelines, standards and regulations for trade in non-timber forest products (NTFPs) and botanicals.* Version 1.0. – New York, Rainforest Alliance. Retrieved from www.rainforestalliance.org/news/archives/ news/news44.html.

Pinheiro, C.U.B. (1997). Jaborandi (*Pilocarpus* sp., Rutaceae). A wild species and its rapid transformation into a crop. *Economic Botany,* 51: 49–58.

Prescott-Allen, R. and Prescott-Allen, C. (1996). *Assessing the sustainability of uses of wild species. Case studies and initial assessment procedure.* Occasional Paper of the IUCN Species Survival Commission 12. Gland and Cambridge, IUCN.

Robbins, C.S. (1998). *American ginseng. The root of North America's medicinal herb trade.* TRAFFIC USA. Washington, DC. USA.

Roling, N. and Wagemakers, A. (1998). *Facilitating sustainable agriculture: participatory learning and adaptive management in times of environmental uncertainty.* Cambridge University Press, Cambridge, UK.

Schippmann, U. (1997). Plant uses and species risk. From horticultural to medicinal plant trade. In: *Planta Europaea*. Proceedings of the first European Conference on the conservation of wild plants, Hyères, France, 2–8 September 1995. Newton, J. (ed.) pp. 161–165. Plantlife, London.

Shan-An, H., and Sheng, N. (1997). Utilization and conservation of medicinal plants in China with special reference to *Atractylodes lancea*. In: *Medicinal plants for forest conservation and health care*. Bodeker, G., Bhat, K.K.S., Burley, J., and Vantomme, P. (eds.) pp. 109–115. FAO. Rome, Italy.

Subrat, N. (2002). *Ayurvedic and herbal products industry: an overview*. In: Workshop on wise practices and experiential learning in the conservation and management of Himalayan medicinal plants. Ministry of Forest and Soil Conservation, Nepal, the WWF-Nepal Program, MAPPA and PPI. Kathmandu, Nepal.

Uniyal, R.C., Uniyal, M.R., and Jain, P. (2000). *Cultivation of medicinal plants in India. A reference book.* TRAFFIC India and WWF India. New Delhi, India.

Verlet, N., and Leclercq, G. (1999). The production of aromatic and medicinal plants in the European Union. An economic database for a development strategy. In: *Medicinal plant trade in Europe*. Proceedings of the first symposium on the conservation of medicinal plants in trade in Europe, 22–23.6.1998, Kew. TRAFFIC Europe, (ed.), pp. 121–126, Brussels, Belgium.

WEB SITES: http://www.bgci.org/resources/news/0525/.

WHO, IUCN and WWF. (1993). *Guidelines on the conservation of medicinal plants.* Gland and Geneva, Switzerland.

WHO. (2006). *Traditional medicine strategy 2002–2005.* Retrieved from WHO website, www.who.int/medicines/ library/trm/trm_strat_eng.pdf

In: Medicinal Plants and Sustainable Development
Editor: Chandra Prakash Kala

ISBN 978-1-61761-942-7
© 2011 Nova Science Publishers, Inc.

Chapter 3

Setting Conservation Priorities for Medicinal and Other Ethnobotanical Resources: Case Study of Kachchh District, Gujarat (India)

*Arun M. Dixit[1] * and Chandra S. Silori[2]*
[1]Centre for Environment and Social Concerns (CESC),
Ahmedabad, Gujarat, India
[2]RECOFTC-The Centre for People and Forest, Bangkok, Thailand

Abstract

This chapter deals with the documentation of traditional ethnobotanical knowledge of rural communities and phyto-sociology of ethnobotanical resources of district Kachchh in western India with a major objective of setting up conservation priorities of ethnobotanical resources. We recorded the ethnobotanical knowledge from about 900 respondents spread across various age groups, gender, educational and socio-economic strata. We documented more than 10200 information 'units' on medicinal and non-medicinal (i.e. domestic) uses of plants. While 259 species were reported for 16 human and 10 veterinary disease classes, 193 plant species were reported for 18 domestic uses. In total 320 species were reported useful by the local communities. The availability of these species was recorded by sampling 24 representative locations in the district. Based on reports of 'purpose-part used' combinations of species, two different indices (the Use-Value Richness, and Use-Value Diversity) were computed to record overall ethnobotanical use-values of each species.

Finally, the use-values and the availability of the species at regional level were integrated to set the conservation priorities. Accordingly, 51 species were grouped under 'high' conservation priority, 38 of them solely threatened by the destructive mode of extraction, justifying immediate attention for their conservation.

* G-3, Sameep Apartment, Nr. Shreyas Bridge, Manekbaug, Ahmedabad, Gujarat, India – 380015. E-mail: arunmdixit@cesc-india.org . Ph: 079-26401571

Keywords: Ecology, Plant Availability, Quantitative Index, Traditional Knowledge, Use Value.

Introduction

Past decades witnessed growing interest on conservation and development of ethnobotanical resources (Arnold and Ruiz Perez, 1998) owing to their significant contribution in local economy, livelihood security and maintenance of biological diversity (de Beers and McDermott, 1989). In India, over 9500 plant species are reported within the domain of traditional knowledge system, for variety of uses such as for food, medicine, beverages, dyes, clothing, shelter, ritualistic practices etc. (MoEF, 1994). About 700 Scheduled Tribes are the main custodian of such rich and diverse knowledge of plant uses. Importantly, it is also recognized that vast majority of knowledge are yet to be documented or codified.

Conversely, high cost of bio-prospecting through formal scientific approaches embarks industries for ethnobotanical leads. In a rapidly globalizing world, where trade is emerging as one major barrier-free economic force, Intellectual Property Rights (IPR) can provide some sort of protection to the exploitation (or theft) of traditional ethnobotanical knowledge and resources. Documentation and protection of such a wealth is prerequisite for accruing the IPR and other benefits to the 'poor but knowledgeable' tribal as well as other rural communities. It is also recognized that the decline of plant resources and erosion of traditional knowledge of various uses of plants are complimenting each other's and form a downward spiral of ecological as well as economical degradation (Gupta, 2001). A workable conservation strategy for ethnobotanically important species, therefore, needs to be relied on (a) meaningful inferences from the traditional knowledge of local communities and (b) ecological status of plant species in the wild. Ironically, the integration of these two elements has seldom been attempted to devise conservation strategies (Kala et al, 2004). Kachchh district in the western Indian state of Gujarat is quite diverse in its ecological settings and thus supports quite a rich plant resource base (Anon, 2002). These plant resources are used for different purpose by various socio-culturally distinct communities. First documentation of plant uses in Kachchh was made by Thackar (1926) who reported medicinal and other economic uses of about 500 flowering plant species. Recently, however, there were several studies conducted to document the domestic and medicinal uses of plants of Kachchh (e.g. Rolla, 1970; Rao, 1970; Silori and Rana, 2000; Master, 2000; Joshi, 2002). While, most of these studies mainly focused on documenting various uses of plants, they generally overlooked basic information about the availability of such species in the wild. Considering such a gap in knowledge in view, this article attempts to presents an analytical approach where traditional knowledge system of plant species and their ecological status is integrated for setting conservation priorities of ethnobotanical resources in Kachchh district.

Study Area

Kachchh district is the second largest district of the country, encompassing an area of 45,652 km^2, forms international border with Pakistan on its northern sides (Figure 1). Almost 50% of the total landmass of the district is covered by two saline desert landscapes- Great and Little Rann of Kachchh. It is characterized by arid to semi-arid climatic conditions with 366 mm of average annual precipitation and high inter-annual variation (~60% CV). Biogeographically, Kachchh is categorized as one of the Biotic Provinces (viz. 3A– Kachchh Desert) within the larger Bio-geographic Zone – the Indian Desert (Rodgers and Panwar, 1988). It consists of a mosaic of three major physiographical regions viz. (a) saline flats of Ranns and Banni (b) coastal regions and (c) mainland. These regions support a range of habitats including the grasslands, savannas, thorn forests and mangroves. According to 2001 census, human population of the district is reported about 15.26 lakhs. Dryland agriculture and animal husbandry are predominant livelihoods for majority of rural population.

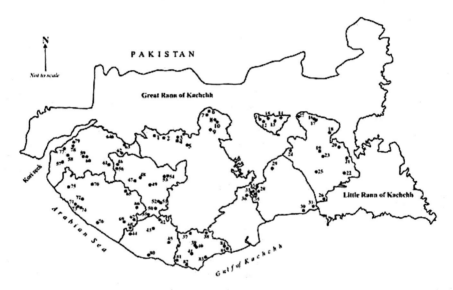

Figure 1. Location Map of Kachchh District. Small Dots Indicate Sample Villages.

Approach and Methodology

Knowledge Documentation

This study was conducted between 2001 and 2003. As per the demographic census of 1991, Kachchh district had 884 villages. For traditional knowledge documentation, we randomly selected and sampled 85 villages distributed across length and breadth of the district. In order to capture the variation in socio-cultural settings and resource use pattern, care was taken to avoid sampling of closely located villages and with similar community composition. Further at household level, respondents were randomly selected from different socio-economic strata. Variation across age, sex, caste and occupation were other important criteria while selecting respondents.

For documenting the traditional knowledge of plant uses, structured questionnaires were developed through iterative process involving several rounds of field testing. The documentation on the uses of plants for medicinal and non-medicinal purposes captured detailed information on the plant part used, mode, season and source of extraction/collection, and methods of administration (for medicinal plants). Documentation of knowledge was done in the local 'Kachchhi' dialect. The interviews were conducted for both individual as well as group respondents. Thus, in 85 sample villages (Figure 1), we recorded ethnobotanical knowledge of about 900 respondents comprising of 273 individual and 181 group interviews.

Ecological Assessment

For ecological assessment, a total of 24 sites representing different ecosystems, habitats and land use types were identified. Vegetation sampling in the selected sites was conducted in monsoon and post-monsoon seasons for three consecutive years (2001-2003). In each site transects of varying length ranging from 1 to 2.5 km, were laid for sampling of tree, shrub and herbaceous species. For sampling tree species, plot of 10 m radius were laid at an every interval of 200m. Within the larger plot for tree sampling, one sub plot of 5 m radius was laid for sampling shrub species, while 3 quadrats of $1m^2$ each were laid for sampling grass and herbaceous species. Thus, a total of 410 plots each were sampled for tree and shrub layers while 1230 quadrats were sampled for the herbaceous layer. In each sampling area, species wise total numbers of plants were enumerated, besides recording other phytosociological parameters.

Data Analysis

Use Value Assessment

In ethnobotanical research, use value of species is defined either as the 'number' of purposes a species is used for (e.g. Dhar et al. 2000, Dixit and Geevan, 2000; Kala et al, 2004) or through some quantitative indices (Philips and Gentry, 1993a, b; Benz et al, 2000; Gomez-Beloz, 2002, Martinez et al, 2006, Uniyal et al, 2006).

In this study, we attempted to analyze this by employing two different indices (a) the 'use-value richness, UVR' and (b) 'use-value diversity, UVD'. We described the use-value of a species by its 'richness' of distinct 'purpose-parts used' combinations (PPC). In quantitative terms, UVR is similar to Marglef's species richness formula (Magurran, 1988) and thus is used for its measurement, as follows:

$$UV_R = (S-1)/\ln N$$

Where, UV_R = Use-Value Richness of a species; S= total number of PPCs reported for the species, and N= total number of information reported for the species.

It is also realized that for UVR estimation, PPC with few reports and that with more reports are not weighted and therefore not adequately differentiated. To incorporate both the richness of uses and the proportional abundance of different PPCs, we contemplated UVD. For a given species, computation of UVD is similar to Shannon-Wiener diversity index, as follows:

$$UV_D = -\sum [(n_i/N)*\log (n_i/N)]$$

Where, UV_D = Use value diversity of species, n_i = Frequency of reports of PPC_i for the species and, N= total number of information reported for the species.

In order to prepare a list of plant species with overall high use-values, the values of two indices were rescaled between 1 and 100 and finally added. Based on the aggregate score (range from 2-200), species were grouped into five use-value rank classes.

Availability of Useful Species

In the context of this study, plant availability is an important variable, determining plant use-pattern. To define these, all the recorded/reported species were first categorized for their distribution (wide or patchy) and local abundance (high or low) based on frequency and density of plants obtained through vegetation sampling. This is also supported by discussion with subject experts who are working in the area. To get a final picture of availability of plants of a particular species, both the distribution and plant abundance classes were arranged in a matrix and each species was grouped into one of the four availability classes (i) very frequent (ii) frequent (iii) less and, (iv) very less.

Results

Use Values

During the survey, respondents furnished a total of 10220 pieces of information: 5548 related with medicinal and 4672 with non-medicinal uses. Present vegetation survey and old records collectively listed 746 plants species from the district, while respondents reported various uses of 320 plant species i.e. on overall basis about 43% species were considered useful.

Importantly, while 193 species were described for their 18 non-medicinal uses, 259 species were reported for their medicinal value for treating 16 human and 10 veterinary diseases classes (Table 1).

Results also indicate that of 193 species with 18 non-medicinal values, about 44% species reported for single use, 47% for 2-5 uses and only 9% for more than 5 uses. Similarly, for 259 medicinal value species 81 (31%) were used for treating only one disease, 110 (42%) were reported for treating 2-5 diseases, 43 (17%) had properties of treating 6-8 disease, and the remaining 25 species reported with medicinal properties for treating more than 8 diseases (Figure 2). Thus overall 157 species were reported only for 1-2 ethnobotanical uses, while 57 species were reported for more than eight ethnobotanical purposes, and thus considered as species with high multipurpose values.

Table 1. Various Uses of Plant Species in District Kachchh

#	Non-medicinal use		Medicinal use		
	Use category	No.of species	Disease classes	No. of species (Human uses)	No. of species (Veterinary uses)
1	Edible	95	Antivenom	43	
2	House Construction	69	Blood Related	19	
3	Fodder	57	Dental	36	
4	Craft	39	Dermatological	36	2
5	Religious	32	ENT	45	
6	Datun (Chewing sticks)	30	Ophthalmic	38	3
7	Pickle	25	Gastrointestinal	141	36
8	Fuel	24	Health Tonic	66	2
9	Dye	23	Gynecological	14	29
10	Fencing hedge	15	Infection	120	36
11	Fibre	13	Nervous	9	1
12	Poison	12	Fever	52	7
13	Agri. Implements	11	Respiratory	73	2
14	Timber	10	Skeleto-muscular	100	
15	Oil	6	Urogenital	28	19
16	Narcotic	6	Others	48	
17	Beverage	4			
18	Musical instruments	5			

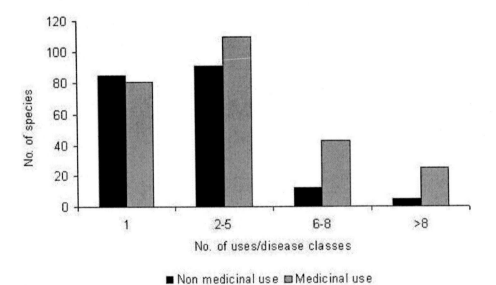

Figure 2. Frequency of Usage of Plant Species for Different Ethnobotanical Purposes.

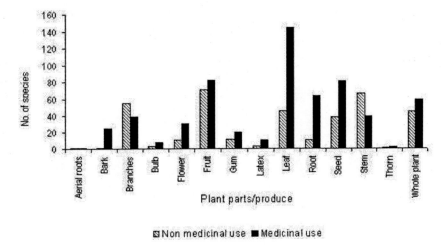

Figure 3. Frequency of Usage of Plant Species with Different Parts.

Respondents reported use of 13 different plant parts for various purposes. Leaves, fruits, seeds and roots topped the frequency of use for medicinal uses, while the fruits, stems and branches were commonly used for other domestic uses (Figure 3). Of the total 320 ethnobotanical species, 98 species were reported with single purpose-part combination (PPC) which effectively produced 'zero' values of UV_R and UV_D. For the remaining 222 useful species with multiple use values, the UV_R and UV_D values recorded substantial variation. Thus, the values of two indices ranged from 0.23 to 9.32 and from 0.07 to 2.89, respectively. Furthermore, out of 222 species, only 28 species recorded higher UV_R values of more than 4.0, while 46 species recorded UV_D values more than 2.0 (Figure 4 and 5). Species with higher index estimates are considered important for local communities.

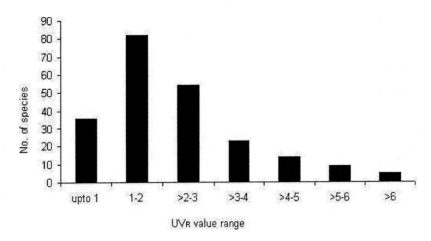

Figure 4. Frequency Distribution of UV_R Value of Ethnobotanical Species.

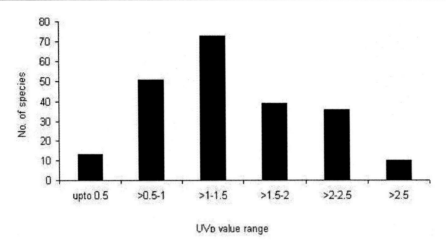

Figure 5. Frequency Distribution of UV_D Value of Ethnobotanical Species.

Conservation Prioritization

For setting the conservation priorities of each useful species, the use value scores were used along with the availability of plants. For easy and better comprehension, the use-value scores and plant availability classes (as described above) were regrouped into two broad classes each- the high and low. The use-value and plant availability classes were collectively placed in a two way matrix and four conservation priority classes were defined (Table 2). Thus the species with high use value and low availability were considered for top conservation priority (Priority-I), while the species with low use values and high availability were grouped under least priority (Priority IV).

Table 2. Conservation Priority based on Use Values and Plant Availability

		Species Availability	
		High	Low
Use Value	High	Priority II	Priority I
	Low	Priority IV	Priority III

It is imperative to emphasize here that this prioritization of species is limited to the Kachchh region and does not take into account whole of state, national or global level of species conservation concerns.

Nonetheless, it is equally important to recognize that the availability of a plant species to local users is key determining factor for setting conservation priorities, especially in the context of ethnobotanical uses.

Accordingly 19, 32, 98 and 171 species were grouped under priority I to IV, in that order. Interestingly, 51 species under Priority I and II constitute only about 16% of the total 320 useful species but they carry around 50% information in the form of total reported PPCs.

Also, 44 of such high conservation demanding species are wild in nature and thus assume greater significance for their management. A list of these 44 high ranked species is presented in Table 3.

Table 3. Reports and Use Values of High Priority Species of Kachchh District

#	Species	No. of Uses	No. of Parts Used	Total No.of Reports	No. of PPC	UV$_R$	UV$_D$
	Herbs/Climbers/Twiners						
1	Achyranthes aspera*	12	7	42	22	5.45	2.65
2	Aerva lanata*	10	5	35	13	3.25	2.1
3	Aristolochia bracteolate*	9	4	37	13	3.15	1.91
4	Boerhaavia diffusa*	8	3	15	12	4.06	2.43
5	Citrullus colocynthis*	19	6	141	28	5.17	2.43
6	Eclipta prostrate*	5	4	14	9	2.95	2.03
7	Launaea procumbens*	8	3	14	10	3.32	2.21
8	Ocimum americanum	11	6	42	16	3.85	2.32
9	Ocimum basilicum*	8	4	12	10	3.41	2.14
10	Solanum nigrum	7	4	24	11	3.15	2.13
11	Tribulus terrestris*	13	5	105	22	4.44	1.85
12	Trichodesma amplexicaule*	7	5	39	13	3.23	2.02
13	Vernonia anthelmintica	11	3	25	13	3.68	2.34
14	Pergularia daemia	15	6	100	25	5.16	2.08
15	Tinospora cordifolia*	12	4	68	20	4.47	2.13
	Shrub/Undershrub						
16	Abutilon fruticosum*	11	5	23	14	4.04	219
17	Abutilon indicum	8	4	12	10	3.62	2.25
18	Aerva persica*	9	6	24	15	4.12	2.36
19	Aloe barbadensis	18	4	153	21	3.76	2.31
20	Asparagus racemosus*	11	4	61	15	3.39	2.25
21	Calotropis gigantica*	12	7	33	16	4.04	2.47
22	Calotropis procera*	24	8	253	44	7.3	2.56
23	Capparis cartilaginea	11	4	63	24	4.99	2.67
24	Capparis deciduas*	23	8	260	42	6.7	2.14
25	Clerodendron phlomidis*	14	5	33	18	4.67	2.33
26	Commiphora wightii*	16	7	138	30	5.49	2.53
27	Crotalaria burhia*	13	5	32	15	3.85	2.06
28	Euphorbia caudicifolia*	19	5	76	23	4.91	2.71
29	Indigofera oblongifolia*	10	7	22	14	4.04	2.38
30	Leptadenia pyrotechnica*	14	6	93	19	3.74	1.99
31	Propospis stephaniana*	9	5	15	12	3.97	2.39
32	Prosopis juliflora	23	7	215	32	5.2	2.4
33	Tephrosia purpurea*	5	3	10	8	3.04	2.03
	Trees						
34	Acacia nilotica*	26	9	354	52	762	2.72
35	Acacia senegal*	21	6	132	26	4.9	1.98
36	Azadirachta indica*	28	10	312	60	9.32	2.77
37	Balanites aegyptiaca	6	3	13	8	2.73	1.99
38	Ficus benghalensis*	14	9	106	23	4.46	2.38
39	Moringa concanensis*	13	7	40	22	5.45	2.68
40	Parkinsonia aculeate	7	6	18	11	3.4	2.26
41	Propospis cineraria*	16	8	109	28	5.43	2.47
42	Salvadora oleoides*	23	7	238	33	5.44	2.02
43	Salvadora persica*	22	7	109	33	6.47	2.7
44	Tecomella undulata*	12	6	27	20	5.7	2.89

*Species indicating destructive harvesting.

Further, it was recorded that the proportion of perennial woody species was more among such species, as compared to the ephemeral herbs. This seems quite logical in view of the climatic variability of the region where availability of perennial woody species for domestic and medicinal uses is much more reliable than for the rainfall dependent ephemeral species.

Extraction of Useful Plants

Respondents reported wild areas as major source of collection of useful plants. Of the total useful species, 77% species with non-medicinal uses and 71% species with medicinal uses were sourced from the wild areas, mostly forest lands. Also, about 4% and 6% species for non-medicinal and medicinal use purpose were either bought from market or imported from outside the district. Demand of remaining species was however met from cultivated lands, such as agriculture fields and fruit orchards (Figure 6).

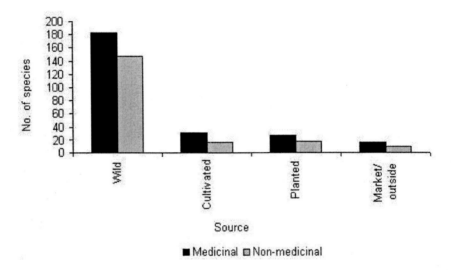

Figure 6. Source Wise Extraction of Number of Ethnobotanical Species.

It is important to note here that the extraction mode of plants and their different parts can have serious implications on the population and conservation status of species. In this context, the use of whole plant and underground parts such as root, bulbs and tubers was considered as 'destructive' mode of extraction. Of the total 320 species, 135 species (42%) were identified with such destructive mode of extraction.

Interestingly, the proportions of number of species with reported destructive modes of use are higher within the high priority species and recorded a declining trend in the lower priority species (Table 4).

Table 4. Number of Species with Destructive Use-mode Across Priority Classes

Priority Class	Total Species	Species with Destructive Use-mode	% of Total
I	19	16	84.2
II	32	22	68.8
III	98	39	39.8
IV	171	58	33.9
Total	320	135	42.2

In a sense, out of total 51 high priority species, 38 species (i.e. about 75%) were found threatened solely by the mode of their extraction (see Table 3) and thus calls for targeted conservation measures. In a sense, the result indicates, although not conclusively, that high use values of a plant often attract destructive mode of extraction which ultimately affect the population of such species leading to their poor availability. Dixit and Rao (2000) reported a similar decline in the population of *Commiphora wightii* in Kachchh region, due to historically heavy exploitation of oleoresin. Currently, this species is included in the lists of rare and endangered plants (WCMC 1994).

Discussion

This chapter successfully attempted a quantitative documentation of floral species of district Kachchh, with an objective to prepare a near complete list of ethnobotanically useful species and prioritize them for conservation measures. Documentation of traditional knowledge of plant uses was quite voluminous, as reflected by the fact that around 900 persons from 85 geographically dispersed villages provided more than 12000 pieces of plant use related information. Representatives from different age, sex, educational status, socio-economic classes and occupational types were adequately covered during the interview. More importantly, this information was collected from the representative common rural population so that other than commonly reported knowledge many unique uses and applications of plants are also recorded.

The methodologies and analytical frameworks employed in this chapter is a major departure from the traditional ethnobotanical studies, which generally focus on documentation of traditional knowledge of local herbal healers or key informants and thus in most of the cases actually document the already codified knowledge. The results obtained using an integrated approach in this study adequately emphasize the importance of orienting and designing the ethnobotanical studies in such a way that could mutually compliment conservation of plant resources as well as traditional knowledge system (Gupta, 2001).

By applying two simplistic use-value indices the results obtained through this study for identifying multipurpose species in the region seem to be logically conclusive. Thus the results in this chapter sufficiently advocate taking up more studies with quantitative ethnobotanical approaches. The fundamental information on plant density and distribution are found quite useful in determining conservation priorities. Since, the availability of plant influences the use pattern of community as well as the future state of traditional knowledge system; the field survey results provide a fairly good picture of the availability of ethnobotanically useful species in the region. More importantly such information was effectively used in identifying conservation priorities for ethnobotanically useful species. It is, however, important to highlight here that the availability of plants of a species to local users and their multi-utility is a crucial factor in determining the conservation priorities. Therefore, the prioritized species identified through this study do not necessarily match with the species of state or national level importance, though majority of them are representative of flora of arid tracts of the country.

Conclusion

This chapter highlighted that, despite many constraints and problems, inflicted by rapidly changing socio-economic setups under market influence, the local people are still a key repository of knowledge about the various uses of plants, majority are in the domain of traditional knowledge system. Nevertheless, it can safely be assumed that the volume of traditional knowledge, documented during this study, can only be a small fraction of the total 'mass' of ethnobotanical knowledge in the region and still lying within uncodified folk knowledge system. At the same time, frequent reports of various uses of many recently invaded exotic plant species like *Prosopis juliflora* also suggests that the knowledge system is quite dynamic and continuously evolving. Documentation, protection and promotion of such knowledge, therefore should be a top priority in the conservation arena.

Acknowledgments

Financial assistance to a larger study was provided by the Ministry of Environment and Forests, Govt. of India (Grant No. 14/33/98-MAB-RE). We sincerely acknowledge the assistance provided by Ms. Nisha Mistry and Ms. Leena Gupta during field data collection and compilation of the same. The cooperation and hospitality extended by villagers during field survey is sincerely acknowledged and appreciated.

References

Anon. (2002). *Kachchh sub-state biodiversity strategy and action plan.* Prepared under National Biodiversity Strategy and Action Plan, Ministry of Environment and Forests, Govt. of India, New Delhi. Gujarat Institute of Desert Ecology, Bhuj 123 pp.

Arnold, J.E.M. and Ruiz Perez, M. (1998). The role of non-timber forest products in conservation and development. In: *Income from the Forest: Methods for the Development and Conservation of Forest Products for Local Communities.* W. Wollenberg and A. Ingles, A. (eds.), pp. 17-42. CIFOR/IUCN, Indonesia.

Benz, B. F., Cevallos, J. E., Santana, F. M., Rosales, J. A. and Graf, S. M. (2000). Losing knowledge about plant use in the Sierra de Manantalan Biosphere Reserve, Mexico. *Economic Botany,* 54: 183-191.

de Beer, J. H. and McDermott, M. J. (1989). *Economic Value of Non-timber Forest Products in Southeast Asia.* International Union of the Conservation of Nature and Natural Resources-World Conservation Union (IUCN).

Dhar, U., Rawal, R. S., and Upreti, J. (2000). Setting priorities for conservation of medicinal plants - a case study in the Indian Himalaya. *Biological Conservation,* 95: 57-65.

Dixit, A. M. and Geevan, C. P. (2000). Quantitative analysis of plant use as a component of EIA: Case study of Narmada Sagar Hydroelectric Project in central India. *Current Science,* 79: 202-210.

Dixit, A. M., Silori, C. S., Gupta. L. and Mistry, N. (2004). *A study on traditional knowledge of ethnobotanical resources of district Kachchh – An approach to the natural resource conservation through creation of ethnobotanical database.* Final project report. Gujarat Institute of Desert Ecology, Bhuj pp. 150.

Dixit, A. M. and Rao, S. V. (2000). Observation on distribution and habitat characteristics of Gugal (Commiphora wightii) in the arid region of Kachchh, Gujarat (India). *Tropical Ecology,* 41: 81-88.

Gomez-Beloz, A. (2002). Plant use knowledge of the Winikina Warao: The case for questionnaires in Ethnobotany. *Economic Botany,* 56: 231-241.

Gupta, A. K. (2001). (Ed). *Criteria and indicators of sustainability in rural development: a natural resource perspective.* UNESCO and Oxford IHB Publ. New Delhi, 424 pp.

Joshi, P. N. (2002). *Study of ethnobotanical angiosperms of Bhuj and Mandvi talukas of Kachchh, Gujarat.* Unpublished PhD Thesis, Bhavanagar University, Bhavanagar.

Kala, C. P., Farooquee, N. A. and Dhar, U. (2004). Prioritization of medicinal plants on the basis of available knowledge, existing practices and use value status in Uttaranchal, India. *Biodiversity and Conservation,* 13: 453-469.

Magurran, A. E. (1988). *Ecological diversity and its measurement.* Chapman and Hall, UK.

Martinez, G. J., Planchuelo, A. M., Fuentes, E. and Ojeda, M. (2006). A numeric index to establish conservation priorities for medicinal plants in Paravachasca valley, Cordoba, Argentina, *Biodiversity and Conservation,* 15: 2457-2475.

Master, I. (2000). *Pachchham Bet ni Vanaspatiyo* (In Gujarati). Sahjeevan Bhuj.

MoEF (1994). *Ethnobiology in India – A status report.* All India Co-ordinated Research Project on Ethnobiology (AICRPE). Ministry of Environment and Forests, Govt. of India, New Delhi.

Phillips, O. and Gentry, A. H. (1993a). The useful plants of Tambopata, Peru: I. Statistical hypotheses tests with a new quantitative technique. *Economic Botany,* 47 (1): 15-32.

Phillips, O. and Gentry, A. H. (1993b). The useful plants of Tambopata, Peru: II. Additional hypothesis testing in quantitative ethnobotany. *Economic Botany,* 47 (1): 33-43.

Rao, R. S. (1970). Studies on the flora of Kutch (Gujarat State) and their utility in the economic development of this semi arid region. *Annals of Arid Zone,* 9: 125-142.

Rodgers, W. A. and Panwar, H. S. (1988). *Planning a wildlife protected area network in India.* Vol. I and II. Wildlife Institute of India, Dehradun.

Rolla, S. K. (1970). Studies on the flora of Kutch (Gujarat State) and their utility in the economic development of this semi-arid region. *Annals of Arid Zone,* 9 (2): 125-142.

Silori, C. S. and Rana, A. R. (2000). Indigenous knowledge on medicinal plants and their use in Narayan Sarovar Sanctuary Kachchh. *Ethnobotany,* 12: 1-7.

Thacker, J. I. (1926). *Plants of Kutch and their utility* (in Gujarati). Unpublished Mimeo.

Uniyal, S., Kumar, A., Lal, B. and Singh, A. B. (2006). Quantitative assessment and traditional uses of high value medicinal plants of Chhota Bhangal area of Himachal Pradesh, Western Himalaya, *Current Science,* 91 (9): 1238-1242.

WCMC (1994). *Status report as of 24 November 1994, Gujarat.* World Conservation Monitoring Centre, USA.

In: Medicinal Plants and Sustainable Development
Editor: Chandra Prakash Kala

ISBN 978-1-61761-942-7
© 2011 Nova Science Publishers, Inc.

Chapter 4

Cultivation of *Saussurea costus* and *Inula racemosa* in Cold Desert of the Lahaul Valley: Revival of Cultivation Needed for their Conservation and Protection

Yashwant S. Rawat [*] *and Subhash C. R. Vishvakarma*
G.B. Pant Institute of Himalayan Environment and Development,
Kosi-Katarmal, Almora, 263 643, Uttarakhand, India

Abstract

Cultivation practice, status and reasons of decline of cultivation of *Saussurea costus* (*kuth*) and *Inula racemosa* (*manu*), the two endangered medicinal plants, were studied in four different agro-ecosystems namely Kuthar (2600 m), Hinsa (2700 m), Jahlma (3000 m) and Khoksar (3200 m), representing the entire Lahaul valley in the cold desert of the north west Himalaya. Cultivation of *kuth* and *manu* were initiated by some progressive farmers in the beginning of the 20th century as the first cash crop in the Lahaul valley. The findings, as discussed in this chapter, reveal that area under cultivation of *kuth* and *manu* has declined sharply due to shift from traditional food cropping to cash cropping (*i.e.* high yielding varieties (HYVs) of pea, potato and hop). These crops got popularity among local farmers due to their early maturity, comparatively higher economic returns and fitting their growth and maturity duration within short growing season of the cold desert environment of the Lahaul valley. The longer cultivation cycle (3 years), small land holdings, continuously fluctuating market rates and option of seasonal cash crops in place of perennial crop were some of the reasons that discouraged farmers to cultivate these crops. About 60-80% seeds of *kuth* and 50-60% seeds of *manu* germinated in the farmers' field. Energy and monetary efficiencies revealed output/input ratio of 0.8 and 7.5 for *kuth* and 0.69 and 5.91 for *manu*, respectively. Providing technical support for scientific cultivation, value addition centre at local level, strengthening existing market

---

[*]E-mail: yas_rawat@yahoo.com

and granting of easy permit for cultivation and export are some of the suggestions for revival of the cultivation of *kuth* and *manu.*

Keywords: *Saussurea costus; Inula racemosa;* endangered medicinal plants; cultivation; cropping efficiency; cold desert agro-ecosystems; Lahaul valley; Indian Himalaya.

Introduction

Saussurea costus (Falc.) Lipsch. (locally called *kuth)* and *Inula racemosa* Hook. f. (locally called *manu*) of the family of Asteraceae are two important Himalayan medicinal plants cultivated in cold desert of the Lahaul valley, between 2400-3600 m altitudinal ranges and in the few places of districts Kinnaur, Chamba and Kullu of Himachal Pradesh (Aswal and Mehrotra, 1994). *Kuth* is an endemic herb in the parts of Jammu and Kashmir (north western Himalaya) from 2500 to 3000 m and neighboring valleys (Anonymous, 1976). Distribution of *manu* extends from eastern Afghanistan (north western Himalayas) to Nepal (central Himalaya) between 1500-2500 m altitudes (Qaiser and Abid, 2003). Over extraction of these species from the natural habitat had led them to their critically endangered status in the wild (IUCN, 1993; Wani et al., 2006). *Kuth* and *manu* have been listed in the Red Data Book of Indian Plants as endangered ones (Nayar and Shastry, 1987, 1988, 1990); both are critically endangered high value medicinal herbs. *Kuth* is enlisted in Appendix I of CITES (Convention on International Trade in Endangered Species of Wild Fauna and Flora) and is among the 214 Himalayan endangered medicinal and aromatic herbs (Anonymous, 1973; Nayar and Shastry 1987, 1988, 1990). Khoshoo (1993) prioritized *kuth* and *manu* along with other 35 Himalayan endangered medicinal plants for *in situ* and *ex situ* conservation. Due to a resource base bottleneck, the Ministry of Commerce, Government of India, has prohibited export of 29 medicinal and aromatic species either in crude form or in processed products that could be separated (Anonymous, 2000). Few years earlier *kuth* was part of this list; now *kuth* of agriculture origin can be exported with due permit. Prior to the 1920s, natural habitats of *kuth* were the exclusive sources of its extraction for pharmaceutical uses (Kuniyal et al., 2005). However, due to increase of requirement and shortage of its availability in the wild few innovative and progressive farmers of the Pattan sub-valley area of the Lahaul valley started its large scale cultivation in agriculture fields as mono crop side by side with traditional food crops like buckwheats, maize, and several varieties of pulses (Singh et al., 1997; Kuniyal et al., 2004; Rawat et al., 2004). In past, *kuth* has contributed high monetary income to the farmers and met high demand of the pharmaceutical industries (Arora et al., 1980); it was the first cash crop of the Lahaul valley. However, after introduction of HYVs of cash crops such pea (*Pisum sativum* L.), potato (*Solanum tuberosum* L.) and hop (*Humulus lupulus* L.) in recent years, the cultivation area of *kuth* and *manu* has declined (Singh et al., 1997; Kuniyal et al., 2004; Kuniyal et al., 2005). Thus the area which was devoted for cropping of *kuth* and *manu* in recent past, on the same land HYVs of cash crops is cultivated now.

HYVs of cash crops obtained popularity due to their early maturity in one growth season as compared to 2-3 years maturity cycle of *kuth* and *manu* and early economic returns in one growth season (Kuniyal et al., 2004). Farmers were less interested towards *kuth* cultivation due to lengthy cultivation cycle, small land holdings, early profits with HYVs of cash crops, permit formalities both for cultivation and export from the valley and fluctuating and relatively low market prices (Kuniyal et al., 2005). Cumulative profit of the *kuth* and *manu* on the unit area land is higher than the seasonal cash crops but returns are late and some time if market rate is less farmer has to wait for other season. The Himalayan Mountains are known to be the storehouses of natural resources, cultural diversity as well as susceptible to biotic and other interferences (Anonymous, 2001). Despite worldwide opportunities for domesticating wild medicinal plants, problems associated with cultivation and extension of wild medicinal plants such as *kuth* and *manu* existing are seldom considered an economic opportunity. The present study is an attempt to analyses various problems associated with cultivation of *kuth* and *manu* and identification of preventive measures to be taken up for the revival of these high values endangered Himalayan medicinal plants.

Materials and Methods

Study Area and Climate

The present study was carried out in 4 altitudinal villages namely Khoksar (3200 m), Jahlma (3000 m), Hinsa (2700 m) and Kuthar (2600 m) in cold desert of the Lahaul valley, district Lahaul-Spiti of Himachal Pradesh, India. The district is situated in between $31^\circ\ 44'\ 34''$ N to $32^\circ\ 59'57''$ N latitudes and $76^\circ\ 46'\ 29''$ E to $78^\circ\ 41'\ 34''$ E longitudes. The total geographical area of the Lahaul valley is 6244 km^2, with a population of 22,545 (Census, 2001). The Lahaul valley is a landlocked area and approachable only during summer months through surface route via Rohtang Pass (3978 m). Geographically, the Lahaul valley can be further divided into three major sub-valleys: Chandra, Bhaga, and Pattan on the names of the rivers flowing in that area (Figure 1).

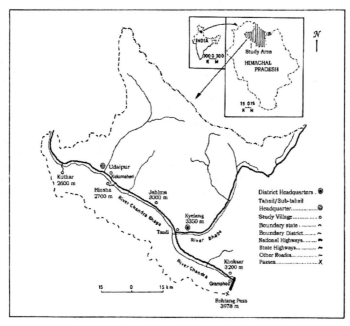

Figure 1. Map of the study area in the cold desert of the Lahaul valley.

The catchment area of river Chandra is called the Chandra sub-valley, similarly the catchment area of river Bhaga is the Bhaga sub-valley. Both the rivers Chandra and Bhaga meet at Tandi, and form the river Chandra-Bhaga in Himachal Pradesh or Chenab in Jammu and Kashmir. The area afterwards Tandi up to a few kilometres beyond Kuthar is called the Pattan sub-valley. The Lahaul is one fourth of the total geographical area of the Himachal Pradesh; its revenue area only occupies 3.9% of total revenue area of the state and 15.6% of the district. Forest land in the district is 7.9% of the total district but at very few places degraded forests can be seen in relict patches in Lahaul. Nearly 69% of the geographical area of the district Lahaul-Spiti comes under non-reported area of land classification category, this is mainly stony out crop and snow bound areas during winters and some of the area comes under perpetual snow and glaciers and the concerned department lacks any proper records till date for this category (Anonymous, 1994; Anonymous, 1995). Only 0.39% of the land is devoted to agriculture/forestry use (i.e. forestry, barren land, current fallow and net sown area) (Anonymous, 1995). The land utilization process of net sown area is broadly divided into three utilization categories, *i.e.*, cash crops, traditional crops and medicinal plants (Table 1).

Agriculture is the prime activity for livelihood in the Lahaul valley (Singh et al., 1997; Kuniyal et al., 2004; Oinam et al., 2005, 2008). Nowadays, in the Lahaul valley, HYVs of cash crops (pea, potato and hop), of high market demand, are cultivated at large scale; these cash crops were introduced few decades back, only a small area of the agriculture land is devoted to less-preferred, traditional food crops like barley (*Hordeum vulgare* L.), wheat (*Triticum aestivum* L.), maize (*Zea mays* L.), varieties of buckwheat (*Fagopyrum esculentum* Moench. and *Fagopyrum tataricum* L.), and medicinal plants such as *kuth* (*Saussurea costus* (Falc.) Lipsch.) and *manu* (*Inula racemosa* Hook. f.) (Kuniyal et al., 2004; Rawat et al., 2004; Rawat, 2006). The agricultural activities begin in the month of April each year, soon after snow melts from the fields and ends up in the month of September.

Table 1. Land utilization under agriculture crops (ha) in cold desert in the Lahaul valley

Land utilization	Khoksar (3200 m) n=12	Jahlma (3000 m) n=41	Hinsa (2700 m) n=52	Kuthar (2600 m) n=17
a. Cash crops				
Pea	3.70 (56.06)	16.99 (46.80)	8.86 (43.43)	-
Potato	2.90 (43.94)	13.98 (38.51)	7.47 (36.62)	0.63 (10.00)
Hop	-	4.54 (12.51)	0.30 (1.47)	-
b. Traditional crops				
Amaranths	-	-	0.11 (0.54)	0.18 (2.86)
Barley	-	-	0.86 (4.22)	0.63 (10.00)
Maize	-	-	1.24 (6.08)	2.41 (38.25)
Wheat	-	-	0.77 (3.77)	0.95 (15.08)
Buckwheat	-	-	0.65 (3.19)	0.67 (10.63)
Kidneybeans	-	-	0.06 (0.29)	0.56 (8.89)
c. Medicinal herbs				
Kuth	-	0.14 (0.39)	0.03 (0.15)	0.27 (4.29)
Manu	-	0.65 (1.79)	-	-
Total land	6.60 (100)	36.30 (100)	20.40 (100)	6.30 (100)

n=number of family heads interviewed from a household.
Values in parentheses are the per cent of the total cultivated area.

Climatically, the Lahaul valley is in cold and arid zone with extremely low rainfall but high snowfall; here winters are prolong and harsh. Broadly, the valley has two seasons: short lived summer and prolonged severe winter. Maximum temperature reaches up to 27.8° C in the month of July, while the minimum temperature drops to -13.2° C in the month of January. The average annual rainfall varies from 241.5 to 272.4 mm and average annual snowfall ranges 466.2 to 693.2 mm. The two months, February and March, received more than 50% of the snowfall.

Rainfall is scarce and mild showers can be noticed during the months of May to September. The high velocity cold winds are common climatic feature of the area. Basically, there are two types of vegetation zones in the Lahaul valley: (i) temperate zone (2400 to 3300 m), and (ii) alpine zone (above 3300 m) (Aswal and Mehrotra, 1994). Forest resources in the entire Lahaul valley are very sparse and scanty. The Chandra sub-valley has very few scattered trees of *Betula utilis, Pinus wallichiana, Juniperus communis, J. indica, S. lindleyana* and *S. pycnostachya* on almost denuded northern slopes; southern slopes are almost barren. In the Pattan sub-valley, both the slope aspects have some patches of open forests. *Juniperus macropoda* is the most important tree species found on the south facing slopes.

Methods

The data and information were generated with the field surveys and primary sources. Derivation of energy and monetary values are based on the primary information collected and secondary sources to strengthen the facts and figures, *etc.* Field surveys were conducted through structured questionnaires and direct interviews with the head of the farmers' family pertaining to a variety of aspects like land holding size, crops sown in an area, utilization, cultivation practices, monetary and energy input and output parameters for *kuth* and *manu*, problem associated with *kuth* and *manu* cultivation, *etc.* After selecting four villages from low altitude (Kuthar 2600 m) to high altitude (Khoksar 3200 m), as well as, from northwest (Kuthar) to southeast (Khoksar) part of the study region to represent the entire Lahaul valley, the techniques of random stratified sampling during selection of the households from each of the villages. Head of a household was selected for interview. Energy efficiencies (output/input ratio) of *kuth* and *manu* were measured by adopting the methods of Kuniyal et al. (2004) for cold desert of the Lahaul valley. Based on values suggested by Michtell (1979) and Gopalan et al. (1985), human and bullock working days were determined 10 hours day^{-1} on account of working for more hours by the local people keeping in mind the shorter growth period; while 8 hours day^{-1} were reported from the adjacent Kullu valley (Kuniyal et al., 2004). Likewise, energy values for different farm inputs applied in an unit area and output obtained from the agricultural system was measured. Agriculture activities were considered in the category of heavy work. Calculation of energy and monetary values of input (human labour, bullock labour, seeds, *etc.*) and output (agronomic yield and by-products) were determined separately. Assessment of labour hours was made by extensive queries from heads of the *kuth* and *manu* growing families for the actual requirement on activities like seed sowing, weeding, irrigation, root harvesting and drying, *etc.* Monetary efficiency (output/input ratio in terms of INR; ₹) was also derived through extensive interview of the family heads of *kuth* and *manu* growers. Prevailing village market rates for monetary inputs and outputs were considered for calculations. Labour cost was considered on the basis of recent wages during the field study, which was ₹60 day^{-1} with one meal and refreshment in a day. For animal power price for a pair of bullock was ₹500 day^{-1} pair^{-1} with fodder for a day. As the gender participation ratio of human labour in performing agricultural activities in a region was 2 males to 3 females, the per hour caloric value collectively for human labour in the present study region after following Kuniyal et al. (2004) was calculated as under:

$$\text{Per hour human labour} = \frac{(2\times M) + (3\times F)}{5}$$

Where: M= Per hour energy value for one male (0.679 MJ hr^{-1})

F= Per hour energy value for one female (0.523 MJ hr^{-1})
5= Workforce ratio in context to present study (2 males + 3 females)

Description of Kuth and Manu

Kuth (Asteraceae) is an erect pubescent perennial herb, grows up to 2 m height. Basal leaves are long triangular and stalked. Upper leaves are large clasping pubescent, toothed with long petioles, base auricled. Flowers are in heads, purple, sessile, axillary or terminal clusters. Involucral bracts are ovate-lanceolate, acuminate, recurved. Achene fruit are compressed, curved upwards and greyish in colour. Seeds are 9.01 mm long and 2.85 mm wide (Aswal and Mehrotra, 1994). *Manu* (Asteraceae) is an erect pubescent perennial herb, grows up to 2 m height. Basal leaves are long triangular, rough above, densely hairy beneath, toothed and stalked. Flowers are in heads, hermaphrodite, purple, sessile, axillary or terminal clusters, yellow in colour and arising in terminal recemes. Achene fruit is 0.4 cm long, slender with radish puppus, compressed, curved upwards and grayish in colour (Aswal and Mehrotra, 1994). Flowering of these species occurred in the months of July-August and fruiting in the months of September-October.

Results and Discussion

Distribution

Kuth and *manu* are endemic and critically endangered medicinal plants of the northwestern Himalaya and its neighbouring regions between 2000-3600 m altitudes (Sharin, 1996; Kalloo and Shah, 1997; Anonymous, 1998; Siddique et al., 2001; Sood et al., 2001; Wani, 2006). The distribution of these species is reported from Eastern to Western Himalaya particularly in Jammu and Kashmir and Himachal Pradesh. In nature, these species are found in Uttarakhand (Pithoragarh, Bhilangana valley, Bhagirathi and Alaknanda valleys) Himachal Pradesh (Kinnaur, Lahaul and Spiti) and Jammu and Kashmir (Aswal and Mehrotra, 1994; Oleg and Adum, 1997; Chauhan et al., 1998; Uniyal, 1998). Both the species are under cultivation in Lahaul-Spiti district of Himachal Pradesh between 2400-3600 m and a few places in Kinnaur, Chamba and Kullu districts for their medicinal roots (Aswal and Mehrotra, 1994). *Kuth* cultivation was on peak during 1960s before introduction of HYVs of cash crops like potato, pea and hop. Though, *kuth* and *manu* are harvested after 2-3 years, yet its monetary efficiency in the past was more than cumulative efficiency of introduced HYVs of seasonal cash crops like potato and pea (Kuniyal et al, 2004, 2005).

Utilization

Kuth and *manu* are widely used in Ayurveda, Unani, and other systems of medicine. The roots of *kuth* is considered as tonic, stomachic, carminative, stimulant, spasmodic in asthma, alternative in chronic skin disease and rheumatism, cough and cold besides, having various uses in cough, cholera, bronchitis, bronchial asthma, dyspepsia, oedema, gas, jaundice, leprosy, phlegm, and skin diseases. Roots contain resinoides, essential oil, alkaloids and other minor constituents like tannins and sugars. The remedial actions of Costus oil in leprosy have obtained recognition since time immemorial, therefore, the name *kushta* (cf. to leprosy in Sanskrit, an ancient Indian Vedic language) has been given to it. The dried leaves are smoked as tobacco. *Kuth* roots are indigenously used for cough, fever and stomachache. The pounded roots of *manu* is used as expectorant and resovlent and use in curing rheumatism, anti-spasmodic, hyptensive, cardiac asthama, cardiovascular and liver troubles, respiratory tract disorder, antiseptic, pulmonary infections, skin diseases and gastrointestinal disorders and in veterinary medicine as tonic and stomachic (Gupta et al., 1981; Anonymous, 1986; Sarin, 1996; Kaul, 1997). It is also used in fever and body pain. It has a sweet, bitter and acrid taste with a neutral potency and antipyrectic/antiseptic, anti-inflammatory, antiasthmatic, anthelmintic and diuretic properties. It has hypoglycaemic activity (Gholap and Kar, 2005). The seeds are bitter and aphrodiac. Apart from the medicinal properties, leaves are also used as fodder and stem as fuelwood. The flowers are used as offering to various deities in religious ceremonies (Koelz, 1979). The people keep a piece of root in between the clothes to save them from the warms.

Bio-Chemical Constituents

Stout tuberous roots of *kuth* are characterized by a penetrating aroma. Pale yellow or brownish viscous oil or costus oil is obtained from the roots either by steam distillation or through extracting with solvents. The oil contains resinoids (6%), essential oil (1.5%), Saussurine and other alkaloids (0.05%). Biological actions of costus oil are hyposensitive, bronchiodialatory, and antiseptic against streptococcus and streptophylococcus (Anonymous, 1976).

The roots of *manu* contain *inulin* (10%), essential oil containing isoalantolactone, alanlolides and di-hydralactone, alkaloids and other minor constituents like tannins and sugars. Alantolactone, β sislosterol, daucosteral and its glucosides have been found in alcoholic extract of roots (Anonymous, 1986; Tan et al., 1998; Kalsi et al., 1989). Isoalantolactone is a major lactone; it has anti-fungal properties against human pathogenic fungi (Tan et al., 1998; Kalsi et al., 1989). The essential oil from the roots has a strong aroma and contains sesquiterpenes aplotaxene (Bokadia et al., 1986).

Cultivation Practices

a) Kuth

Kuth performs well in sandy loam and alluvial soil, but it gives better yields in blackish sandy loam. Agro-climatic conditions like low temperate and sub-alpine climatic condition are more suitable for *kuth* cultivation. *Kuth* can be propagated both through seeds and roots. Two type of sowing are in practiced *viz.*1). Line sowing, and 2). Broadcast sowing. The seed sowing is done during October-November before snowfall; it is very rarely done in the months of April-May. In line sowing plant to plant distance of 4x6 inches are maintained. For cultivation of one ha areas about 34.02 kg seeds are required (Thakur et al., 1998). The manure is spread in the field, after ploughing. The weeds and stone particles are removed and soil is leveled, rows are prepared for the sowing of seeds; seeds are sown in rows. The irrigation schedule ranges from 3-5 times seasonally. Proper and timely weeding and cleaning are essential for healthy plant and better production. Weeding requirement depends on the growth stage of the plants. Generally, 2-3 times weeding is needed in the first year and 1-2 times in second and third years, respectively.

About 5890 kg ha^{-1} farmyard manure is needed to maintain soil nutrient under moraine soil conditions of the Lahaul valley. The manure is applied in two doses: the first dose is applied before seed sowing and second just before snowfall. Some farmers use chemical fertilizers also. The harvesting is done after three years of sowing. Sometimes farmers harvest the root after 2 years, even though, it produces lesser quantity as compared to 3 third years old crop. The harvesting is generally carried out after flooding the field to make the soil loose and soft for easy digging. The roots are dug out using picket. The soil and unwanted scales were removed by sieving through a locally prepared coarse sieve, soil and scale free roots are dried completely and packed in gunny bag for safe storage in a cool and dry place. There are few incidents of wide spread diseases infestation in *kuth*. Sometimes a variety of caterpillar feeds the leaves destroying the plant. Decay and hollowing of the roots occur with frequent watering or water logging near the plants. The farmers used *Nivan* (2 ml in 20 litres of water) to mitigate and protect from this disease. Pest attack occurs mostly in initial stage of cultivation but such infestation is rarely seen in the Lahaul valley. Still, there is a wide perception among the local farmers that traditional night soil compost is useful to obtain better root yield. Yield of *kuth* was estimated 4.65 MT ha^{-1} for roots and 1.7 MT ha^{-1} for fodder. The root production is higher in high altitude valley area as compared to sloppy mountainsides.

b) Manu

Manu is cultivated in moist heavy clay, sandy loam and alluvial soil, but blackish sandy loam is useful to obtain better growth and yield. It requires similar climatic conditions like *kuth*. The propagation is done normally through root cuttings; exceptionally sometimes it is cultivated through seeds also in the months of October-November. *I. racemosa* can be easily propagated both through roots and seeds (Arora et al., 1981). The sowing is done during October-November before snowfall. The distance between plant to plant should be 4x6" (inches) and 2-3" (inches) deep in soil for the better yield and seed quality. The distance may be changed according to plant growth during first year. The irrigation schedule ranged from 3 to 5 times in a season. The proper and timely weeding and cleaning are essential for healthy growth of plants and better production. The first weeding is required after 20-30 days of germination. Once plant is grown well, only one weeding can be done in a month. The manure is spread in the fields after ploughing and land is tilled deeply 2-3 times for better penetrating the roots up to a depth of 30 cm in the soil. Usually, the fields are ploughed during October-November. The weeds, stone and pebbles are removed and soil is leveled; rows are prepared for the planting of root cuttings. Like *kuth, manu* also required farm yard manure of nearly 5890 kg ha^{-1} in moraine soil conditions. This manure is applied two times in a year with two different doses. Roots are harvested after 2-3 years; however, three years old plant produces better return. After harvesting of *I. racemosa* either potato or pea are cultivated in rotation. All the procedure and processes for digging, cleaning, drying and packing of roots are similar like *kuth*. However, when roots are stored as propagules, they are stored in a pit and covered with soil to protect them from moisture. The closed surface of the pit is covered with potato and willow leaves soil is piled up there 1 ft soil to check out the contact moisture. The roots are dug out in the months of March-April after melting the snow from the agricultural fields and planted them as a new crop. M*anu* yields about 4.26 MT ha^{-1} of roots and 1.6 MT ha^{-1} fodder, respectively.

Seed Production and Seed Germination:

a) Kuth

The seeds of healthy plant are used for cultivation. Achenes (capsules) are picked up from 3 years old mature plants. Then, seeds are kept under sun till complete drying. Dried seeds are stored in an air passing container for further sowing. Nearly, 80 kg ha^{-1} seeds are produced from a 3 years old crop; seeds remain viable for a period of 4-5 years. The seeds collected during September-October months performance is better in terms of seed germination, plant growth and root production. Usually, seeds collection from first and second year plants is avoided. The *kuth* is successful sexual breeder and produces enormous quantity of seeds (Sidhique et al., 2001). *Kuth* can produces 81.66-910.71 seeds per 3-capitulate plants and 265.71-284.5 per q- capitulates. The total number of seeds per capitulam ranges between 25.6±2.56 and 33.66±2.6. More than 80% seeds remain viable for a period of 3-4 years (Siddique et al., 2001). *Kuth* seeds can be easily germinated without using any hormonal and mechanical treatments. This property of *kuth* seeds makes this crop much easier for cropping and acceptable to farmers. The maximum germination percentage has been reported in the month of June (99±1.33%), followed by May (95±3.53%) and lowest in the month of September (45±9.61%) when seed treated in hot chamber at 30°C. Chauhan et al. (1998) reported 96% germination in *kuth* seeds treated with 25-PPM IAA and 88% in control. Chauhan et al. (1998) reported 96% seed germination in *kuth* treated with 25 ppm IAA (Indole Acetic Acid) and 88% in control. Jabeen et al., (2007) found maximum seed germination (100%) after 13 days of inoculation under continuous illumination of 40 µM m^{-2} sec^{-1} at a temperature of 25±2°C. In cold chamber at 20°C maximum (81±2.67%) germination was observed in the month of July and lowest (4±0.00%) in the month of December. An identical trend has been noted in seeds sown in hot chamber at 30°C in respect to first germination initiated after 2 to 4 days of seed sowing. Seeds sown in cold chamber at 20°C take more time in seed germination; germination starts after 5 to 14 days after seed sowing where as in hot chamber seed starts germinating after 2-3 days. In general, observation in cold chamber could not show better germination as compared to comparison to hot chamber at 30°C (Rawat et al., 2004).

b) Manu

The seeds of healthy plant are used for cultivation. Achenes are picked up from 3 years old matured plants in the months of September-October. Then, seeds are kept under sun till its complete drying. After that it is stored in air passing container for sowing. The seed production of 3 years old crop was measured 55 kg ha^{-1}. The seeds collected during September-October months perform better in terms of overall yield; per capitulam number of seeds ranges between 400-600. Seeds germinate easily without any hormonal and mechanical treatments. The maximum germination of 71.12±2.11% in hot chamber was recorded in the month of June followed by May (67.62±2.71%) and September (65.43±7.51%). In cold chamber, low seed germination was recorded at 20° C. Seed sown in cold chamber at 20° C taken more time in seed germination starts after 5 to 14 days of sowing, whereas, in hot chamber it germinates much early after 2-3 days. Jabeen et al., (2007) found maximum seed germination (100%) after 13 days of inoculation under continuous illumination of 40 µM m^{-2} sec^{-1} at a temperature of 25±2° C. Whereas, Chilling>GA$_3$ is best treatment of *I. racemosa* (Sharma et al., 2006).

Monetary and Energy Efficiency

The total monetary input for cultivation of one hectare of *kuth* was ₹40937 and ₹36868 for *manu* (Table 2). The value of human labour for both the crops stood highest (₹20991) followed by organic manure (₹8305) and bullock labour (₹2286). The seed input of ₹9356 for *kuth* and ₹5286 for *manu* were needed. *Manu* and *kuth* are labour intensive crop; about 56.94% for *kuth* and 51.28% for *manu* of total monetary inputs were in the form of human labour for ploughing, land preparation, mixing of organic manure, seeds sowing, weeding, irrigation, harvesting and drying of roots and their packing, *etc.* (Table 2). Total energy inputs applied for *kuth* and *manu* cultivation were 45387 MJ ha^{-1} and 45398 MJ ha^{-1}, respectively. The energy input was recorded maximum for organic manure (42936 MJ ha^{-1}), followed by human labour (2050 MJ), bullock labour (276 MJ) for both species, and seeds (136 MJ for *kuth* and 125 MJ for *manu*).

In terms of energy, 95% input was for the organic manure. Maintenance of soil fertility status of moraine soil in cold desert is a very tedious job; here annually maximum nutrient leaches out along with prolong snow melt flow exhausting soil nutrient, subsequently a regular nutrient supplement is needed (Kuniyal et al., 2004; Rawat et al., 2004). The total monetary output of ₹305153 ha-^{1} and energy output of 38531 MJ ha-^{1} for *kuth* were recorded. Values for *manu* were ₹218031 ha-^{1} for monetary output and 31091 MJ ha^{-1} for energy output, which were relatively lower values for both the monetary and energy outputs than the *kuth* (Table 2). In *kuth*, the agronomic yield (root) generated maximum monetary output of ₹279090 followed by seeds (₹21929) and by-products (₹4134), whereas, in *manu,* the agronomic yield (root) generated maximum monetary output of ₹202930 followed by seeds (₹11210) and by-products (₹3891). Roots contributed 91.46% of total monetary output in *kuth* and 93.07% in *manu*. Contribution of seed for *kuth* and *manu* were, respectively 7.19% and 5.14% of total monetary output. Contribution of vegetative parts which is used as husk for both the species was quite less. Seeds are sold to other farmers as propagules. Energy output values were maximum for by-products of both the medicinal crops (19606 MJ ha^{-1} for *kuth* and 17375 MJ ha^{-1} for *manu*) followed by energy output of roots (18606 MJ ha^{-1} for *kuth* and 13511 MJ ha^{-1} for *manu*) and seeds (319 MJ ha^{-1} for *kuth* and 205 MJ ha^{-1} for *manu*) (Table 2). In term of total energy output contribution, the highest output contribution was of by-products (50.88% for *kuth* and 55.88% for *manu*), contribution of roots ranked on second position (48.29% for *kuth* and 43.46% for *manu*) and seed ranked on third position. Cropping efficiencies, which is a ratio of output/input, was 7.5 in terms of monetary value and 0.8 in terms of energy value for *kuth*. Monetary and energy efficiencies of *manu* were, respectively 5.9 and 0.69, lower than the cropping efficiencies of *kuth*.

Table 2. Energy (MJ h^{-1}) and monetary (₹ h^{-1}) efficiencies of *kuth* and *manu* crops in the Lahaul valley (values in parenthesis are percentage of total)

Attributes	Kuth		Manu	
	Monetary ha^{-1}	Energy ha^{-1}	Monetary ha^{-1}	Energy ha^{-1}
Input total	40937	45398	36868	45387
Human labour	20991 (51.28)	2050 (4.52)	20991(56.94)	2050(4.52)
Bullock labour	2286 (5.58)	276 (0.61)	2286(6.20)	276(0.61)
Seeds	9356 (22.85)	136 (0.30)	5286(14.34)	125(0.28)
Organic manure (FYM)	8305 (20.29)	42936 (94.58)	8305(22.53)	42936(94.60)
Output	305153	38531	218031	31091
Agronomic yield	279090 (91.46)	18606 48.29)	202930(93.07)	13511(43.46)
By-products	4134 (1.35)	19606 (50.88)	3891(1.78)	17375(55.88)
Seeds	21929 (7.19)	319 (0.83)	11210 (5.14)	205(0.66)
Net profit/loss	264215	-6868	181163	-14296
Output Input ratio	7.45	0.85	5.91	0.69

In other word, *kuth* cultivation is more profitable than that cultivation of *manu* in the cold desert of the Lahaul valley. Though, *kuth* and *manu* are harvested after three years, their monetary efficiency was more than cumulative monetary efficiency of HYVs of potato, pea and potato or pea, potato, pea as per then prevalent crop rotations in the recent past. The monetary efficiency of 7.5 estimated during present study for *kuth* is quiet lower than 11.8 monetary efficiency of *kuth* in 1995-96 (Kuniyal et al., 2004). Lower market rates of roots and increase in market rates of input are the main reasons for the lower monetary efficiency in the present.

Setback in the Cultivation

In the Lahaul valley, the changes from traditional subsistence agriculture to cash crops based agriculture have advanced in between 1970s to 1980s. Consequently, the ecological and economic security of the traditional agro-ecosystem of the region appears to be in jeopardy. In 1960s, the cultivation of *kuth* and *manu* were at peak. This farmer's practice supported the rural economy immensely till 1960s.

During this period India was a major *kuth* exporter to France and Hong Kong (Anonymous, 1976). In due course, HYVs of cash crops received a special attraction in the cold desert agriculture due to its shorter maturation period that fits in the growth period of cold desert and early monetary return as compared to very late monetary return from *kuth* and *manu* (after 2-3 year) (Singh et al., 1997).

Table 3. People's perception (%) for a setback in *kuth* and *manu* cultivation in the Lahaul valley

| Problems | Villages | | | | | | | |
| | Khoksar (12)[a] | | Jahlma (42)[a] | | Hinsa (52)[a] | | Kuthar (17)[a] | |
	Kuth	*Manu*	*Kuth*	*Manu*	*Kuth*	*Manu*	*Kuth*	*Manu*
Lengthy cultivation cycle	72.7	69.0	71.4	72.0	29.4	35.0	10.0	15.0
Small land holdings	18.2	22.0	18.6	16.0	35.3	45.0	30.0	45.0
Low and fluctuating price	9.1	9.0	10.0	10.0	11.8	12.0	10.0	19.0
Others	-	-	-	-	2.9	3.0	-	5.0
No response	-	-	-	2.0	20.6	5.0	50.0	16.0
Total	100	100	100	100	100	100	100	100

[a]Indicates number of households.

As a result, the pioneer cash crops of the Lahaul valley *i.e. kuth* and *manu* and traditional food crops like barley (*Hordeum vulgare* L.), native variety of wheat (*Triticum aestivum* L.) and many more were either replaced by HYVs of seasonal cash crops or being cultivated just with a purpose to maintain seed bank of trusted varieties of the cold desert environment. The area under *kuth* cultivation was approximately 400 to 600 hectares (ha) during the early 1960s, while in recent past it has been reduced to ~ 80 hectares (Thakur et al., 1998). The cultivation has decreased sharply from 1980s to 2000s, as cash crops established their secured position in the market. Findings of the questionnaire based survey are presented in table 3. A total of 72.7% households at Khoksar for *kuth* and 72% households for *manu* at Jahlma said that cultivation was a lengthy practice and people get monetary return quite late as compared to pea, potato and hop. Smaller land holding was another reason of lesser preference of *kuth* and *manu* cultivation among larger numbers of farmers and only farmers of moderate and larger land holding can afford to cultivate crops of 3 years maturation cycle like *kuth* and *manu* (Table 3); numbers of farmers of the smaller land holding is more in the Lahaul valley as compared to farmers of moderate and larger land holdings. Small land holding was a major problem to the farmers of Hinsa and Kuthar for *kuth* and *manu* cultivation nowadays when farmers have options for shorter maturation HYVs of cash crops. About 18.2% households were not cultivating *kuth* due to small land holding and 9.1% households were discouraged with the fluctuating and relatively low market prices. Other problem faced by the villagers in cultivating of *kuth* is that permit was required from the state forest and revenue departments for cultivation and export from the Lahaul valley (Kuniyal et al., 2005). The retail rates of *kuth* and *manu* at village level need to be updated to the extent that it could be profitable as compared to pea and potato in modern scenario (Kuniyal et al., 2005). The farmers are still maintaining the seed bank of these species in a small pocket in the Lahaul valley.

Conclusion

Farmers are gradually replacing the *kuth* and *manu* with HYVs of introduced cash crops like potato, pea and hop due to higher economic return in short duration. Easier and simpler permit procurement procedure for cultivation and export, establishment of stable market, easy export and technical inputs for scientific cultivation, value addition at local level could be some of the positive approaches in a direction of revival of cultivation, *ex-situ* conservation and protection of endangered but domesticated medicinal crops like *kuth* and *manu*. Experiments on mixed cropping of *kuth* and *manu* with food crops like pea may also be a scientifically tested for obtaining better profits as it has been tested in case of *Picrorhiza kurrooa* (Nautiyal et al., 2001). Revival of this farmers innovated cropping of *kuth* and *manu* certainly requires an integrated approach involving local administration, indigenous communities and regional technical institutions (Kuniyal et al., 2005). This overall management will be a viable strategy or a kind of adaptive management (Armitage, 2003). It is encouraging that farmers are still maintaining the seed bank of *kuth* and *manu* at least in small pockets in a hope of better tomorrow.

Acknowledgments

The authors are thankful to Dr. L.M.S. Palni, Director, G.B. Pant Institute of Himalayan Environment and Development, Kosi-Katarmal, 263 643, Almora (UK) for providing the necessary facilities. Thanks are also due to the Ministry of Environment and Forests for providing financial support and Council of Scientific and Industrial Research (CSIR) Govt. of India, New Delhi for awarding senior research fellowship.

References

Anonymous. (1973). *Convention on International trade in endangered species of wild fauna and flora.* Signed at Washington D. C. on 3 March, 1973 and amended at Bonn on 22 June 1979.

Anonymous. (1976). *Wealth of India: Raw Materials.* Publication and Information Directorate, Council of Scientific and Industrial Research, India, New Delhi, Vol. XI. P. 241.

Anonymous. (1994). *Statistical Outline,* Department of Economics and Statistics, Himachal Pradesh, H.P., Shimla.

Anonymous. (1995). *Sankhyikeey Pustika: Jan Jateey Kshetra, Himachal Pradesh*, Govt. of Himachal Pradesh, Shimla.

Anonymous. (2000). *Report of the task force on conservation and sustainable use of medicinal plants.* Planning Commission, Government of India, New Delhi, India.

Anonymous. (2001). Herbal heist. *Down to Earth*, January 31, 2001 pp. 29-41.

Anonymous. (1986). *The useful plants of India.* CSIR, New Delhi.

Anonymous. (1998). *Threatened medicinal plants of Himalaya-A check list.* CAMP, Workshop, Lucknow.

Armitage. D. R. (2003). Traditional agro-ecological knowledge, adaptive management and the socio-politics of conservation in central Sulawesi, Indonesia. *Environmental Conservation,* 30 (1): 79-90.

Arora, R.K., Maheshwari, M.L., Chandel, K.P.S. and Gupta, R. (1980). Mano (*Inula racemosa*): Little known aromatic plant of Lahul valley India. *Economic Botany,* 34 (2): 175-180.

Aswal, B.S. and Mehrotra, B.N. (1994). *Flora of Lahaul-Spiti.* A Cold desert in North West Himalaya. Bishen Singh, Mahendra Pal Sigh, Dehradun, India.

Bokadia, M.M., Macleod, A.J., Mehta, S.C., Mehta, B.K. and Patel, H. (1986). The essential oil of *Inula racemosa*. *Phytochemistry,* 25: 2887-2888.

Census of India. (2001). Series 3 of Himachal Pradesh, Provisional Population Total. Paper No.1 of 2001, Directorate of Census Operation, Himachal Pradesh.

Chauhan, J.S., Tomar, Y.K. and Vashist, D.P. (1998). Effect of various levels of IAA on the seed germination of *Saussurea costus* (Falc.) Lipschitz (*S. lappa* (Decne.) Sch.-Bip.). *J. Indian Botanical Society*, 77: 175-177.

Gholap, S. and Kar, A. (2005). Regulation of cortisol and glucose concentration by some plant extract in mice. *J. Medicine Aromatic Plant Science,* 27: 478-482.

Gopalan, G.B., Ramasastri, V. and Balasubraminiam, S.C. (1978). Nutritive Value of Indian Foods. National Institute of Nutrition, Hydrabad, India, 204p.

Gupta, O.P., Srivastava, T.N., Gupta, S.C. and Badola, D.P. (1981). Ethanobotanical screening of high altitude plants of Ladakh- II. Bull. *Medico-ethanobotany Research,* 2: 67-88.

IUCN. (1993). *Draft IUCN Red List Categories,* Gland Switzerland.

Jabeen, N., Shawl, A.S., Dar, G. N., Jan, A. and Sultan, P. (2007). Micropropagation of *Inula racemosa* Hook f. A valuable medicinal plant. *International J. of Botany,* 3 (3): 296-301.

Kaloo, Z.A. and Shah, A.M. (1997). Plant regeneration from shoot apical tips of *Inula racemosa*-A threatened medicinal plant species. *J. Oriental Science,* 2: 17-22.

Kalsi, S.R., Goyal, K.K., Talwar and Cabra, B.R. (1989). Sterostructures of two biologically active sesquiterpen lactones from *Inula racemosa*. *Phytochemistry,* 28: 2093-2096.

Kaul, M.K. (1997). *Medicinal plants of Kashmir and Ladakh.* Indus Publications, New Delhi.

Khoshoo, T. N. (1993). Himalayan biodiversity conservation: an overview. In: *Himalayan Biodiversity. Conservation Strategies.* U. Dhar (ed.), pp. 5-38. G.B. Pant Institute of Himalayan Environment and Development, Almora.

Koelz, W.N. (1979). Notes on the ethanobotany of Lahul, a province of the Punjab. *Quar. J. Crude Drug Research,* 17: 1-56.

Kuniyal, C.P., Rawat, Y.S., Oinam, S.S, Kuniyal J.C. and Vishvakarma, S.C.R. (2005). *Kuth* (*Saussurea lappa*) cultivation in the cold desert environment of the Lahaul Valley, northwestern Himalaya, India: Arising threats and need to revive socio-economic. *Biodiversity and Conservation,* 14 (5): 1035-1045.

Kuniyal, J.C., Vishvakarma, S.C.R. and Singh, G.S. (2004). Changing crop biodiversity and resource use efficiency of traditional versus introduced crops in cold desert of northwestern Indian Himalaya: A case of Lahaul valley. *Biodiversity and Conservation,* 13(7): 1271-1304.

Mitchell, R. (1979). An analysis of Indian agro-ecosystem, New Delhi, Interprint, 1870p.

Nautiyal, B. P., Prakash, V., Chauhan, R. S., Purohit, H. and Nautiyal, M. C. (2001). Assessment of germinability, productivity and cost benefit analysis of *Picrorhiza kurrooa*, cultivated at lower altitudes. *Current Science,* 81 (5): 579-585.

Nayar, M. P. and Shastry, A. R. K. (1987, 1988 and 1990). Red Data Book of Indian Plants. 3 volumes, Botanical Survey of India, Kolkata, India.

Oinam, S.S., Rawat, Y.S., Khoiyangbam, R.S., Gajananda, K., Kuniyal, J.C. and Vishvakarma, S.C.R. (2005). Land use and Land changes in Jahlma watershed of the Lahaul valley, cold desert region of the northwestern Himalaya, India. *Journal of Mountain Science,* 2 (2): 129-136.

Oinam, S.S., Rawat, Y.S., Kuniyal, J.C., Vishvakarma, S.C.R. and Pandey, D.C. (2008). Thermal supplementing soil nutrients through biocomposting night-soils in the cold desert of the Lahaul valley, northwestern Indian Himalaya. *Waste Management,* 28: 1008-1019.

Oleg, P. and Adam, S. (1997). Flowers of the Himalaya. Delhi Oxford University Press. pp. 207.

Qaiser, M. and Abid, R. (2003). Flora of Pakistan. Ateraceae (II) Inuleae, Plucheeae and Gnaphalieae. S.I. Ali and M. Qaiser (eds.). No. 210: 1-215. Department of Botany, University of Karachi and Missouri Botanical Press. Missouri Botanical Garden St. Louis, Missouri, U.S.A.

Rawat, Y.S. (2006). Vegetational analysis, Socio-economic and Cultural aspects of *Salix* sp. in Cold Desert Environment, North-Western Himalaya (HP). *Ph.D. Thesis,* HNB, Garhwal University Srinagar (Garhwal), Uttarakhand, 270+xiii pp.

Rawat, Y.S., Oinam, S. S., Vishvakarma S.C.R. and Kuniyal, J.C. (2004). *Saussurea costus* (Falc.) Lipsch: a promising medicinal crop under cold desert agro-ecosystem in north-western Himalaya. *Indian Journal of Forestry,* 27 (3): 297-303.

Sarin, Y.K. (1996). Illustrated manual of herbal drugs used in Ayurveda National Institute of Science Communication (CSIR). Dr. K.S. Krishnan Marg. New Delhi, India.

Sharma, R.K., Sharma, S. and Sharma, S.S. (2006). Seed germination behavior of some medicinal plants of Lahaul and Spiti cold desert (Himachal Pradesh): implications for conservation and cultivation. *Current Science,* 90 (8): 1113-1118.

Siddique, M.A.A., Wafai, B.A., Mir, R.A. and Sheikh, S.A. (2001). Conservation of *Kuth* (*Saussurea costus*)- A threatened medicinal plant of Kashmir Himalaya. In: *Himalayan Medicinal Plants: Potential and Prospects*. HIMVIKAS Occasional Publication No. 14. S.S.Samant, U. Dhar and L.M.S. Palni (eds.). Gyanodaya Prakashan, Nainital. 197-204.

Singh, G. S., Ram, S. C. and Kuniyal, J. C. (1997). Changing traditional land use pattern in Great Himalaya: a case study of Lahaul valley. *Journal of Environmental System,* 25 (2): 195-211.

Sood, S.K., Nath, R. and Kalia, D.C. (2001). Ethnobotany of Cold Desert Tribes of Lahoul-Spiti (N.W. Himalaya), Deep Publication, New Delhi. 228p.

Tan, R.X., Tang, H.Q., Hu, J. and Shuai, B. (1998). Lignans and sesquiterpenes Lactones from Artemisia sieversiana and *Inula racemosa*. *Phytochemistry,* 49: 157-161.

Thakur, K.C., Raina, K. K., Bhagwan, S. and Pratap, T. (1998). Agro-biodiversity values and issues related to the domestication and farming of *Kuth* (Costus) by highland farmers in

Lahaul valley, Himachal Pradesh, Indian Himalaya. In: T. Pratap and B. Sthapit (eds.). *Managing Agro-biodiversity: farmers changing perspectives and Institutional Responses in the Hindu Kush-Himalayan Region.* ICIMOD and IPGRI. Kathmandu, Nepal, pp. 379-389.

Uniyal, M. (1998). Agriculture of Medicinal Plants in India. pp. 1-174.

Wani, P.A., Ganaie, K.A., Nawchoo, I.A. and Wafai, B.A. (2006). Phenological episodes and reproductive strategies of *Inula racemosa* (Asteraceae)- a critically endangered medicinal herb of North West Himalaya. *International J. of Botany,* 2 (2): 388-394.

In: Medicinal Plants and Sustainable Development   ISBN 978-1-61761-942-7
Editor: Chandra Prakash Kala   © 2011 Nova Science Publishers, Inc.

Chapter 5

Propagation and Cultivation Techniques for *Heracleum candicans* Wall: A Himalayan Medicinal Resource in Peril

Jitendra S. Butola[1], S. S. Samant[2],
Rajiv K. Vashistha[3] and A. R. Malik[4]

[1]G.B. Pant Institute of Himalayan Environment and Development, Kosi- Katarmal, Almora-263643 (Uttarakhand), India
[2]G.B. Pant Institute of Himalayan Environment and Development, Mohal-Kullu-175 126 (Himachal Pradesh), India
[3]HAPPRC, Post Box No -14, HNB Garhwal University Srinagar Garhwal – 246174 (Uttarakhand), India
[4]Division of Forestry, SKUAST-K, Shalimar, Srinagar-191121 (Jammu and Kashmir), India

Abstract

Heracleum candicans Wall. (Apiaceae), an endangered Himalayan native medicinal herb, is commercially useful as a major source of Xanthotoxin. Natural populations of the plant are exclusive source of raw materials being supplied to drug industries. Due to indiscriminate over-harvesting and several other biotic pressures, a speedy decline in populations of the plant has been registered in north-west Himalaya. *Ex-situ* cultivation of threatened medicinal plant species is unanimously accepted as viable option for sustainable supply of homogenous quality raw materials and their conservation management. Through present communication we provide a simple, low cost and proven propagation protocol, agro-and post harvesting technologies for this species. Additionally, comprehensive information on local names, market value, natural distribution, IUCN status, cultivation status, taxonomic description, phenology, active ingredients, traditional and contemporary uses of the species has been given. Extensive relevance of the present information for economically viable cultivation, sustainable utilization and effective conservation management of this species is discussed.

Keywords: Patrala, medicinal plant, threatened, propagation, cultivation, post harvesting process, Himalaya.

Introduction

Family Apiaceae (formerly known as Umbelliferae), one amongst the largest families of Angiosperms, is recognized for diverse group of species of medicinal value (Rawat and Rodger, 1987). The family comprises of about 450 genera and 3,700 species worldwide (Pimenov and Leonov, 1993). In India, of the total 186 species (representing 55 genera) of the family, 150 (80.6%) species representing 45 genera (81.8%) are Himalayan (Mukherjee, 1978). According to Samant et al. (1998), over 25% of total representatives of this family in the Indian Himalayan Region are of medicinal value and >70% of these confined to subalpine-alpine zones. The family is mostly characterized by alternate leaves, widening at the base into a sheath that clasps the stem, often furrowed. Flowers are usually compound, almost concentrated in flat-topped umbels. Flowers have 5 petals, usually uneven, and 5 stamens. Fruit is two-chambered, separating into two, single-seeded structures at maturity. Some parts of the plant usually have strong aroma, primarily due to various oil producing glands.

Diversity and Distribution of Heracleum Species

Genus *Heracleum* of Apiaceae is well known for various traditional and modern uses. *Heracleum* is a derivative of Latin word, *Herâclêus* or belonging to *Hercules* (itself derived from the Greek) means 'glory of Hera'. The genus, widely distributed in temperate Europe, Asia (109 spp.), North America and Abyssinia, comprises of 120-125 species worldwide (Pimenov and Leonov, 2004). However, Schmidt (2004) reported 70 species from north temperate regions and tropical mountains. India and adjoining countries like Nepal, Bhutan, Sri-Lanka, Burma, Pakistan and Bangladesh represent 21 species (Hooker, 1879). These species mainly occur in northern, northeastern and southern parts of the India (Table 1). Out of the 15 species reported from the Himalayan region, 6 species occur in North-west Himalaya, 2 in Trans Himalaya, 3 in Central Himalaya and remaining 4 in Eastern Himalaya (Hooker, 1879; Nasir, 1972). Samant et al. (1998) have reported four species in Indian Himalayan Region. This is a widespread, taxonomically complex genus and many species are morphologically similar. Mandenova *et al.* (1978) has removed 15 taxa of this genus originated from southern Asia (India and the Himalaya) and placed them into a new genus *Tetrataenium* (DC.) Manden. According to these authors, *Heracleum* species distributed in North-west and Central Himalaya are much more homogeneous and the expansion and propagation of this genus as a whole occurred distinctly in Northern part of Himalaya. *H. candicans* and *H. pinnatum* are of common occurrence in Northwest and Trans Himalayan regions (Kaul, 1989).

Table 1. Diversity of *Heracleum* species in India (Modified after Hooker, 1879)

Northern and North-eastern India	Southern India and Ceylon
H. barmanicum Kurz	*H. aquilegifolium* Cl.
H. brunonis Benth.	*H. ceylanicum* Gardn.
H. cachemiricum Cl.	*H. concanense* Dalz.
H. canascens Lindl.	*H. hookerianum* Wt. and Arn.
H. candicans Wall.	*H. panda* Dalz. and Gibs.
H. jacquemontii Cl.	*H. pedatum* W.
H. nepalense D. Don	*H. rigens* Wall.
H. nubigenum Cl.	*H. sprengelianum* Wt. and Arn.
H. obtusifolium Wall.	
H. pinnatum Cl.	
H. sublineare Cl.	
H. thomsonii Cl.	
H. wallichii DC.	
13	8

Heracleum Candicans Wall: Distribution, Economic Potential and Population Status

The whole genus is rich in furanocoumarins which are converted into xanthotoxin through a chemical process (Handa and Rao, 1970). The xanthotoxin is widely used in the treatment of leucoderma as a component of sun-tan lotion. It has been isolated from many Himalayan and non-Himalayan plant species of *Heracleum*, *i.e.*, *H. mantegazzianum* Somm. and Lev., *H. spondylium* L., *H. yunngningense* HAND.-MASS, *H. rapula* Franchet, *H. lanatum* (Michx.) Dorn, *H. persicum* L., *H. sibiricum* L. and other Apiaceae species, *i.e.*, *Ammi majus* L. and *Angelica japonica* A. Gray. Among the Himalayan species, *H. candicans* Wallich ex de Candolle (Figure 1) has maximum percentage of xanthotoxin (1.5%) followed by *H. cachemiricum* Cl. (0.05%), *H. canescens* Lindl. (0.005%) and *H. pinnatum* Cl. (0.005%) (Banerjee et al., 1979; Kaul, 1989). *H. candicans*, a Himalayan native species, is found in montane and alpine zones of west Pakistan, Nepal, Bhutan, Afghanistan, south-west China and north India (Table 2).

Being major source of xanthotoxin, it has constant demand in pharmaceutical industries and amongst the medicinal plants exported from India (BCIL, 1996). The commercial demand of its raw materials is solely met through indiscriminate harvesting of natural populations. Kaul (1989) estimated that during 1980-85, about 150 tonnes of fresh roots of the plant had been harvested every year from the wild sources in Kashmir Himalaya.

More recently in Himachal Pradesh (H.P.), 186.0 tonnes in 2004-05 and 101.0 tonnes in 2005-06 were extracted which was fairly higher than that of 68.3 tonnes in 2002-03 (Source: Forest Department, H.P.).

Table 2. Distribution of *Heracleum candicans* Wall in different states of India*

World	West Pakistan, Nepal, Bhutan, Afghanistan, south-west China along 1800-4500 m asl
India	Himachal Pradesh, Jammu and Kashmir, Sikkim and Uttarakhand
Himachal Pradesh	
Distribution range (m)	1800-5000
Average Density (ind./m^2)	1-1.65
Districts (Locality)	Kullu (Rohtang pass, Banjar valley (Jalodi pass, Hirb and Shojha catchments), Parvati valley (Kanawar Wildlife Sanctuary, Malana), Manali Wildlife Sanctuary, Great Himalayan National Park, Khokan Wildlife Sanctuary); Mandi (Jaidevi forest division, Kamrunag, Jwalapur, Churag valley, Nargu Wildlife Sanctuary); Lahaul and Spiti (Khoksar, Mulling, Trilokinath, Hinsha, Gosal, Tindi, Jalma, Yangla, Gondla, Nalda, Raape, Rasil, Bihadi, Dasrath, Jahlma, Sansha, Pin valley); Chamba (Pangi valley, Bharmour, Dharwas valley); Kinnaur (Sangla valley, Rispa, Sarahan-Chora); Shimla (Rohru forest division and Mahaso) and Kangra (Treuend and Titarcha hills)
Uttarakhand	
Distribution range (m)	2000-4000
Average Density (ind./m^2)	1-2
Districts (Locality)	Chamoli (Kunwari pass, Rudranath, Bednibugyal, Nanda Devi Biosphere Reserve (Valley of Flowers, Lata), Bakkibugyal, Auli, Garpak, Dronagiri); Rudraprayag (Madmaheswar, Vashukital); Pouri (Bharsar, Binser forest (Chakisain); Tehri (Panwali Kantha); Uttarkashi (Harkidun); Nainital (Mukteshwar, Tipin Top; Bageshwar (Pindari valley); Almora (Morunala Reserve Forest, Near Bhimtal, Doonagiri); Pithoragarh (Ghandhuru) and Dehradun (Mussoorie)
Jammu and Kashmir	
Distribution range (m)	1700-3100
Average Density (ind./m^2)	2-3
Districts (Locality)	Jammu (Khan *et al.* (2009) reported its distribution between 800 and 1500 m in Sewa river catchment area which is an exception over other reports on distribution ranging from 1700-5000 m); Leh (Drass, Ladakh); Kargil (Kargil); Gandbral (Boniyar, Harwan, Drang, Dachigam Sanctuary); Kupwara (Lolab valley, Machile, Sadhna valley, Budinimal, Mudhum-Zurhuma, Jumgund, Bungus, Keran, Rajwar); Baramulla (Uri, Tangmerg, Gulmerg) and Bandipora (Guraz valley)
Sikkim	
Distribution range (m)	2000-3500
Average Density (ind./m^2)	1-2
Locality	Kangchenzonga Biosphere Reserve

*Based on available reports and extensive surveys of the authors on threatened medicinal plants in Himachal Pradesh, JandK and Uttarakhand.

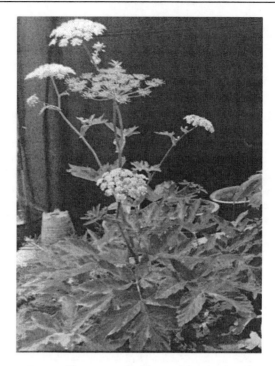

Figure 1. Mature individual of *Heracleum candicans* Wall. under cultivation.

In H.P., local people have rights to harvest Minor Forest Produce by paying a certain amount of royalty; it is only Rs. 25 per quintal for *H. candicans*.

Due to unsustainable *in-situ* harvesting, human excessive interference, habitat loss and fragmentation and grazing pressure, it has become endangered in Northwest Himalaya (Khan et al., 2005; Butola, 2009). Sastry and Chaterjee (2000) prioritized it among the species of high conservation concern.

Now, it is globally accepted and well proved concept that harvesting pressure on natural populations of medicinal plants can be mitigated by bringing them under large scale cultivation.

However, systematic cultivation of nearly all the threatened Himalayan medicinal plants excluding *Saussurea lappa* and *Inula racemosa* has not been done so far. Lack of standardized propagation and cultivation technology is one of the prominent reasons of this malady.

Previously, very few studies were carried out on phyto-chemistry, propagation and agrotechnology of *H. candicans* (Bhat and Kaul, 1979; Kaul, 1989; Joshi and Dhar, 2003; Joshi et al., 2004).

The present report contains several new information on propagation and cultivation of this species and is comprehensive addition to the existing literature (Badola and Butola, 2003; Butola and Badola, 2004; Badola and Butola, 2005; Butola and Badola, 2006a,b,c, 2007, 2008a,b; Butola, 2009).

This species is very variable, particularly in the size and dissection of the leaves and the shape of the leaflets. Under experimental trials in Kashmir, Kaul (1989) has identified two races of the species on the basis of flowering pattern, *i.e.*, early flowering race and late flowering race.

Early flowering race is further categorized into two types, *i.e.*, early flowering broad-leaved type and early flowering narrow-leaved type.

The present study was conducted on broad-leaved type race of the species. An introductory profile of the species has been given in table 3.

Table 3. Introductory profile of *Heracleum candicans* Wall

Family	Apiaceae
Local names	Tukar, Sukar and Chhetaro in Nepal; Folla in Pakistan; Hakh Bul in Andhra Pradesh and Tamil Nadu; Radara, Padara, Tunak, Gojihwa, Tukar, Rasal, Padara, Patrala, Patishan and Patlain in Himachal Pradesh; Kakriya, Raswal and Arwa in Uttarakhand; Hirakali, Gurkrandal, Patrali, Hirwi and Ramthianthen in Kashmir; Hogweed and *Heracleum* in English.
Trade name	Patishan roots, Patrale, Heracleum
Synonymous or taxonomically similar species	*H. lanatum* Michx., *H. nepalense* D. Don and var. *H. obtusifolium* Wallich ex de Candolle
Market value	Roots- Rs. 20-22 (Kullu); 35-40 (Amritsar); Xanthotoxin (>50,000/kg) is exported to foreign countries (Europe, America and other affluent countries).
IUCN-Threat status	Endangered for the Indian Himalayan Region, particularly in northwest Himalaya. The reduction in population of at least 50% over the last 10 years.
Cultivation status	Under experimental trials by some research institutions of the country.
Habitats	Mostly grows in open slopes, open meadows, rocky crevices, along water channels, riverbeds, shrubberies, slopy marshy lands and near cultivated fields, between 1800-4300 m amsl.
Taxonomic Description	Perennial erect, robust herb; stem 0.5-2m high, fistular, striate, pubescent. Leaves large, 20-40cm long, glabrous to pubescent, 1-pinnate or pinnatifid; lobes oblong-lanceolate, 8-12cm long, irregularly sharply toothed, upper surface usually glabrous, lower densely white tomentose; petioles 6-12cm long. Flowers pale-white, polygamous, in terminal, 8-15cm across, compound umbels. Rays 15-40, unequal, pubescent, 8.5cm long. Bracts 0; bracteoles 5-8, linear to lanceolate. Calyx teeth minute, linear. Petals 5, ovate, deply notched, incurved. Fruits 4-12 mm long, pyriform or obovate, minutely pubescent; dorsal and intermediate ridges filiform, lateral winged. Fruit (a schizocarp) consists of two one seeded mericarps that separate during ripening. Each mericarp is a seed.
Phenology	Flowering: June-July; Fruiting: August-September; Senescence: October-November
Active ingredients	Roots are rich source (6-16%) of furanocoumarins (8-geranoxypsoralen, imperatorin, heraclenin, heraclenol) (Handa and Rao, 1970), sphondin, bergapten, candicanin, candicopimaric acid and xanthotoxol). These can be converted by a chemical process into xanthotoxin (1.5%). Roots are a major source of xanthotoxin after the seeds of *Ammi majus*. Roots also provide about 0.1% essential oil.
Indigenous Uses	In Himalayan region, its delicate shoots and young leaves are eaten, mostly by shepherds and tribes, and also used as good fodder, especially for increasing the milk production of cows. The natives use its root paste for skin disease, eczema and itches and relieving from joint pain. '*Amchis*' (traditional herbal doctors) of Ladakh region use its roots for liver complaints, arthritis and toothache. '*Amchis*' of Nepal use this plant in curing phlegm, earache, stomach disorders, infection, bleeding, leprosy, fever due to wounds and blood pressure. The roots contain coumarin. The plant powder is given in giddiness in '*Malanis*' peoples of Kullu district, Himachal Pradesh. Seeds are orally given in abdominal, colic, other digestive and flatulence complaints. Its fruits are used as spice or flavouring agent in cooking.
Pharmaceutical uses	Xanthotoxin produced from the roots is widely used in the treatment of leucoderma as a component of sun-tan lotion. Its pubescent, obovate, flattened fruits are used as aphrodisiac and nerve tonic. Roots also show antimicrobial and anti-inflammatory properties.
Taste/Potency/Toxicity	Bitter and acrid/Neutral/Slightly toxic
Research ongoing	G.B. Pant Institute Himalayan Environment and Development, Almora and its Units; IIIM, Jammu (JandK); YSPUHandF, Solan (H.P.); NBRI, Lucknow (U.P.)
Products	Sun-tan lotion; Oxsoralenultra caps

Propagation and Agrotechnology

Climate and Soil

H. candicans can be cultivated in a fairly wide range of soils varying in texture from sandy loam to clay loam and altitude ranging from 2000 to 4500 m. It has branched root system, therefore, loose textured soil is conducive for proliferation of roots. In Kashmir, this species has been successfully grown on degraded land having less fertile soil. Overall, temperate climate is the best suited for the luxuriant growth of the plant. The slopes are suitable for optimum growth and survival of the plant.

Field Preparation and Manuring

This species requires deep ploughing or digging for profuse growth of its roots. 20 t/ha forest humus or FYM is required. Water logging is detrimental for growth of plant. Proper drainage system is required in the cultivated field.

Propagation and Cultivation

H. candicans can be propagated through seeds and rhizome divisions. Seeds are collected in September-October. Seed viability is moderate and germination is erratic. Seeds require chilling to initiate germination. In natural condition, the seeds undergo chilling during December-March and germinate well in spring. This chilling requirement can be met through dry chilling at $2\text{-}5^0C$ for 14 days. Germination occurs in a wide range of temperature regime, *i.e*, from 5 to 30^0C. Seed viability can be maintained by storage of seeds at low temperature (4^0C). Seeds loose viability rapidly after 3 years of collection and storage at room temperature. Seeds are sown during October-November for developing seedlings in nursery. Direct seed sowing in the field is not a suitable practice owing to low germination in this species. Sandy loam soil and forest humus or vermicompost in 1:1 ratio is used as growing media/potting media. Seeds are treated with Sodium hypochlorite for 30 minute or Potassium Nitrate (100 μM) for 24 hrs to enhance germination, reduce mean germination time and develop healthy seedlings. After treatments, seeds are washed under running tap water and sown in the polybags at a distance of 5×5 cm and 0.5-1.0 cm depth. Seeds start germinating after 10-15 days and germination completed within 35 days of sowing. Greenhouse condition can also be used for higher and early germination. After germination, the polybags/pots are transferred to the partially shady condition. Seeds from the plants cultivated at low lying areas contain low viability as well as germination as compared to that from wild plants. Different phenophases in *H. candicans* are shown in figure 2.

Minimum four months' old seedlings are transplanted to the field during May-June before onset of monsoon. Approximately 90,000 plants or 2.5-3 kg seeds are required for one hectare land.

Vegetative propagation is not preferred due to poor rooting, higher chances of decaying of roots and subsequent low yielding. However, rooting can be increased by the treatment of IBA (0.25 mM). Multiplication can also be done through *in-vitro* techniques (Wakhlu and

Sharma, 1998; Sharma and Wakhlu, 2003; Joshi et al., 2004), however, it require extra technical inputs, necessary infrastructure and expertise and thus, not feasible for marginal farmers in Himalayan region.

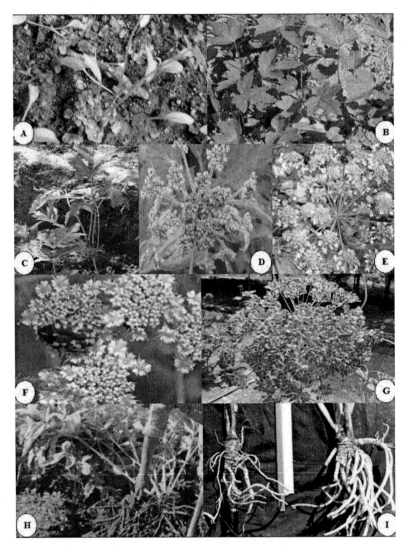

Figure 2. Different stages of growth in *Heracleum candicans*: field emergence (A); true-leaf initiation (B); vegetative growth (C); flowering initiation (D); blooming (E); pollination by insect (F); fruiting (G); final growth (H); and harvested rhizome (I).

Irrigation and Weeding

Watering is required every day up to two-leaf stage in seedlings. Subsequently, watering is done twice or thrice in a week. During summer and rainy season weeding is done at least thrice in a month. During remaining months, monthly weeding is sufficient. Proper drainage system is required to avoid the water-logging in the cultivated field.

Insect/Pest Management

High moisture cause different diseases in this species. Leaves are invaded by Aphids. The roots are susceptible to root rot (caused by *Pythium* spp.) and root galls (caused by root nematodes). Root rot can be controlled in the initial stages by drenching the plant as well as soil with 5% copper sulphate solution. Roots are treated with formaldehyde (10% solution) for 15 minutes before planting to overcome root galls. The fields can be also fumigated with nematicides like DD (1, 2 dichloropropane) @ 250 litres/hectare before planting. The infected plants show symptoms of wilting and drying (for details *see* Kaul, 1989).

Phenology

Rhizome segments propagated in March sprout within 10 to 15 days of propagation. Floral buds commence in early May and bloom by the end of the same month. Fruiting starts in June end and seed maturation continues throughout the July. Seeds start shedding during amidst August and stem senescence commences during September end which extends till October end. The commencement period of pheno-phases in cultivated plants is very early as compared to those in wild habitats. Generally, the plants developed through seeds give flowering during second year of cultivation. Exceptionally, Butola (2009) has recorded flowering in seed-raised plants during the first year of cultivation while using vermicompost as field manure.

Harvesting Period

Detail studies on suitable harvesting period of the species were conducted by Bhat and Kaul (1979) and Kaul (1989). Roots of two year old plants are harvested during September-October. The coumarin content is found more or less same at pre- (7.0%) and post- (6.6%) flowering stages of growth. However, the roots harvested in late autumn season contain high percentage of total coumarins (9.30%). The root yield and percentage of coumarin (>1.5) is considerably increased in the second year of growth. The average content of total coumarins ranged from 6 to 9% which could be converted into 1-1.5% xanthotoxin. The coumarin percentage in early flowering race (9%) is higher than that in late flowering race (6%) (Kaul, 1989).

Productivity and Economic Viability

In agriculture fields with sandy loam soil, yield of fresh roots is about 4.3 t/ha using FYM, 6.2 t/ha using forest humus and 9.3 t/ha using vermicompost. In orchard with clay soil, the estimated yield is about 1.6 t/ha. After two years, the monetary gain is Rs. 48,837/ha for the plants cultivated in orchards. The profit can be further increased if the plants are cultivated in agricultural fields. The above productivity and monitory gain are based on cultivation between 2200 to 2500 m altitudes. It may vary while cultivating the plant at other altitudinal zones and climatic conditions.

Post Harvest Processes

Harvested roots are washed properly under running tap water and cut into small pieces (4-5 cm) for grading. These are dried in mild sunlight for one month. The roots contain 70-80 % moisture contents. After complete drying, roots are packed in cloth/jute bags and stored in dry places to avoid insect/pest infestation. The roots are delicate and susceptible to insect/pest invasion. In view of this, long time storage should be avoided or time to time monitoring of the stored roots is crucial to ensure safe storage for long time.

Conclusion

We propose a simple, low cost and proven propagation protocol (conventional), agro-technology and post harvesting technology for *Heracleum candicans*. Further, for economically viable cultivation and sustainable utilization as well as conservation management of natural populations and to ensure regular supply of homogenous quality raw materials of this species, the following issues need to be immediately addressed:

(1) Extensive field trials should be conducted at various agro-climatic zones (2000-4500 m amsl) to explore suitable sites for nursery and cultivation;
(2) Populations of the species need to be assessed through standard ecological methods to quantify existing stock and explore elite populations;
(3) Sustainable harvesting methods should be developed to regulate rampant harvesting of the wild stock;
(4) Chemical properties of other species of *Heracleum* need to be investigated, so that the sources of the xanthotoxin could be increased;
(5) To promote its cultivation among different stakeholders, a proper technological demonstration and dissemination of its economic potential should be initiated. Particularly, local communities and indigenous people those who are engaged in collection and trade of medicinal plants should be encouraged for *in-situ* conservation and cultivation and;
(6) The Government and Non Government Organizations are required to offer financial, technical and marketing support and supply quality planting materials to the stakeholders.

Acknowledgments

We are grateful to the Director of G.B. Pant Institute of Himalayan Environment and Development for providing necessary facilities and consistent encouragement. The first author is grateful to Dr. Mohinder Pal, former Director of the Institute for his guidance and moral support. We extend our gratitude to Dr. Arvind Bhatt and Dr. Sanjay Gairola for providing information on distribution of the species in Uttarakhand.

References

Badola, H.K. and Butola, J.S. (2003). Cultivation production trials of *Heracleum candicans*, a threatened high value medicinal Herb, in Himachal Himalaya. *Umbellifereae Improvement Newsletter,* 13: 6-10.

Badola, H.K. and Butola, J.S. (2005). Effect of ploughing depth on the growth and yield of *Heracleum candicans*: a threatened medicinal herb and a less-explored potential crop of the Himalayan region. *Journal of Mountain Science,* 2 (2): 173-180.

Banerjee, S.K., Rao, P.R., Sarin, Y.K., Jamwal, P.S. and Atal, C.K. (1979). *Heracleum* spp. as sources of furanocoumarins. Paper presented in symposium on *Production and Utilization of Forest Products*, held at RRL, Jammu, March 5-7, 1979.

BCIL (1996). *Sectoral study of Indian Medicinal Plants- status, perspective and strategy for growth.* Biotech Consortium India Ltd., New Delhi.

Bhat, B.K. and Kaul, M.K. (1979). Prospectus of *Heracleum candicans* Wall. cultivation in Kashmir. *Herba Hungarica,* 18: 59-62.

Butola, J.S. and Badola, H.K. (2004). Seed germination improvement using chemicals in *Heracleum candicans* Wall, a threatened medicinal herb of Himalaya. *Indian Forester,* 130 (5): 565-572.

Butola, J.S. and Badola, H.K. (2006a). Effects of growing medium on vegetative propagation of Himalayan endangered medicinal plants, *Angelica glauca* and *Heracleum candicans*, using rhizome segments. *Journal of Hill Research,* 19 (2): 65-70.

Butola, J.S. and Badola, H.K. (2006b). Chemical treatments to improve seedling emergence, vigour and survival in *Heracleum candicans* Wall. (Apiaceae): a high value threatened medicinal and edible herb of Himalaya. *Journal of Plant Biology,* 33 (3): 215-220.

Butola, J.S. and Badola, H.K. (2006c). Assessing seedling emergence, growth and vigour in *Angelica glauca* Edgew. and *Heracleum candicans* Wall. under different growing media and environments. *Journal of Non-Timber Forest Products,* 13 (2): 141-153.

Butola, J.S. and Badola, H.K. (2007). Vegetative propagation of *Angelica glauca* and *Heracleum candicans*. *Journal of Tropical Medicinal Plants,* 8 (1): 85-91.

Butola, J.S. and Badola, H.K. (2008a). Himalayan threatened medicinal plants and their conservation in Himachal Pradesh. *Journal of Tropical Medicinal Plants,* 9 (1): 125-142.

Butola, J.S. and Badola, H.K. (2008b). Propagation conditions for mass multiplication of three threatened Himalayan high value medicinal herbs. *International Plant Genetic Resource Newsletter,* 153: 43-47.

Butola, J.S. (2009). *Propagation and field trials using conventional methods, of some threatened medicinal plant species of Himachal Pradesh.* PhD Thesis submitted to Forest Research Institute University, Dehradun, India.

Handa, K.L. and Rao, P.R. (1970). Xanthotoxin from *Heracleum candicans. Research and Industry,* 15: 164.

Hooker, J.D. (1879). *Flora of British India*, Vol. 2. L. Reeve and Co. England.

Joshi, M. and Dhar, U. (2003). Effect of various pre-sowing treatments on seed germination of *Heracleum candicans* Wall. Ex DC.: a high value medicinal plant. *Seed Science and Technology,* 31: 737-743.

Joshi, M., Manjkhola, S. and Dhar, U. (2004). Developing propagation techniques for conservation of *Heracleum candicans*–an endangered medicinal plant of the Himalayan region. *Journal of Horticulture and Biotechnology*, 79: 953-959.

Kaul, M.K. (1989). Himalayan *Heracleum* Linn (Hogweed)- a review. CSIR, Jammu, India.

Khan, S.K., Karnat, N.M. and Shankar, D. (2005). India's Foundation for the Revitalization of Local Health Traditions Pioneering In Situ Conservation Strategies for Medicinal Plants and Local Cultures. *HerbalGram*, 68: 34-48.

Khan, M., Kumar, S. and Hamal, I.A. (2009). Medicinal Plants of Sewa River Catchment Area in the Northwest Himalaya and its Implication for Conservation. *Ethnobotanical Leaflets*, 13: 1113- 1139.

Mandenova, I.P., Carbonnier, J., Cauwet Marc A.M., Guyot, M., Molho, D. and Reduron, J.P. (1978). Contribution A L'etude Du Genre Tetrataenium (DC) Manden. In: Actes du 2 eme Symposium international sur les Ombelliferes "Contribution Pluridisciplinaries a la sustematique", Peripignan, 1977.

Mukherjee, P.K. (1978). *A Resume of Indian Umbelliferae*. Actes du Zeme Symp. Inter. Sur. Les. Ombelliferes, pp. 47-70.

Nasir, E. (1972). *Umbelliferae in Flora of West Pakistan*. (Eds., Nasir, E. and Ali, S.I.), Rawalpindi, Pakistan.

Pimenov, M.G. and Leonov, M.V. (1993). *The genera of Umbelliferae*, Royal Botanical Gardens, Kew.

Pimenov, M.G. and Leonov, M.V. (2004). The asian umbelliferae biodiversity database (ASIUM) with particular reference to South-West Asian taxa. *Turkish Journal of Botany*, 28: 139-145.

Rawat, G.S. and Rodger, H.S. (1987). *Alpine meadows of Uttar Pradesh*. An ecological review. *Proceeding of Natural Rangeland Symposium*, pp. 119-137.

Samant, S.S., Dhar, U. and Palni, L.M.S. (1998). *Medicinal Plants of Indian Himalaya: Diversity, Distribution Potential Values*. HIMAVIKAS Publication. No. 13, Gyanodaya Prakashan, Nainital, p. 163.

Sastry, A.R.K. and Chattergee, S. (2000). Prioritization of medicinal plants of India. In: *Setting biodiversity conservation priorities for India*, (Eds., Singh, S., Sastry, A.R.K., Mehta, R. and Uppal, V.), Vol. II. World Wildlife Fund, 467–73.

Schmidt, R.J. (2004). Umbelliferae (Umbellifer or Carrot family). - http://BoDD.cf.ac.uk/BotDermFolder/BotDermU/UMBE.html.

Sharma, R.K. and Wakhlu, A.K. (2003). Regeneration of *Heracleum candicans* Wall. plants from callus cultures through organogenesis. *Journal of Plant Biochemistry and Biotechnology*, 12: 71-72.

Wakhlu, A.K. and Sharma, R.K. (1998). Micropropagation of *Heracleum candicans* Wall.: a rare medicinal herb. *In-vitro Cellular and Developmental Biology of Plants*, 35: 79-81.

B. Medicinal Plants: Technological and Scientific Interventions

In: Medicinal Plants and Sustainable Development
Editor: Chandra Prakash Kala

ISBN 978-1-61761-942-7
© 2011 Nova Science Publishers, Inc.

Chapter 6

Influence of Pre-Sowing Dormancy Breaking Treatments on the Germination of Medicinally Important Species of the Family Solanaceae

Zubaida Yousaf[1]*, Uzma Hussain[2] and Aisha Anjum[2]
[1]Department of Botany, Lahore College for Women University,
Lahore, Pakistan
[2]Department of Botany, Pir Mehr Ali Shah Arid Agriculture
University Rawalpindi, Pakistan

Abstract

Solanaceae is one of the economically important families and seed dormancy has been observed in some species of this family. Seeds of some medicinally important plant species of Solanaceae, collected from different areas of Pakistan, were subjected to various treatments viz; distilled water (control), pre-chilling, NaNO3 (1 % and 0.5%), CaNO3 (1 % and 0.5%), hot water treatment (3hrs, 24hrs) and 100ppm GA3. Treatments were given to seeds in germinating chamber and at the room temperature. Species showed different response to various treatments. All the species responded well to 100ppm GA_3 and 0.5 % $CaNO_3$. However, the percentage germination was low in case of 0.5 % $CaNO_3$. Five species germinated by prechilling treatment. *Solanum erianthum*, *S. melongena* and *S. incanum* showed the 100% germination, whereas 20% germination was observed in *Withania coagulans*. Seeds of *H. pusillus*, *S. surattense* and *D. innoxia* were germinated when treated with calcium and sodium nitrates (0.5%), suggesting the presence of strong primary dormancy.

Keywords: Dormancy, Germination, Solanceae, Pre-chilling, NaNO3, CaNO3, and GA3.

---

* z4zubaida@yahoo.com, 9201950 ext 250.

Introduction

Solanaceae is a cosmopolitan family. Though the species are distributed throughout the world, they occur, in greater concentrations, in tropical and warm temperate regions with centers of diversity occurring in the Southern Hemisphere, particularly in South America. Other center of speciation occurs in Australia and Africa, with relative few and less diverse species being found in Europe and Asia (Symon, 1981; D'Arcy, 1991; Hawkes, 1992).

Among angiosperm families, the Solanaceae rank as one of the most important to human beings. Various species of Solanaceae are used for food (e.g. *Solanum tuberosum* L. (potato), *S. lycopersicum* L. (tomato), *S. melongena* L. (eggplant), for drugs (e.g. *Solanum nigrum* and *Atropa belladonna* L. (deadly nightshade), *Mandragora officinarum* L. (mandrake), *Duboisia* spp. sources of commercial alkaloids) and as ornamentals (e.g. *Petunia hybrida* Hort.).

Wild existence of species is one of the biggest sources for collecting medicinal plants. With increasing pressure of extensive utilization there is a need to bring these plant species into cultivation. However, physical dormancy is one of the biggest problems for germination of some species belonging to the Solanaceae. The dormancy is due to presence of three to five layers of rather thick-walled endosperm cell layers and thick testa, which prevent entry of water to the embryo (Leubner-Metzger, 2001).

Primary dormancy in freshly collected seeds was also observed in the Solanaceae species. Primary dormancy inhabits the germination of seeds immediately after the shading (Rahman et al., 2001). Physical and primary dormancy can be over come by chemical and temperature shocks. A solution of Nitrates with different concentration has been used for the different species of *Solanum* showed very good results. This accelerates the germination rate and emergence of seedlings (Bithell et al., 2002). Temperature shocks in the form of pre-chilling or hot water treatment also help in breaking dormancy.

Bithell et al., 2002 determined the germination requirement of laboratory stored seeds (at 5°C) of *Solanum nigrum* and *Solanum physalifolium*. For this purposes they collected the fresh seeds and stored them at 5°C for almost two months. In the first experiment, seeds were germinated in 24hrs light at constant temperature of 10, 15, 20 or 25°C after 14 days all material was transferred to 20/30°C with 16:8h light: dark for 7 days.

The second experiment was designed to test the pre germination chilling level for 5 days at 5°C. In third experiment, seeds were treated with 0.2% KNO_3, 0.05% GA_3 and water prior to sowing. They concluded that alternate temperature, pre germination chilling and light were all required to germinate the seeds of black night shade seeds. Based on the treatment of potassium nitrate they concluded the presence of primary dormancy in *Solanum* species.

Koornneef et al., 2002 published a review article on seed dormancy and germination. Higher plants have complex adaptive traits of seed dormancy and germination. These two genes influence by large number of genes and environmental factors.

On the basis of genetical and physiological studies it was concluded that plants hormones like abscisic acid and gibberelline play an important role in the regulation of dormancy and germination. They suggested molecular techniques for further investigation related to these two phenomena.

The main objective of the present investigations was to evaluate different dormancy breaking techniques for medicinally important species of the family Solancaeae.

Materials and Methods

Experiment was conducted at the Plant Genetic Resource Institute of the National Agricultural Research Center, Islamabad. Seeds of selected medicinally important species of Solanaceae were sown in pots and kept in green house to provide appropriate germination conditions.

Seeds of *Solanum anguivii, S. pseudo-capisucm, S. nigrum, S. villosum, S. americanum, Datura stramonium, Hyoscyamous niger, Capsicum frutescense* and *Withania somnifera* were germinated but the seeds of *S. torvum, S. erianthum, S. surattense, S. melongena* and *S. incanum, D. innoxia , W. coagulans* and *H. pusillus* did not germinate. Then the seeds of these species subjected for germination test. Paper towel method was used for this purpose. Three pre soaked paper towels were laid on one and other. Ten seeds of each species were placed on top of the upper most sheet in a fairly regular pattern.

Fourth paper towel was placed on top of them. Paper towel were rolled gently to form a tube. Rolled papers were placed in suitable container in upright position covered with polyethylene bags and kept in germinating chamber on recommended temperature 20-25°C (Jennifer and James, 1997). Germination was not observed in any of the species. These dormant seeds were subjected to different dormancy breaking treatments.

Dormancy Breaking Treatments

Ten seeds from each dormant species were subjected to different dormancy breaking treatments. Seeds were given nine different treatments as following:

1. Distilled water treatment
2. Pre-chilling (0°C in refrigerator for one week)
3. Hot water treatment for three hours
4. Hot water treatment for 24 hours

Seeds were soaked at 60°C in hot water for different time periods (3hrs and 24hrs). Tubes were kept in water bath to maintain the temperature.

1. Treatment with 0.5% $NaNO_3$
2. Treatment with 1% $NaNO_3$
3. Treatment with 0.5% $CaNO_3$
4. Treatment with 1% $CaNO_3$
5. Treatment with GA_3

For all these chemical treatments Seeds were soaked in respective solution for one day before sowing.

Seed Sowing

Treated seeds were placed in Petri dishes for germination. All Petri dishes were placed in two different temperature conditions. One was in germinating chamber where the temperature was 20-25°C. Second set of all treatment was kept at the room temperature 15-20°C. One set of all treatments was placed on room temperature and other in seeds germination chamber with the fluctuation of temperature from 20-25°C.

Results and Discussion

Solanaceae is an important source of alkaloids, yet germination is suppressed by seed coat imposed dormancy. Methods for breaking dormancy of medicinally important species of this family were investigated. Seeds collected from different areas of Pakistan were subjected to various treatments viz; distilled water (control), prechilling $NaNO_3$ (1% and 0.5%), Ca NO_3 (1% and 0.5%), hot water treatment (3hrs, 24hrs) and 100ppm GA_3 (Table 1). Treatments were given at room temperature and germinating chamber.

All selected species showed different behavior towards different dormancy breaking treatments (Figure 1-8). *Solanum incanum* and *S. melongena* showed response to maximum number of treatments, whereas response of *Datura innoxia* recorded only for a few treatments. *Solanum erianthum, S. melongena* and *S. incanum* have 100% germination, following pre-chilling and 80%, 100%, 90%, respectively after GA_3.

Hyoscyamous pusillus and *Datura innoxia* were not germinated when hot water and prechilling treatments were given. Both of these species showed maximum responses to GA_3, which was 70% and 50%, respectively. Overall best germination results were obtained with GA_3. Pre-chilling also gave high germination but not equivalent to GA_3. Nitrates of sodium and calcium (concentration 0.5%) proved good dormancy breaking treatments. *Solanum melongena* significantly responded to these treatments (Figure 3). This species showed the 90% and 70% germination after the treatment of 0.5% NaNO3 and 0.5% CaCO3. *Datura innoxia, W. coagulans, Solanum eriantum* and *S. torvum* showed only 10% germination by following these treatments (Figure 6-8). When treatments are given at room temperature no species except *Solanum incanum* germinated. In *S. incanum* 10% germination is observed following pre-chiling treatments.

The effect of various dormancy breaking treatments on medicinally important species of Solanaceae was greatly variable (Figure 1-8). Gibberellic acid considers growth promoting chemical. It functions by promoting the induction of cell wall hydrolases and promote endosperm weakening (Leubner, 2000), which is the main cause of dormancy in this group of plants.

All species germinated when treated with GA_3 solution of 100-ppm. Ibrar and Hussain (2002) also found it as growth promoting agent in *Atropa accumiata,* another species of same family. They treated it with 1-ppm solutions of gibberellic acid (GA_3) for 20 hrs; it resulted in 38% germination. *Withania coagulans* resulted in 80% germination with GA3, it was also observed by the Verma et al. *(2001)* in other species, *Withania somnifera* of same genus.

Treatment of *W. somnifera* seeds with 100-ppm gibberellic acid resulted in improved percentage germination, speed of germination, emergence, coefficient of velocity of germination, and a reduced mean germination time, compared with control seeds. *S. torvum* showed the minimum germination by this treatment. Percentage germination of this species is 20.

Table 1. Effect of dormancy breaking treatments on percentage germination of different Species of family Solanceae

Treatments	Percentage germination							
	1	2	3	4	5	6	7	8
Distill water	0	0	0	0	0	0	0	0
Hot water (24 hrs)	7	0	100	0	32	15	0	0
Hot water (3hrs)	40	20	67	0	42	40	20	0
Pre-chilling	100	0	100	0	80	20	100	0
100ppm GA3	90	20	100	70	70	80	80	50
0.5% NaNO3	70	40	90	50	60	40	10	10
1% NaNO3	0	0	10	0	10	0	30	50
0.5% CaNO3	50	10	70	20	70	10	20	10
1% CaNO3	10	0	0	10	40	50	0	0

1: S. incanum 2: S. torvum, 3: S. melongena, 4: H. pusillus, 5: S. surattense, 6: W. coagulans, 7: S. erianthum, 8: D. innoxia

Nitrates of sodium and calcium with different concentration proved very good dormancy breaking treatments. Kattimani et al. (2001) observations were similar. They soaked seeds of *Withania somnifera* in 0.5 and 1.0% solutions each of nitrates of potassium, ammonium, cobalt, sodium, calcium and zinc for 24 h, followed by air drying under a fan for 0.5 hrs at ambient temperature 25.5 to 27.5°C. Seed soaking in 1.0% sodium nitrate for 24 h significantly reduced the number of days taken for germination (9 days), increased the germination percentage (92.13%). Soaking of seeds in sodium nitrate (1.0%) germinated only *S. melongena, S. surattense S. erianthum* and *D. innoxia.* Kattimani et al. (2001) observed that these treatments resulted in the highest root and shoot lengths at the time of harvest.

It was also observed that 1% sodium nitrate gave the most rapid germination and highest percentage germination (92% compared with 26% in untreated controls). Kattimani et al. (2001) concluded that seeds soaked with nitrates of sodium and calcium at 1.0% for 24 h produced more vigorous seedlings, higher dry matter accumulation and root length as compared to unsoaked and water soaked seeds.

Nitrate solution of sodium and calcium with two different concentrations were used in this experiment and it was found that these treatments produced the rapid germination but reduced the percentage germination of species. Treatments of 0.5% nitrates of sodium and calcium resulted in germination of all species used in experiment. But *S. incanum, S. torvum, H. pusillus* and *W. coagulans* did not show any response to treatment of 1% nitrate of sodium. Similarly *S. torvum, S. melongena, S. erianthum* and *D. innoxia* remained inert by the treatment of 1% nitrates of calcium.

Hot water treatments also help to soften the testa and improve the intake of water. Except *D. innoxia* and *H. pusillus* all other species show germination when this treatment provided only for three hrs. When this period is extended to 24hrs various behaviors observe in different species (figure 3-10).

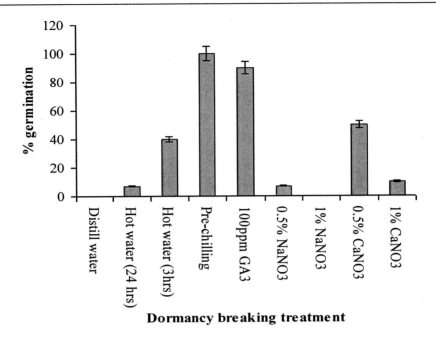

Figure 1. Response of *Solanum incanum* toward different dormancy breaking treatments.

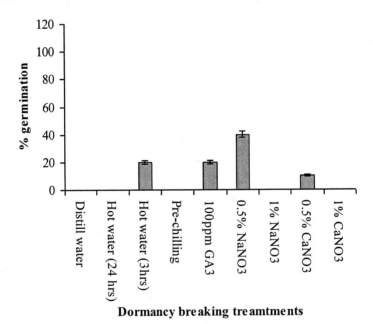

Figure 2. Response of *Solanum torvum* toward different dormancy breaking treatments.

Germination of *S. melongena* became 100% while *S. torvum* and *S. erithanum* became zero. Considerable reduction in the germination of *S. surattense*, *S.incanum* and *W. coagulans* is occurred. When Suryawanshi et al. (2001) treated seeds of *S. viarum* with hot water for about twenty-four hrs there was no sign of germination.

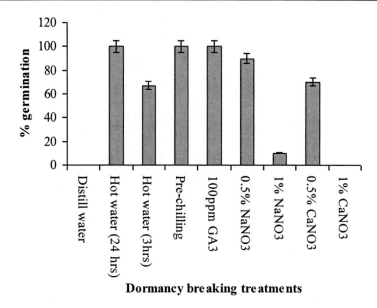

Figure 3. Response of *Solanum melongena* toward different dormancy breaking treatments.

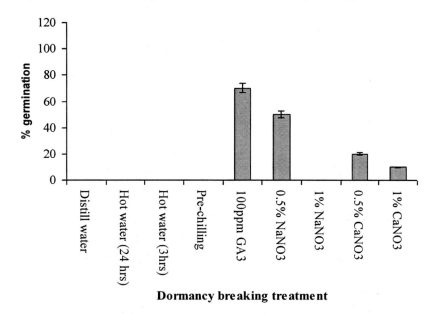

Figure 4. Response of *Hyoscyamous pusillus* toward different dormancy breaking treatments.

Kattimani et al. (2001) observed increased germination when seeds of *W. coagulans* soaked in water before sowing. Pre-chilling is another important factor for the breakdown of dormancy. *S. torvum, H. pusillus* and *D. innoxia* remained ungerminated while *S. erianthum, S. surattense, S. melongena* and *S. incanum* showed about 100% germination after this treatment. This result was same as obtained by Tikhonova and Kruzhalina (1997). They were studying the effect of deep freezing of seeds on growth and development of some medicinal plants. *Datura innoxia* showed response to only four treatments.

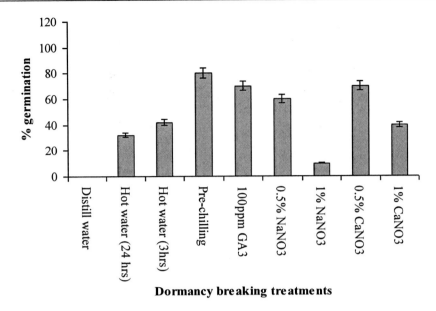

Figure 5. Response of *Solanum surattense* toward different dormancy breaking treatments.

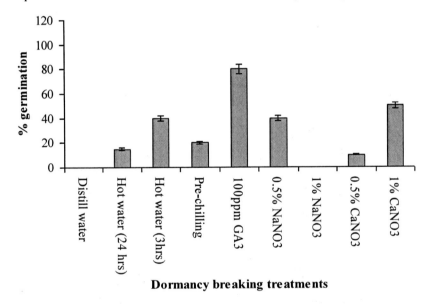

Figure 6. Response of *Withania coagulans* toward different dormancy breaking treatments.

By the treatments of GA_3 and 1% NaNo$_3$ this species germinated 50%. This percentage is highest for this species in all treatments. 0.5% NaNo$_3$ broke dormancy of *D. innoxia* but the percentage germination was only 10%. Afridi et al. (1999) Germinated seeds of *D. innoxia* by using vitamin B1, B6 and C. They treated seeds for 18 hrs at 20°C with 0, 250, 500, 750 or 1000 ppm, of these 3 vitamins as well as B-complex incubated in petri dishes for 5 weeks. They found that B6 and a dose of 500 ppm were best at promoting seed germination and accelerating early seedling growth.

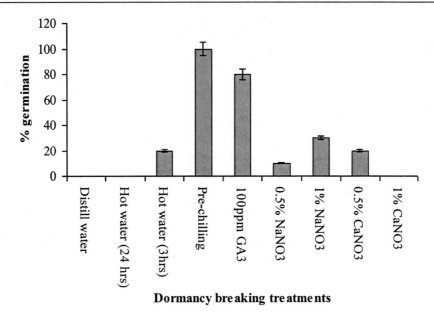

Figure 7. Response of *Solanum erianthum* toward different dormancy breaking treatments.

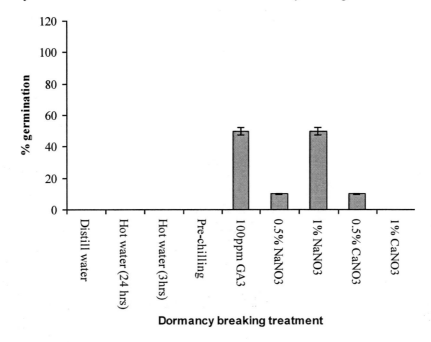

Figure 8. Response of *Datura innoxia toward* different dormancy breaking treatments.

The result suggested that the best treatment in order to break dormancy and promotion of germination in species of Solanaceae is of GA_3. Prechilling, 0.5% nitrates of sodium and calcium treatments are good. For best results seeds should be treated with GA_3 for one day before sowing.

Good germination results could be obtained by pre-chilling treatment for almost one week and treatment with different concentration of nitrates for one day. Temperature range for the germination of the Solanaceous species is 20-25°C.

Conclusion

Solanaceae is an economically and medicinally important family in which most of the species produce physically dormant seeds. Studies on Solanaceae have shown that physical dormancy is due to presence of three to five layers of rather thick-walled endosperm cell layers and thick testa, which prevents entry of water to the embryo. Primary dormancy in freshly collected seeds was also observed in the various species of Solanaceae. Primary dormancy inhabits the germination of seeds immediately after the shading. Physical and primary dormancy can be overcome by chemical and temperature shocks. The present investigations suggested that the best treatment for breaking the dormancy and to promote the germination in species of Solanaceae is of GA_3. Prechilling, 0.5% nitrates of sodium and calcium treatments are good. For best results seeds should be treated with GA_3 for one day before sowing. However, the good germination results could be obtained by pre-chilling treatment for almost one week and treatment with different concentration of nitrates for one day. Temperature range for the germination of the selected species of Solanaceae is 20-25°C. Since the species of Solanaceae contain rich source of medicinally important alkaloids, which has wide applicability, to reduce the pressure on wild plant resource it is important to bring them into cultivation. The present study is a step ahead in this direction.

References

Afridi, S.H., Wasiuddiun A. and Khalique, A. (1999). Effect of nitrogen on growth and alkaloid content of Datura innoxia L. *Indian Journal of Pharmacy*, 6: 165-166.

Bithell, S.L., Mckenzie, B.A.,. Bourdot, G.W., Hill G. D. and Wralten, S.D. (2002). Germination requirements of laboratory stored seeds of *Solanum nigrum* and *S. physalifolium*. New Zealand. *Plant protection*, 55: 222-227.

D' Arcy, W.G. (1991). The Solanaceae since 1976, with the Review of its Biogeography. In: *Solanaceae III; Taxonomy, Chemistry and Evolution*. Hawkes J. G., Lester, R. N., Nee M. and Estrada N. (eds). pp 75-137. Academic press, London.

Hawkes, J.G. (1992). Biosystematics of the potato. In The Potato crop. Harri P.M. (ed.). pp.909. Chapman and Hall, London.

Ibrar, M. and Hussain, F. (2002). Germination studies on A*tropa acuminata* Royle ex Lindley. *Pakistan Journal of Botany*, 34 (4): 341-344.

Jennifer, M.E. and James A.C. (1997). Black nightshades, *Solanum nigrum* L. and related species. pp 113. Plant Genetic Research Institute, Italy.

Kattimani, K.N., Reddy, Y.N., Rao, B.R. and Rakesh, T. (2001). Influence of pre-sowing seed treatments on seedling vigour, root length and dry root yield of ashwagandha *(Withania somnifera)* under semi-arid tropical climate of Hyderabad In: Proceedings of the National Seminar on the Frontiers of Research and Development in Medicinal Plants Lucknow, India. J. of Medicinal and Aromatic Plant Sciences, pp 221-223.

Koornneef, M.L., Bentsink, L. and H. Hilhorst (2002). Seed dormancy and germination. Urr. Opin. Plant. Biol. 5(1): 33-36.

Leubner-Metzger, G. (2000). Brassinosteroids and gibberellins promote tobacco seed germination by distinct pathways. *Planta,* 213, 758–763.

Rahman, A., James, T.K., Mellsop, J.M. and Grbavac, N. (2001). Weed seed bank dynamics in maize under different herbicide regimes. N. Z. Plant Prot. 54: 168-173.

Symon, D. E. (1981). A revision of genus *Solanum* in Australia. *Journal of Adelaide Botany Gar.* 4: 1-367.

Suryawanshi, Y.B., Patil, R. B. and Moholkar, N. D. (*2001*). Study on seed germination procedures in some medicinal plant species. *Seed Research.* 29 (2): 141-144.

Tikhonova V. L. and Kruzhalina, T. N. (1997). The effect of deep freezing seeds on growth and development of some medicinal plants. *Phytochemistry* 46 (8): 1313-1317.

Verma, S., Sharma R.K and Shrivastava, D.K. (2001).Seed germination, viability and invigoration studies in medicinal plants of commercial value. In: *AICRP on medicinal and aromatic Plants.* Sushill, K.S., Hassan, A., Samresh, D. Kukreja, A.K, Ashok, S., Singh, A.K. and Srikant, S. (eds). College of Agriculture, Indore, India.

In: Medicinal Plants and Sustainable Development
Editor: Chandra Prakash Kala

ISBN 978-1-61761-942-7
© 2011 Nova Science Publishers, Inc.

Chapter 7

In vitro Cytotoxicity of Some Medicinal Plants Used in Traditional Medicine in Tanzania

D. P. Kisangau[*1], *H. V. M. Lyaruu*[1], *K. M. Hosea*[2], *C. C. Joseph*[3], *L. N. Bruno*[4], *K. P. Devkota*[4], *T. Bogner*[4] *and N. Sewald*[4]

[1]Department of Biological Sciences,
South Eastern University College, Kitui, Kenya
[2]Department of Molecular Biology and Biotechnology,
University of Dar es Salaam, Dar es Salaam, Tanzania
[3]Department of Chemistry, University of Dar es Salaam,
Dar es Salaam, Tanzania
[4]Department of Chemistry, Organic and Bioorganic Chemistry,
Bielefeld University, 33501, Bielefeld, Germany

Abstract

Plants used in traditional medicine in Tanzania were screened for their cytotoxicity using the brine shrimp and CellTiter-Blue™ cell viability assays. Dichloromethane extracts of *Capparis erythrocarpos, Cussonia arborea, Dracaena steudneri, Lannea schimperi, Pseudospondias microcarpa, Rauvolfia vomitoria, Sapium ellipticum* and *Zehneria scabra* exhibited various cytotoxic activities against brine shrimp larvae. Only semi-purified fractions of *C. erythrocarpos, C. arborea, D. steudneri, Lannea schimperi* and *S. ellipticum* and one pure compound Lup-20(29)-en-3-one (1) from *S.ellipticum* were tested against K562 Leukaemia cell line using the CellTiter-Blue™ cell viability assay method. In the brine shrimp lethality assay, *P. microcarpa* was the most toxic plant with an LC50 value of 1.9 µg/ml (95%CI, 1.6-2.2 µg/ml) , while *Z. scabra* was the least toxic plant with LC50 value of 179.4 µg/ml (95%CI, 156.1-213.9 µg/ml). In the

---
[*] E-mail: kisangau@yahoo.com; Tel: +254 727 225 814.

CellTiter-Blue™ cell viability assay, the mean % cell vitality growth for the fractions of each of the five plant species *C. arborea, C. erythrocarpos, D. steudneri, L. schimperi* and *S. ellipticum* were 43.1%, 67.2%, 82.1%, 52.3% and 87.6% respectively, with P<0.0001 and 95% confidence intervals (CI) of 54.746-81.082 µg/ml. The IC50 concentration for compound Lup-20(29)-en-3-one (1) was $1.747 \times 10{\text -}6$ µM with 95% confidence intervals (CI) of 3.019×10^{-7} to 1.011×10^{-4} µM. Results indicate that most of the extracts tested were relatively non-toxic hence supporting the inherent use of these plants in traditional medicine.

Keywords: Medicinal plants, safety, toxicity, standardized herbal formulations.

Introduction

Medicinal plants from the wild have for centuries been used as sources of medicine in virtually all cultures (Tadeg *et al.*, 2005). Apart from their efficacy, safety of herbal medicines is of paramount importance as a lot still remains unknown about many plants that are used in traditional medicine. (Moshi *et al.,* 2007). Despite their advantages, several studies have established that some medicinal plants are potentially toxic to humans and animals, especially if taken in large amounts. Toxic plant chemical compounds are produced as part of the plants defence mechanism against being eaten by pests and herbivores or to gain an advantage over competing plants (Orech *et al.,* 2005). Plant poisons are highly active substances that may cause acute effects when ingested in high concentrations and chronic effects when accumulated (Pfander, 1984; Kofi-Tsekpo, 1997). Most medicinal plants are relatively unpalatable and their digestibility may be limited hence toxic. Usually, unpalatability comes from allelochemicals in plants and these chemicals may be toxic. In addition, traditional medicines prepared from medicinal plants may not always be safe (Orech *et al.,* 2005). Toxic principles in plants usually fall into various phytochemical groups which include alkaloids, glycosides, oxalates, phytotoxins (toxalbumins), resins, essential oils, amino acids, furanocoumarins, polyacetylenes, proteins, peptides, coumarins and flavonoids (Nkunya, 1996; 2002). For example, toxalbumins are poisonous proteins, usually irritant in nature and mainly found in the seeds of plants (Kokwaro, 1993). *Datura stramonium* contains alkaloids hyoscine, as well as atropine, hyoscyamine, apohyoscine, and meteloidine. Thus it is poisonous and hallucinogenic as well as acting as a pain killer (Alarcon and Pinedo, 2000). *Lycopersicon esculentum* leaves and stem contain the toxic solanidan alkaloids, µ-solanine and demissine and their aglycones.

The toxic pyrrolizidine alkaloids are a large group of related compounds which occur in plants, mainly in species of *Crotalaria, Senecio, Heliotropium, Trichodesma, Symphytum* and *Echium* and are poisonous (Brown, 2003; Orech *et al.,* 2005).

Brine shrimp lethality and cell line culture assays are the most frequently used in estimating preliminary toxicity potential of different biological agents. In this study, brine shrimp and CellTiter-Blue™ Cell Viability Assays were used in evaluating the cytotoxity potential of different plant extracts.

Material and Methods

Preparation and Extraction of the Plant Material

The test plant material used in this study were dichloromethane extracts of Capparis erythrocarpos roots (CER), Cussonia arborea bark (CAB), Dracaena steudneri bark (DSB), Lannea schimperi bark (LSB), Pseudospondias microcarpa leaves (PML), Rauvolfia vomitoria bark (RVB), Sapium ellipticum bark (SEB) and Zehneria scabra leaves (ZSL). Extraction of the test plant materials, fractionation and isolation of one pure compound was done according to Kisangau et al. (2007). Briefly, plant were pulverized using a grinder and concentrated in vacuo using a rotary evaporator at temperature not exceeding 40°C. Fractionation of C. erythrocarpos, C. arborea, D. steudneri, L. schimperi and S. ellipticum crude extracts was done using vacuum liquid chromatography (VLC). Column chromatography (CC) was used to isolate a pure compound from crude extract Sapium ellipticum.

Brine Shrimp Lethality Assay

Dicholoromethane extracts of *C. erythrocarpos, C. arborea, D. steudneri, L. schimperi, P. microcarpa, R. vomitoria, S. ellipticum* and *Z. scabra* were tested for their toxicity against brine shrimp larvae according to Meyer *et al.,* (1982). Artificial seawater was prepared by dissolving 38.0 g of sea salt in 1 litre of distilled water. The seawater was put in a small tank and a teaspoon of brine shrimp eggs added to one side of the divided tank, which was covered. The other side was not covered so as to allow light that would attract the newly hatched phototropic larvae (nauplii). The tank containing the brine shrimp eggs was left at room temperature for 48 hours to allow the eggs to hatch. About 20mg of each plant extract was prepared in test tubes using dimethyl sulfoxide (DMSO) in duplicates, and in decreasing concentrations ranging from 240 µg/ml to 1 µg/ml. The nauplii were counted macroscopically in the stem of a pipette against a lighted background and 10 nauplii added to each test tube. All test tubes were kept in the dark at room temperature for 24 hrs. After this period, the number of the dead and the surviving larvae were recorded including those in the control (sea water without extracts).

Celltiter-Blue™ Cell Viability Assay

CellTiter-Blue™ Cell Viability Assay method was used according to Yang and Balcarcel (2004) and Nateche *et al.* (2006) to determine the cytotoxicity potential of plant extracts against selected human cell lines. The 23 semi-purified fractions and compound Lup-20(29)-en-3-one (**1**) were screened against K562 Leukaemia cell lines from a 53-year old female. The cell lines were maintained as exponentially growing cultures in RPMI 1640 culture medium with L-Glutamine (®PAA Laboratories GmbH) supplemented with 10% foetal bovine serum, PH 7.4. 40mg of each of the extracts were dissolved in DMSO and diluted in the RPMI 1640 culture medium to give a final concentration of 100µg/ml in 0.25% v/v DMSO (Monks *et al.,* 2002). 180µl of the extracts were dispensed in quadruplets into flat-bottomed 96-well microtitre plates. Control wells contained uninoculated and cell-inoculated Medium in 0.25% v/v DMSO. Compound Lup-20(29)-en-3-one (1) was however serially diluted to give concentration ranges of $10^{-5}\mu M$ to $10^{-7}\mu M$. Approximately 15ml of viable cell lines were dispensed in centrifuge tubes and centrifuged at 750 rpm orbital for 6 minutes using an ®Eppendorf 580R centrifuge (Eppendorf-Netherlands-Hinz GmbH). The medium suspension was discarded and the cell pellets resuspended in 10ml of HBSS buffer (Hanks' balanced salt solution with calcium and magnesium, 10 mM HEPES, and 1% fetal bovine serum) to maintain the PH levels of the basal medium between 7.2-7.6. The cell suspension was recentrifuged at 750 rpm orbital for 6 minutes and the buffer discarded, and then resuspended in 10ml of the RPMI 1640 medium. Viable cell count was done using Haemocytometer (0.100mm depth x $0.0025m^2$, ®Neubaur assistent) and the total cell density estimated at 3.2×10^6 cells/ml. About 4 µl of the cell suspension were added into each of the wells with the tests at and the plates incubated for 36 hrs at 37^0C in 5.3% CO_2 and 100% humidity in ®Forma Scientific CO_2 incubator (HEPA filter).

After 36 hrs, 20µl of CellTiter-Blue™ Reagent containing Resazurin indicator dye reagent (Promega Corporation, USA) were added into all the wells. The plates were incubated for further 6 hours and then put into a Fluorometer microplate reader with an Excitation of 530nm and Emission of 580 nm ($530_{Ex}/580_{Em}$) filter set. The end point percentage vitality readings were determined using Tecan I-Control™ software (Tecan Group Ltd. Switzerland).

Data Analysis

The brine shrimp lethality assay was subjected to Probit Analysis (Neyer, 1991; Throne, *et al.,* 1995) and the lethal concentration values that kill 50% of the shrimps (LC50) determined using ®PoloPlus version 1.0 software. The preliminary screening data of the 23 semi-purified fractions were subjected to Wicoxon signed rank test. The IC_{50} (concentration which inhibits cellular growth by 50%) was analyzed using GraphPad-Prism programme (©1992-2005 GraphPad software Inc; Version 4.03).

Results

Brine Shrimp Lethality Test

The plant extracts tested exhibited various levels of toxicity against Brine shrimp larvae as shown in Table 1. The results shown however are for six plant species (*C. erythrocarpos, C. arborea, D. steudneri, P. microcarpa, S. ellipticum* and *Z. scabra*) since extracts of *L. schimperi* and *R. vomitoria* did not dissolve well in DMSO to allow serial dilutions for the experiment.

Table 1. Toxicity of plant extracts to *Artemia salina* larvae and their LC$_{50}$ and 95% Confidence intervals (CI)

Plant species	Part	% Mean mortality after 24 hrs at different extract concentrations (µg/ml)									LC$_{50}$ (µg/ml)	95%CI (µg/ml)
		240	120	80	40	24	8	4	2	1		
C. erythrocarpos	Root	100	100	90	35	5	0	0	0	0	46.6	43.3-50.0
C. arborea	Bark	80	80	70	35	15	0	0	0	0	62.5	38.9-98.8
D. steudneri	Bark	95	90	45	15	5	0	0	0	0	73.8	57.0-95.5
P. microcarpa	Leaves	100	100	100	100	100	90	80	45	30	1.9	1.6-2.2
S. ellipticum	Bark	90	85	35	5	0	0	0	0	0	88.6	64.1-120.9
Z. scabra	Leaves	60	35	20	5	5	0	0	0	0	179.4	156.1-213.9

The LC$_{50}$ values of the plant extracts ranged between 1.9 and 179.4 µg/ml. *P. microcarpa* was the most toxic plant with an LC$_{50}$ value of 1.9 µg/ml (95%CI, 1.6-2.2 µg/ml) , while *Z. scabra* was the least toxic plant with an LC$_{50}$ value of 179.4 µg/ml (95%CI, 156.1-213.9 µg/ml). The LC$_{50}$ for *C. erythrocarpos*, *C. arborea*, *D. steudneri* and *S. ellipticum* were 46.6 (95%CI, 43.3-50.0 µg/ml), 62.5 (95%CI, 38.9-98.8 µg/ml), 73.8 (95%CI, 57.0-95.5 µg/ml) and 88.6 (95%CI, 64.1-120.9 µg/ml) respectively.

Celltiter-Blue™ Cell Viability Test

Fractionation of extracts of the five plant species yielded a total of 23 semi-purified fractions. Figure 1 shows the percentage cell vitality against the 23 semi-purified fractions at a concentration of 100μg/ml. The most cytotoxic fractions were CAB2, CAB4, CAB5 (from *C. arborea*), CER2 (from *C. erythrocarpos*), LSB1, LSB2 (from *L.schimperi*) and SEB5 (from *S.ellipticum*) as they reduced the mean cell vitality to less than 50%. Eleven fractions out the 23 had a weak cytotoxicity effect with more than 80% cell vitality growth. The mean % cell vitality growth for the overall fractions of each of the five plant species, CAB (*C. arborea*), CER (*C. erythrocarpos*), DSB (*D. steudneri*), LSB (*L. schimperi*) and SEB (*S. ellipticum*) were 43.1%, 67.2%, 82.1%, 52.3% and 87.6% respectively.

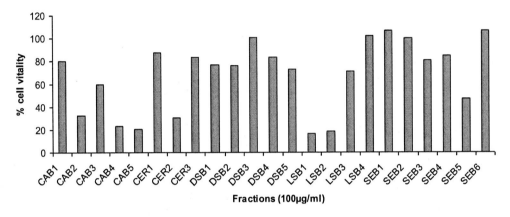

Figure 1. Percentage cell vitality of semi-purified fractions.

Column chromatography of extracts of *S. ellipticum* yielded lup-20(29)-en-3-one (1) compound, a triterpene. The IC_{50} concentration for compound Lup-20(29)-en-3-one (1) was 1.747×10^{-6} μM with 95% confidence intervals (CI) of 3.019×10^{-7} to 1.011×10^{-4} μM (Figure 2).

(1)

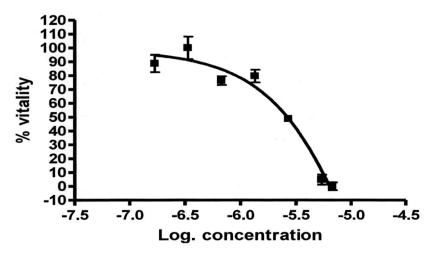

Figure 2. Percentage vitality cell growth against log. concentrations (μM) for compound 1.

Discussion

According to the criteria of the American National Cancer Institute, the LC_{50} limit to consider a crude extract promising for further purification to isolate biologically active (toxic) compounds is lower than 30μg/ml (Suffness and Pezzuto, 1991; Masoko, 2007). From the results, *P. microcarpa* was the most cytotoxic plant as its toxicity against the brine shrimp larvae was far much below the standard cut point of 30μg/ml. On the other hand, *C. erythrocarpos, C. arborea, D. steudneri, L. schimperi, S. ellipticum* and *Z. scabra* were less cytotoxic as their levels were above the cut point. Amongst the five plant species tested for their cytotoxicity against the leukaemia cell line, *C. arborea* was the most cytotoxic since the mean percentage cell vitality for its five fractions was below 50%. The cytotoxicity of this plant species is ascribed to fractions CAB2, CAB4 and CAB5 which reduced the cell vitality to 25.2%. The cytotoxicity effects of these fractions could be due to one toxic compound present in large amounts in the three fractions or several compounds present in various amounts in the three fractions. Two fractions, LSB 1 and LSB 2 of *L. shimperi* exhibited extremely high cytotoxicity effects on the cell lines, with the cell vitality growth reduced to 16.81% and 18.85% respectively. However, the overall mean cell vitality for the four fractions of this plant was 52.3% slightly above the average. This means that there could be neutralizing effects of the less cytotoxic compounds against the toxic ones. A similar situation was observed for *C. erythrocarpos* and *S. ellipticum* fractions. The same reason could explain why compound Lup-20(29)-en-3-one (**1**) was cytotoxic in extremely very low concentration yet the plant (*S. ellipticum*) from which the compound was isolated was found to be non-toxic in both brine shrimp and in the cell viability assays. This observation is consistent with Mtolera (1991) who reported that individual isolates from one crude extract could be more toxic than their crude extracts, while some other isolates could be relatively less toxic. Said (1994) reported that individual compounds may have inhibitory effects on the bioactivity of one another.

There is normally no direct correlation that can be tied up between brine shrimp lethality and cell line toxicity tests or to special types of bioactivities. Exceptions have however been reported by McLaughlin and Rogers (1998) who investigated the usefulness of the brine shrimp assay as an antitumor pre-screen for plant extracts against 9KB cells. These are cells derived from the human carcinoma of the nasopharynx used as an assay for antineoplastic agents. In a related study by Anderson *et al.*, (2007), the brine shrimp assay proved to be superior or equally as accurate as the *in vitro* human solid tumor cell lines. No published work on whether brine shrimp can be used to detect specific activity of antimicrobial agents.

Despite the potential toxicity that could be associated with many medicinal plants, the local people have for centuries been using them as recipes for traditional medicines. They have in many cases been able to effectively control possibilities of toxicity through knowledge handed down from forefathers. One way of eliminating potential toxicity of extracts by the herbal practitioners is by burning their herbal preparations before dispensing. This was evident in the present study where many of the herbal preparations used for skin infections would be burnt into powder first before application.

Conclusion

From the results, most of the extracts tested were relatively non-cytotoxic, which could be an indicator of some safety aspects of the tested plants, hence justifying the generational uses of these plants in traditional medicine. This information could be a basis for development of safe herbal therapies with fewer or no side effects compared to conventional medicines most of which have been reported to have many side effects. Since only a preliminary screening was done for the reported extracts, there would be a need to carry out further studies on their toxicity and safety margins, and develop standardized herbal formulations based on this. There would also be a need to screen the extracts against a panel of more than one cell line as different cell lines exhibit different sensitivities towards various extracts or compounds.

Acknowledgments

We acknowledge financial support from DAAD/NAPRECA, The International Foundation for Science (IFS) in association with Organization for the Prohibition of Chemical Weapons (OPCW) and The Inter-University Council of East Africa Research initiative (VicRes). We are also grateful to the respondents and the general community in Bukoba Rural district from where plant materials were collected. Messrs F.M. Mbago and S. Haji of the Herbarium, Botany department of the University of Dar es Salaam are thanked for identifying plant voucher specimens.

References

Alarcon, S. and Pinedo, A. (2000). *Datura stramonium.* http://medplant. nmsu.edu/datura.html retrieved on Tuesday, 13th November, 2007.

Anderson, J.E, Goetz, C. M, McLaughlin, J. L. and Suffness, M (2007). A blind comparison of simple bench-top bioassays and human tumour cell cytotoxicities as antitumor prescreens. *Phytochemical Analysis*, 2 (3): 107-111.

Brown, D. (2003). *Poisonous plants information database*, Cornell University, http://www.ansci.cornell.edu/plants/toxicagents/index.html retrieved on Saturday, 16th Februray, 2008.

Kisangau, D. P., Hosea, K. M.,Lyaruu, H. V. M., Joseph, C.C.,Mbwambo, Z. H.,Masimba, P. J.,Gwandu, C. B.,Bruno, L. N.,Devkota, K. P. and Sewald, N. (2009). Screening of traditionally used Tanzanian medicinal plants for antifungal activity. *Pharmaceutical Biology*, 47 (8): 708-716.

Kofi-Tsekpo, W.M. (1997). *Pharmaceutical applications of ethnobotany. Conservation and utilization of indigenous medicinal plants and wild relatives of food crops.* United Nations Educational, Scientific and Cultural Organization (UNESCO), Nairobi.

Kokwaro, J.O. (1993). *Medicinal plants of East Africa.* (2nd Ed.). Kenya literature Bureau, Nairobi.

Masoko, P. (2007). *In vitro tests of the developed extracts.* Unpublished Ph.D. Thesis. University of Pretoria, 185-200 pp.

McLaughlin, J.L. and Rogers, L.L. (1998). The use of biological assays to evaluate Botanicals. *Drug Information*, 32: 513-524.

Meyer, B.N., Ferrigni, N.R., Jacobsen, L.B., Nichols, D.E. and McLaughlin, J.L. (1982). Brine Shrimp. A convenient general bioassay for active plant constituent. *Planta Medica*, 45: 35-38.

Monks, N.R., Ferraz, A., Bordignon, S., Machado, K.R., Lima, M.F.S., Rocha, A.B. and Schwartsmann, G. (2002). *In vitro* cytotoxicity of extracts from Brazilian Asteraceae. *Pharmaceutical Biology*, 40 (7): 494-500.

Moon, J.E. (2007). *Herpes zoster,* http://www.emedicine.com/topic1007.htm retrieved on Saturday, 21st July, 2007.

Mtolera, M.S.P. (1991). *Studies of antibacterial and antifungal activities of selected Tanzanian marine algae.* Unpublished MSc. Thesis, University of Dar es Salaam.

Nateche, F., Martin, A., Baraka, S., Palomino, J.C., Khaled, S. and Portaels, F. (2006). Application of the resazurin microtitre assay for detection of multidrug resistance in *Mycobacterium tuberculosis* in Algiers. *Medical Microbiology*, 55: 857-860.

Neyer, B.T. (1991). *Sensitivity testing and analysis.* 16th International Pyrotechnics seminar, June 1991, Sweden.

Nkunya, M.H.H. (1996). Unusual metabolites from Tanzanian Annonaceous plants: The genus *Uvaria.* In: *Chemistry, Biological and Pharmacological properties of African medicinal plants.* Hostettmann, K., Chinyangaynya, F., Maillard, M. and Wolfender, J.L. (Eds.). pp. 268-281. Proceedings of the first International IOCD symposium, Victoria Falls, Zimbabwe University of Zimbabwe.

Nkunya, M.H.H. (2002). *Natural chemicals for disease and insect management.* Professorial inaugural lecture, Department of Chemistry, University of Dar es Salaam, Tanzania.

Orech, F.O., Akenga, T., Ochora, J., Friis, H. and Aagaard-Hansen, J. (2005). Potential toxicity of some leafy vegetables consumed in Nyang'oma Division, Western Kenya. Africa. *Food Nutrition and Science*, 5: 1.

Pfander, F. (1984). *Colour Atlas of poisonous plants: a handbook for pharmacists, doctors, toxicologists and biologists.* Wolfe Publishing Limited, London.

Said, S.A. (1994). *Chemical studies of some biologically active corals from Tanzanian Coasts.* Unpublished M.Sc. Thesis, University of Dar es Salaam.

Suffness, S.M. and Pezzuto, J. (1991). Assays for cytotoxicity and antitumor activity", In: *Methods in Plant Biochemistry*, Hostettmann, K. (Ed.), London Academic Press, Vol 6 pp. 71–133.

Tadeg, H., Mohammed, E., Asres, K. and Gebre-Mariam, T. (2005). Antimicrobial activities of some selected Ethiopian medicinal plants used in the treatment of skin disorders", *Ethnopharmacolology*, 100: 168-175.

Throne, J.E., Weaver, D.K., Chew, V. and Baker, J.E. (1995). Probit analysis of correlated data: Multiple observations overtime at one pesticide concentration In: *Resistant Pest Management*, Caprio, M.A. (Ed.). A Biannual Newsletter of the Pesticide Research Center (PRC) in Cooperation with the Insecticide Resistance Action Committee (IRAC), Vol. 7, No. 2.

Yang, Y. and Balcarcel, R. (2004). 96-Well Plate Assay for Sublethal Metabolic Activity". *Assay Drug and Development Technology*, 2 (4): 353 –361.

In: Medicinal Plants and Sustainable Development
Editor: Chandra Prakash Kala
ISBN 978-1-61761-942-7
© 2011 Nova Science Publishers, Inc.

Chapter 8

Mycorrhizal Inoculation of Some High Value Medicinal Plants: Field Trials and Effect on the Bioactive Phyto-Constituents

Yudhvir K. Bhoon[*]

Sri Venkateswara College, University of Delhi, Dhaula Kuan, New Delhi, India

Abstract

Mycorrhizae are plant symbiont used as Microbial biofertilizers and makes available the undissolved phosphates in the rhizosphere zones to the plants under the symbiotic relation between the plants and the fungus, saves up to 40% of the chemical fertilizers and are the essential and mandatory component of the organic farming. A study was initiated on the mycorrhizal inoculation of the high valued medicinal plants of the sub-tropical region. The selected medicinal plants are in extensive use in Ayurvedic Pharmacies and also traded internationally. Attempts were made to investigate the effects of mycorrhizal inoculation on the quality and bioactive phyto-constituent of the selected medicinal plants, such as, *Centella asiatica, Bacopa monnieri, Silybum marianum, Cassia occidentalis, Asparagus racemosus, Andrograhis paniculata, Ocimum sanctum, Clitoria ternatea, Acalypha indica, Phyllanthus amarus, Lepidium sativum* and *Adhatoda vasica* in view of producing the quality planting material. There was an overall increase in the root biomass, seed weight, number of the feeder roots, early flowering, higher rate of photosynthesis, and in some cases even marginal increase in the bioactive phyto-constituents per gm of the plant in the inoculated medicinal plants than the control. These findings in this chapter are of direct application to the farmers cultivating the medicinal plants and by the use of this technology, the farmers may benefit by receiving up to 20-25 % increase in yields and also retaining the soil fertility.

Keywords: Mycorrhizae, medicinal plants, mycorrhizal inoculation, sustainable agricultural practices

---

[*] Email: ykbhoon@svc.ac.in,ykbhoon@gmail.com

Introduction

The herbal health care systems have attained global acceptability because of the least side effects (Kala, 2005a, 2006). Most of the Traditional Systems of Medicines practiced in different countries of the world are based upon the use of the medicinal plants, which are found to grow in nature. These medicinal plants have been exploited, unscientifically and un-judiciously from their natural habitats because of their heavy demands in the national and international markets. Many of these plants have now been placed in the rare and endangered categories of IUCN (Kala, 2000, 2005b). Efforts have been made to study the medicinal plants by the Government of India by prioritizing 32 species initially in view of their cultivation at large scale (Kala, 2009, 2010). In this regard, Sri Venkateswara College, University of Delhi, has been working on the mycorrhizal inoculation of medicinal plants (e.g., Bhoon, 2005; Kumari et al., 2003, 2004; Bhoon and Prasad, Comm.) in an effort to give the exact cultural practices to be used by the farmers to get not only higher yields but also the quality medicinal plants for the Ayurvedic Pharmacies.

The nature has provided a wide range of the soil microbes for the benefit of plants and these microbes live in the rhizoshere zone. These microbes are responsible for the fertility of the soils. With the advent of Green Revolution in the mid sixties, the excessive use of chemical fertilizers coupled with the various agrochemicals without adding the required quantity of the organic manures there were tremendous harmful effects on the microflora in the soil. In most of the land areas of Indian states of Haryana and Panjab, the "feeding bowl", the lands loose their fertility due to scarcity of nutrients and soil microbes. The micronutrients are in the precipitated form not available to the plants. The organic matter reached to such low level that unless the Urea and DAP is not added in higher quantity, the yield remains very low. In-fact, the yields of the crops per acre are declining in the subsequent years and the farmers of these states are fed up with the high costs involved in the cultivation.

There are more than 40,000 research papers published in various scientific journals but unfortunately, the results have not gone to the farmers (Kumari et al., 2003, 2004. Bhoon and Prasad, Comm.). There are numerous challenges, which have to be adopted, demonstrated and let the farmers in the remotest area get benefited. Keeping in view of the importance of mycorrhizal inoculation, this chapter describes the effects of mycorrhizal inoculation on some selected high valued medicinal plants, such as, *Centilla asiatica, Bacopa monnierie, Silybum marianum, Cassia occidentalis, Asparagus racemosus, Andrograhis paniculata,* Catharanthus roseus, *Ocimum sanctum, Clitoria ternatea, Acalypha indica, Phyllanthus amarus, Lepidium sativum,* and *Adhatoda vasica.*

Methods

How to Use the Mycorrhiza Inoculums

Mycorrhiza inoculum is available in 1 kg packet, which is sufficient for 700 plants. At the time of the plantation of the one year old saplings, 1.5 g of the Mycorrhiza inoculums, which is available either in the fly ash or in the lignite as a carrier, may be added in the micro pit. The micro pit is of the size of the earth ball of the plant. The mycorrhiza inoculum is mixed well and the plant sapling is inserted in the micro pit along with the earth ball, pressed and irrigated lightly. Flood irrigation may be avoided at the time of plantation. After 5 days of the inoculation, the results will be visible.

Raising the Mycorrhized Saplings

Mycorrhized saplings can also be raised either in the polythene bags or in the nursery beds. Mycorrhiza inoculum be directly mixed in the potting mixture at the rate of 1kg of the inoculum per 500 kg of the soil mixture and seeds may be sown. If the saplings have to be raised in the beds, mycorrhiza inoculums be mixed in the beds at the rate of 100g of the inoculum per 500 sq feet area. It may be mixed with the cow dung /vermicompost at the rate of 20 kg and mixed in the bed uniformly so that the spores are distributed uniformly and are made available to each and every plant for better growth. The above described methods were used and applied for the mycorrhizal inoculation of the selected medicinal plant species.

Results and Discussion

This chapter has provided some interesting insights of mycorrhizal inoculation on medicinal plant species. Table 1 depicts the results of comparative status of seeds weight in control and micorrhiza inoculated selected medicinal plants. Table 2 deals with the comparison in control and micorrhiza inoculated tubers, stems, roots and biomass of selected medicinal plants. Table 3 shows the status of bio-active phyto-constituents in selected medicinal plants. The results are discussed species wise as given below.

1. Silybum Marianum

The experiment was conducted in a view of the extensive use of *Silybum marianum* in allopathic system for the treatment of Hepatitis B, which is virus based and is being adopted by Indian System of Medicine also and also because the fact that the plant is being cultivated commercially in India to meet the international market demand. The growth of the plants raised from direct sown seeds, which were inoculated with Ecorrhiza at the time of sowing of the seeds was much satisfactory than non inoculated plants (Figure 1).

The total height of the plants, leaf area, the branching, and collar girth of the plants was higher in inoculated plants. The flowering was observed 10 days earlier in the inoculated plants. The colour of the seeds was dark black in the inoculated plants while in the control, it was light brown and variegated.

The seeds of the inoculated and control plants were subjected to HPLC Analysis for the Silymarin contents and the seeds from the inoculated plants were found to have silymarin contents 1.88 % while the control seeds were having 1.77 %. There is a marginal increase in the silymarin contents as a result of inoculation. The weight of 1000 seeds from inoculated plants was higher by 14.25% to than the control plants and the amount of the seeds harvested from 10 plants was 25% more than the control plants which will be beneficial to the farmers in taking 25% more production than the control plants.

Table 1. Comparison of seed weight in control and micorrhiza inoculated (*Weight of 1000 Seeds (g)*)

Plant	Control	Treated with mycorrhiza	Increase (%)
Silybum marianum	14.7g	16.8g	14.2
Lepidium sativum	3.6g	4.5g	25.0
Linum usitatissimum	4.7g	5.6 g	19.15
Cassia occidentalis	11.4g	14.2g	24.5
Clitoria ternetea	42.3g	56.3 g	33.09

Table 2. Comparison in control and micorrhiza inoculated tubers, stems, roots and biomass of selected medicinal plants

Plant	Plant (part)	Control (*weight, g*)	Treated with mycorrhiza (*weight, g*)	Increase (%)
Asparagus racemosus	Tubers	32.50	64.33	97.94
Euphorbia hirta	Roots Biomass	0.98 10	1.14 16	15.9 60.00
Acalypha indica	Roots Biomass	0.85 10.42	1.07 14.87	25.3 42.7
Achyranthes aspera	Roots Biomass Height	5.23 10.15 110cms	5.68 12.35 114cms	8.6 21.7 3.63
Catheranthes roseus	Stems Leaves	16.5 10.0	36.5 32.5	121.2 225
Phyllanthus amarus	Leaves Biomass Height Stem diameter	1.6 12.70 64cms 3.0 cm	3.0 16.95 84cms 3.5 cm	87.5 34 31.3 16.6
Andrographis paniculata	Biomass	202	310	55

During October 2004 seeds collected from the inoculated and non inoculated plants were sown and the plants raised from the seeds of the inoculated plants were in flowering stage during 3rd week of March 2005 while the plants raised from the seeds of the non inoculated plants were under going vegetative growth only.

Table 3. Status of bio-active phyto-constituents in selected medicinal plants

S. No.	Name of the Plants (part)	Chemical(s)	Control (%)	Mycorrhized (%)
1.	*Bacopa monieri* (WP)	Bacoside A3	0.24	0.65
2.	*Centella asiatica* (WP)	Brahmic acid	0.59	1.49
3.	*Adathoda vasica* (Leaves)	Vasicine	0.166	0.384
4.	*Asparagus racemosus* (Tubers 0.5 years old)	Shatavarin 4	Not detected	Less then 0.1
5.	*Cassia occidentalis*	Total anthraquinones	Seeds 0.084±0.001 Leaves 0.067±0.007	0.103±0.003 0.079±0.005
6.	*Silybum marianum* (WP)	Silymarin	1.77	1.89
7.	*Andrographis paniculata* (WP)	Andrographolide	3.4	3.4
8.	*Phyllanthus amarus* (WP)	Phyllanthin and Hypophyllanthin	1.7	1.7

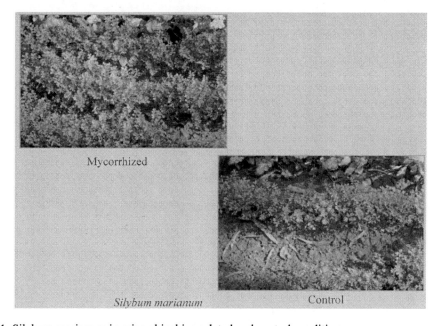

Figure 1. Silybum marianum in micorrhizal inoculated and control conditions.

2. Clitoria Ternetea

One of the interesting observations while doing inoculation of *Clitoria ternetea* was that the leaf area of the leaves of the plants raised from the seeds obtained from the inoculated plants was practically 150 t more than the plants raised from the seeds of the non inoculated plants during monsoon of 2004. The plants after completing the dormancy in Dec-Jan (2004-05) are again sprouting and the leaf area of the plants either inoculated with Ecorrhiza or raised from the seeds of the inoculated plants was 100-200 t more than the control plants.

3. Cassia Occidentalis

The seedlings of *Cassia occidentalis* raised from the seeds collected from the plants growing in the campus of Sri Venkateswara College were inoculated both in the pots and the beds in an effort to undertake the field trials.

Like the results obtained with other plants, the growth of the inoculated plants was much faster than the non inoculated plants (Figure 2).

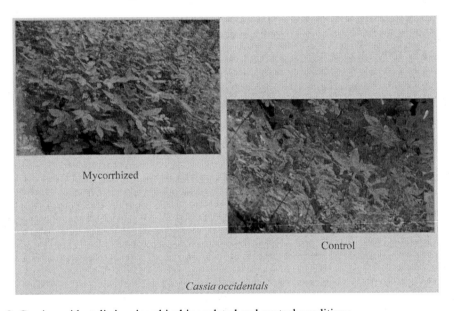

Figure 2. Cassia occidentalis in micorrhizal inoculated and control conditions.

The average collar girth of the inoculated plants was found to be 92% more than the non inoculated plants during December 2004. However, when the measurements were undertaken during March-April, 2004, the collar girth was found to be only 13.20% higher in the inoculated plants. The increase in the height of the plants was noted during the vegetative growth period in June and July 2004. There was an increase of 8.53% in the height of the inoculated plants in mid June while 30.62% increase in the height of the inoculated plants was observed during mid July 2004. The collar girth in the inoculated plants was higher by 30% than the non inoculated plants, more seedpods were formed in inoculated plants and the quantity of the seeds collected from 10 pants was 35% more than non inoculated plants. The leaves and the seeds of the non inoculated and inoculated plants were subjected to the total anthraqinane contents and the inoculated plants were having higher % of the anthraquinone both in the seeds and the leaves in comparison to the non inoculated plants.

4. Acalypha Indica

While doing the inoculation of *Acalypha indica*, some of the interesting observations are as follow:
  i)   The growth of the inoculated plants was much faster
  ii) The leaf viral attack on the inoculated plants was very less
  iii) The total height of the inoculated plants was 15-20% more than the non inoculated plants
  iv) The flowering was early
  v)   The branching in the inoculated plants was more than the non inoculated plants.

The total biomass in the inoculated plants was higher by 20% than non inoculated Plants. The average height of the plants inoculated with Ecorrhiza (taken for 8 plants) as observed on 12.6.04 and 17.7.04 was found to be 39.75 and 78.63 cm for control plants and 47.41 and 89.5 cm for the inoculated plants (average taken for 12 plants). The increase in the average height in the inoculated plants was found to be 19.27% and 13.86% more at those dates as compared to the non inoculated plants.

However, at the maturity stage after 3 months of plantation, the average height of the inoculated plants was 114 cm and non inoculated plant was 110.0 cm. The total average biomass of the aerial plants was 123.5g in inoculated and 101.5g in non-inoculated. There was an increase of 42.68% in biomass as a result of Ecorrhizal inoculation.

The increase in the root weight was 26.47% more in inoculated plants than the control plants. It is interesting to note that the 'Panchang' (whole plant) is used in the Indian System of Medicine.

5. Phyllanthus Amarus

The results of inoculation in *Phyllanthus amarus* are equally encouraging. The inoculated plants were longer in length, collar girth and total biomass.

It is significant because, whole of the plant is used in Indian system of medicine. The increase in the biomass in the inoculated plants was found to be 34.3% more than the non inoculated plants.

The collar thickness was found to be 70% more in the inoculated plants. However, per unit mass, the % of the active ingredient Phyllanthin (1.7%) was found to be exactly the same.

However, per unit area, because there is 34.5% increase in biomass in inoculated plants, one should expect higher yields.

6. Catharanthus Roseus

The results of the Mycorrihzal inoculation in *Catharanthus roseus* are also equally encouraging. The average collar girth of the inoculated plants was found to be 30% more than the non inoculated plants. The average biomass in the inoculated plants was found to be 92.03% more than the non inoculated plants.

7. Lepidium Sativum and Linum Uritatissimum

The weight of the 1000 seeds from inoculated *Lepidium sativum* was found to 4.5 and control plants was only 3.6g and there was increase of 25% increase in size of the inoculated seeds while in case of *Linum uritatissimum*, the 1000 inoculated seeds were weighing 19.15% more than the non inoculated plants. An increase of 25% in the weight of the inoculated seeds will result in overall higher yield per acre.

8. Asparagus Racemosus

After the preliminary results of inoculation on the seedlings of *Asparagus racemosus*, the field trials were undertaken both in the college campus and at Surjeevan Farm of Besar village of Gurgaon, where the soil was sandy. The plants were uprooted after 1.5 years of plantation and comparative morphological studies indicated the following results.

Three and four branches of the inoculated and non inoculated plants were taken for the comparative studies. There was 97.94% increase in the average weight of the tubers from the inoculated plants which are of medicinal importance.

In the bunch of the tubers of the inoculated plants, the thickness of the 168 tubers which were obtained varied from 0.6 cm – 24 mm while in the control plants, the 148 tubers which were obtained, the thickness only was in the range 0.8mm to 10 mm.

The length of the tubes in the inoculated bunch was in the range 5cm to 44cm while in the control plants, it was in the range 4cm – 33cm. The tubers harvested after 1.5 year of plantation were dried after peeling off the thin layer and subjected to HPTLC (M/s Natural Remedies, Pvt Ltd) while in the inoculated plants, Shatavarin IV was found to be <0.1 %, Shatarvarin was so low in the non-inoculated plants that it could not be detected indicating that the Ecorrhizal inoculation helps in the easy synthesis of the higher % of the active ingredient.

9. Andrographis Paniculata

The inoculation of 3 months old saplings was done with Ecorrhiza directly in the fields as Surjeevan Farm during February 2003 and the plants were allowed to grow and the aerial parts of the plants were harvested during Nov 2004.

The inoculated plants in the 5'x20' beds showed good branching, the flowering was earlier by 10 days than the non inoculated plants. The foliage area spread over in the inoculated plants was 20-25% more than the non inoculated plants.

The leaves and twigs were analyzed for Andrographolide and there was no change in the % of the active ingredient per unit mass as a result of inoculation. However, the biomass which is medicinal value was found to be 26% more in the inoculated plants, the inoculation with Ecorrhiza can give higher field.

10. Bacopa Monnieri and Centella Asiatica

Bacopa monnieri (Brahmi) is a very significant plant of Ayurved. The inoculation studies were carried out at the Surjeevan Farma. The plants were inoculated with the mycorrhiza inoculum by putting 1.5 g of the inoculum 2" deep round the root zone during the Ist week of July and allowed to grow for three months.

The plants were uprooted both from the control and inoculated beds. During the growing period, there was enough growth in the inoculated beds to the extent that the soil was not visible and in the control beds, the soil could be seen and it was scanty growth.

The % of Bacoside-A3 was found to be 0.65 in the inoculated plants and was only 0.24 in the control plants. Similar results were obtained in *Centella asiatica* (Mandookparni) where the % of Brahmic acid in the inoculated plant was found to be 1.49 and only 0.59 in the control plants.

11. Adathoda Vasica

The cuttings of Adathoda *vasica* were obtained from the plants growing wild in the Bhondsi village of Aravali Ranges, Gurgaon. The cuttings were rooted by using 2000 ppm sols of IBA following quick deep method and the rooted cuttings were used for the inoculation studies. These were planted in the control and experimental beds adjacent to one another and allowed to grow for one year.

The flowering in the inoculated plants was observed 20 days before the control plants, the plants were harvested, the leaves removed, shade dried and subjected to quantification of Vasicine in the control and inoculated plant leaves. The % of Vasicine was found to be 0.384 in the inoculated plants and was as low as 0.166 in the control plants.

12. Ocimum Sanctum and Andrograhis Paniculata

The experiment was conducted at the Research Farm situated near Denkanikota in Tamil Nadu. This was irrigated land located at 900mts above sea level and is free from the pesticides and chemical fertilizers, with an average rainfall of 900 mm per year.

The soil is of red variety and overall the soil is good for growing *Andrograhis paniculata*. Two experimental beds of 10x10 ft were made, one of which was selected for the experimental and the other one served as control. Seedlings of *Andrograhis paniculata,* which were 6 weeks old, were planted at a distance of 20 to 30 cm apart. The bed was maintained for a period of 3 weeks. A small groove of 4 inch depth was made 2 inches away from each row and of the plant in the experimental bed. The inoculum was applied uniformly in the groove and the groove was covered with the soil mixture. These beds were irrigated at regular intervals and care was taken such that the water did not flow from one bed to another. Two to three rainfalls occurred during the experimental period. The beds were also maintained free from the weeds.

No pesticides and chemical fertilizers were applied during the experiments. *Andrograhis paniculata*, Kalmegh plants grew to an average height of 30-40 cm in a period of 3.5 months after which they were harvested and dried. The results are tabulated below.

Andrograhis paniculata,
Period of Experiment: 111 days.
Date of transplantation: 02.09.08
Date of Mycorrhizal application: 25.9.08
Date of Harvest: 22.12.2008

Experiments	Yield (Wet)	Andrographolide By HPLC	Water soluble extractive	Alcohol solubleextractive
Control	1.940 kg	1.47%	25.25%	13.23%
Treated	2.450 kg	1.51%	23.43	13.14%

Based on the above experiment, it is concluded that there was a considerable increase (12.5%) in the biomass in the treated plants over the control group of plants. However, the increase in the Andrographolide content was found to be insignificant. The increase in the biomass however will be beneficial to the farmers in terms of the more production and higher profits.

Ocimum sanctum
Duration of experiments: 107 days
Date of transplanting: 04/09/08
Date of Mycorrhizal inoculation: 25/09/2008
Date of harvest: 20/12/2008

Experiments	Yield (Wet)	Ursolic acid	Water soluble extractive	Alcohol soluble extractive
Control	5.710	0.645%	27.42%.	12.77%
Treated	6.550kg	0.63	24.78	14.42%

Though there was insignificant increase in the Ursolic acid content as a result of inoculation, the biomass which is of commercial value, increased to 20.81 %.

Uniqueness of Mycorrhiza Over Other Bio-Fertilizers

Mycorrhiza is the only known fungal system, which is categorized as a biofertilizer. Its hyphae can extend much beyond a few meters away the depletion zone and thus can acquire nutrients from a much wider soil area.

In soil, mycorrhiza produces vegetative structures like chlamydospores and zygospores, which become dominant during the period of environmental stress and germinate with the return of favourable conditions (Bhoon, 2005; Kumari et al, 2003). Thus, they are better equipped for combating the unfavorable conditions and have larger shelf lives as compared to bacterial systems.

- Mycorrhiza is a broad spectrum nonspecific organism. A single species is known to colonize 85 % of the land plants.
- It has broad ecological adaptability and is known to occur in deserts as well as arctic, temperate, tropical and other inhospitable habitats.
- It offers upto 50 % reduction in the phosphatic fertilizers application and under organic conditions where organic manure is applied and the only source for N, P, K, will dissolve the combined form of the organic P.
- It facilitates better uptake of nutrients like P and immobile trace elements like Zinc, Cobalt, Manganese, Iron, Copper, and Molybdenum leading to better nutrients for the plants.
- It offers to tolerance against a range of soil stresses like heavy metals toxicity, salinity, drought and high soil temperature. This enhances the chances of plant survival immensely.
- It offers higher resistance to various soil and root born pathogens thus becoming a potential disease control agent.
- It increases the rate of photosynthesis and hence improves plant growth.
- The AM Biofertilizer is known to increase the nitrogen fixing potential of legumes when given together with Rhizobium. The mycorrhiza first stimulates the nodules bacteria in a sequential process by increasing the tissue phosphorous contact, this results in improved nodulation. There are also reports of positive interaction between Azotobacter and AM fungi. AM colonization favorably affects the population of these free living N- fixing bacteria and thus stimulates better growth of the plants. But these dual inoculation effects have to be seen in the medicinal plants.

Conclusion

This chapter highlighted some successful experiments of mycorrhizal inoculation on the improvement of quality and bioactive phyto-constituent of the selected medicinal plants, such as, *Centilla asiatica, Bacopa monnierie, Silybum marianum, Cassia occidentalis, Asparagus racemosus, Andrograhis paniculata, Ocimum sanctum, Clitoria ternatea, Acalypha indica, Phyllanthus amarus, Lepidium sativum* and *Adhatoda vasica*. The overall increase was observed in the root biomass, seed weight, early flowering, and in some cases marginal increase in the bioactive phyto-constituents per gm of the plant in the inoculated medicinal plants than the control. Besides, mycorrhizal inoculation facilitates better uptake of nutrients, and offers higher resistance to various soil and root born pathogens thus becoming a potential disease control agent. By using this technology, as given in this chapter, the medicinal plants growers may benefit by receiving up to 20-25 % increase in yields.

Acknowledgments

The study was carried out under the grant sanctioned by the National Medicinal Plants Board, Deptt. of AYUSH, Ministry of Health and Family Welfare, Govt. of India Research Project No. 87 (2002-2005). Some of the field trials were conducted at the Surjeevan Farm of Akbar village of Gurgaon owned by Devan Srivastava, and I thank him for permitting to carry out these trials. The analysis of the plant material for Phytoactive constituents was carried out in R and D Labs, Natural Remedies, Bangalore and I thank Dr. Amit Aggarwal for his support. Prof. KK Bhutani, Natural Products Division, NIPER, PERD, Ahmedabad and Indian Herbs Saharanpur R and D Labs are thanked for promoting experiments as discussed in this chapter.

References

Bhoon, Y.K. (2005). Biodiversity of AMF in the Medicinal Plants of Aravali Ranges District Gurgaon and Reserved Saraswati Forest, District Kaithal, Haryana; Inoculation of Medicinal Plants with Mycorrhiza and Comparative Phytochemical Investigations. Final Technical Report. Submitted to National Medicinal Plants Board, Government of India. New Delhi.

Bhoon, Y.K. and Prasad, N.V.S.R.K. (Communicated). Effects of Arbuscular Mycorrhizae (AM) and Effective Microorganism (EM) inoculation in Medicinal Plants - Solanum nigrum. *Indian Journal of Microbiology*.

Bhoon, Y.K. and Prasad, N.V.S.R.K. (Communicated). Comparative inoculation studies on Oxalis cernea with Piriformaspora indica and effective microorganism. *Indian Journal of Microbiology*.

Bhoon, Y.K. and Prasad, N.V.S.R.K. (Communicated). Vesicular Arbuscular Mycorrhiza inoculation of an important medicinal plant, Asparagus racemosus: Pot and Field Studies. *Indian Journal of Microbiology*.

Kala, C.P. (2000). Status and conservation of rare and endangered medicinal plants in the Indian trans-Himalaya. *Biological Conservation*, 93 (3): 371-379.

Kala, C.P. (2005a). Current status of medicinal plants used by traditional Vaidyas in Uttaranchal state of India. *Ethnobotany Research and Applications*, 3: 267-278.

Kala, C.P. (2005b). Indigenous uses, population density, and conservation of threatened medicinal plants in protected areas of the Indian Himalayas. *Conservation Biology*, 19 (2): 368-378.

Kala, C.P. (2006). Preserving Ayurvedic herbal formulations by Vaidyas: The traditional healers of the Uttaranchal Himalaya region in India. *HerbalGram*, 70: 42-50.

Kala, C.P. (2009). Medicinal plants conservation and enterprise development. *Medicinal Plants*, 1 (2): 79-95.

Kala, C.P. (2010). *Medicinal Plants of Uttarakhand: Diversity, Livelihood and Conservation*. Biotech Books, Delhi.

Kumari, R., Krishan, H., Bhoon, Y.K. and Varma, A. (2003). Colonization of Cruciferous plants by Piriformaspora indica. *Current Science*, 85: 1672-1674.

Kumari, R., Pham, G.H., Singh. A., Bhoon, Y.K., Srivastava, A.K. and Varma, A. (2004). *Biotechnological Processes for Transfer Technology of Medicinal Plants : Mediated by Symbiotic Microorganisms* (From Lab to Fields Novel Concepts.). Souvenir, World Herbal Expo, Bhopal, India.

In: Medicinal Plants and Sustainable Development
Editor: Chandra Prakash Kala

ISBN 978-1-61761-942-7
© 2011 Nova Science Publishers, Inc.

Chapter 9

Phytoplasma on Medicinal Plants: Detection, Diversity and Management

Yamini Chaturvedi[1], Madhupriya[1] and G. P. Rao[2]*
[1]Sugarcane Research Station
Kunraghat, Gorakhpur 273 008, Uttar Pradesh, India
[2]Division of Plant Pathology, Indian Agricultural Research Institute, New Delhi -
110012, India

Abstract

Medicinal plants constitute a group of industrially important crops which are of great value for domestic use and for export. Phytoplasma cause diseases in several medicinal plant causing serious economic losses. Therefore, phytoplasma diseases are the major constraints in profitable cultivation and production of medicinal plants and lower its quantum and quality. Phytoplasmas are gaining international importance because of unspecific symptoms, various losses and diverse epidemiology throughout the world. Epidemics of these diseases have compelled withdrawal of many medicinal plant varieties from cultivation such as *Catharanthus roseus, Withania somnifera, Rosa alba, Cannabis sativa, Achyranthes aspera, Carica papaya, Cocus nucifera*, etc. General yellowing and stunting of plants, proliferation of shoots, phyllody, virescence and reduced size of flowers and reddening of leaves are the common symptoms observed on medicinal plants all over the world. Knowledge of the diversity of phytoplasmas has been expanded by recent studies and the availability of molecular tools for pathogen identification. Medicinal plants phytoplasmas showed wide geographical distribution. '*Ca.* P. asteris' belonging to 16SrI group is the major group associated with medicinal plants worldwide. So far more than 24 medicinal plant species were reported to be affected with phytoplasma diseases. Based on the sequences retrieved from Genbank identified phytoplasmas on medicinal plants mainly belonged to 16SrI, 16SrII, 16SrIV, 16SrV, 16SrVI, 16SrVII, 16SrVIII, 16SrX, 16SrXII, 16SrXIII, 16SrXIV, 16SrXV, 16SrXVII and 16SrXXX. In this review chapter, detailed information on occurrence, symptomatology, molecular characterization, transmission, taxonomy, genetic diversity and management approaches on medicinal phytoplasmas has been discussed.

---

[*] Email: gprao_gor@rediffmail.com

Keywords: Genetic diversity, identification, management, medicinal plants, molecular characterization and Phytoplasma.

2. Introduction

Phytoplasmas are non-helical mollicutes associated with diseases of several plant species (Bové, 1984; McCoy et al., 1989; Lee et al., 1998; Christensen et al., 2004; Al-Saady and Khan 2006 a,b; Bertaccini, 2007; Bertaccini and Maini, 2007; Harrison et al., 2008 a,b). These disorders are characterized by flower malformation, growth aberrations, yellowing and/or decline, collectively referred to as yellows disease. They were thought to be caused by viruses until a group in Japan (Doi et al., 1967) recognized wall-less pleomorphic bodies in diseased plants. Phytoplasmas have varying sizes ranging from 200 to 800 nm (Figure 1), which, could survive and multiply only in plant phloem or insect emolymph. They are strictly host-dependent, but for some phytoplasma transmissions were reported in insects as transovarially such as for the combinations *Scaphoideus titanus*/aster yellows (Alma et al., 1997); *Hishimonoides sellatiformis*/mulberry dwarf (Kawakita et al., 2000), *Matsumuratettix hiroglyphicus* (Matsumura)/sugarcane white leaf (Hanboonsong et al., 2002), and *Cacopsylla melanoneura* (Tedeschi et al., 2006). The phytoplasma genome is very small (600 to 1,200 kbp) and its phylogenetic studies propose that the common ancestor for phytoplasmas is *Acholeplasma laidlawii* in which the triplet coding for tryptophan (trp) is UGG, while in the other prokaryotes, enclosing mycoplasmas and spiroplasmas, Trp is coded by UGA.

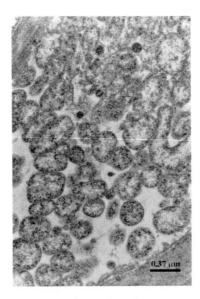

Figure 1. Ultra thin section of *Oxalis acetossa* showing numerous short chain phytoplasma in the infected phloem tissues observed by Transmission Electron Microscopy.

The phytoplasma detection relied for more than last three decades on DAPI staining or electron microscopy. However, in the last 15 years the applications of DNA-based technology allowed to preliminary distinguish different molecular clusters inside these prokaryotes. The Phytoplasma Working Team of the International Research Project for Comparative

Mycoplasmology (IRPCM) adopted the trivial name 'phytoplasma' to identify the prokaryotes belonging to this group. The '*Candidatus* Phytoplasma' genus has been proposed and adopted in order to start formal classification of these prokaryotes (Anonymous, 2004). Up-to-date satisfaction of Koch's postulates has not been achieved, but indirect proof, such as phytoplasma symptoms elimination after tetracycline treatments, confirmed that they are associated with many plant diseases worldwide, several of them being of economical or quarantine importance. It was also demonstrated that genetically undistinguishable phytoplasmas can be associated with diseases inducing different symptoms and/or affecting different plant species; it was also verified that different phytoplasmas can be associated with similar symptoms in the same or in different plant host(s).

3. Phytoplasma Diseases on Medicinal Plants

Many medicinal plants are reported to be infected by phytoplasma showing varieties of symptoms (Samad et al., 2006 a, b; Bertaccini and Marani, 2007; Zhao et al., 2007 Harrison et al., 2008 a,b; Raj et al., 2008 a,b). Yellows, virescence, witches'- broom, chlorosis, little leaf, leaf roll phyllody and generalized decline are very common symptoms (Bertaccini et al., 2005).

3.1. Phytoplasma Diseases in *Cannabis sativa*

Cannabis sativa (Canabinaceae), known as hemp and marijuana, a medicinal plant grown wildly through out Himalayas and is cultivated in some provinces of India as a source of narcotic resin, fibre and edible oil. Properties attributed to it include analgesic hypnotic, antiepileptic–antispasmodic, appetite stimulant, prophylactic and treatment of the neuralgia's, including migraine, anti-depressant tranquilizer, psychotherapeutic aid, antiasthmatic oxytoxic, titussive, topical anesthetic, withdrawal agent for opiate alcohol addition, childbirth analgesia and even an antibiotic (Mikuriya, 1969). A witches'-broom disease on a *Cannabis* sp. has been recently reported to be associated with a phytoplasma of elm yellows group (16SrV) in China Zhao et al. (2007). Raj et al. (2008a) and Mall et al. (2009) observed yellowing, witche's broom, shortening of internodes and little leaf symptoms on *C. sativa* in India. BLAST search analysis of the 16S rRNA sequence of the *C. sativa* phytoplasma showed a 99% identity with *Sesamum* phyllody phytoplasma (DQ431843); *Parthenium* virescence phytoplasma (EU375485) and aster yellows phytoplasma (EU439257); members of aster yellows group (16SrI).

3.2. Phytoplasma Diseases in *Achyranthes aspera*

Achyranthes aspera (family *Amaranthaceae*) is an indigenous medicinal plant of Asia and is commonly used by traditional healers for the treatment of malarial fever, dysentery, asthma, hypertension and diabetes (Girach and Khan, 1992). A root extract is also used to treat scorpion and snake bites by Indian tribes. A typical yellows and small leaves symptoms were noticed on *A. aspera* plants growing as weeds on road sides in Uttar Pradesh, India and found to be associated with phytoplasma (Raj et al., 2008c). BLAST search analysis of the 16S rRNA sequence of the *Achyranthes* phytoplasma showed 99% sequence similarities with the members of '*Candidatus* phytoplasma asteris' (16SrI group phytoplasma): sugarcane yellows (EU423900); periwinkle little leaf (EU375834, DQ381535); onion yellows (AP006628, D12569); carrot phytoplasma (EU215426, EU215425) and aster yellows phytoplasma (EF489024, AY665676). Therefore, the phytoplasma in *A. aspera* has been identified as an isolate of '*Ca*. P. asteris'.

3.3. Phytoplasma Diseases in *Withania somnifera*

Withania somnifera L. commonly known as Ashwagandha is cultivated as an important medicinal cash crop. The whole plant is of great importance in the Indian system of medicine and pharmaceutical industries, but the roots are the main source of active alkaloids. Some of the important alkaloids are tro-pine, pseudotropine, somniferine, colin, withaferin a, withanoides, and a few flavanoides. Phytoplasma disease on this plant has been observed by Samad et al. (2006) in India. The diseased plants showed phyllody, little leaf, dense clusters of highly proliferating branches with shortened internodes and witches'-broom symptoms. Partially sequenced nucleotide sequence analysis of 16SrRNA gene cloned from *W. somnifera* phytoplasma showed high similarity with several isolates of the 16SrVI group of phytoplasmas. The highest nucleotide matching (99 and 98%) of *Withania* phytoplasma was observed with *Centaurea solstitialis* virescence phytoplasma (AY270156) and Periwinkle little leaf phytoplasma (AF228053) reported in Italy and Bangladesh, respectively. Khan et al. (2006) detected phytoplasma associated with little leaf symptoms in *Withania somnifera* in India.

3.4. Phytoplasma Diseases in *Carica papaya*

Carica papaya (papaya) contains a natural pain reliever. A papaya paste was used traditionally for the relief of burns, cuts, rashes and stings. A compound known as papain is derived from the papaya fruit and has long been used as a natural meat tenderizer. It is believed that this enzyme may help the body digest meats and amino acids more efficiently.The whole papaya fruit is an excellent source of dietary fiber, which is also necessary for digestive health. Papaya pills are promoted for use as natural antacids, for ulcer relief and to relieve constipation. Unripe papaya has been used for contraceptive purposes by traditional healers in Pakistan, India and Sri Lanka. Phytoplasma have been reported for papaya diseases in Australia and Israel (Gibb *et al.,* 1996). Arocha et al. (2003, 2007, 2009) observed bunchy top symptom of papaya in Cuba. Arocha et al. (2008) repoted 16SrII group phytoplasma associated with Papaya bunchy top disease in Cuba and the decline disorder of papaya in Ethiopia. The symptoms observed in papaya affected with the decline disorder in Ethiopia was a bright yellowing of the upper young leaves, mosaic, crinkling, leaf tip necrosis and drying of the whole plant death. Symptoms those observed in PBT-like affected papaya in Cuba were characterized by leaf stunting, crinkling and yellowing, short internodes, bunched appearance of the inner crown leaves, rigid petioles extending more horizontally from the main stem than normal, lost or decrease of latex fluid, and reduction of fruit size. The Ethiopian isolate showed the highest similarity (98%) with that of papaya yellow crinkle disease in Australia (Y10097), a member of the 16SrII group, while the Cuban isolate showed the highest sequence homology (99%) with that of *Polygalla* phyllody phytoplasma (AY787140), also a member of the 16SrII group.

3.5. Phytoplasma Diseases in *Cocos nucifera*

Cocos nucifera is an important small-holder's crop in many tropical countries and are used to enhance esthetics of coastal areas. Numerous medicinal properties of tender coconut water reported are- good for feeding infants suffering from intestinal disturbances, oral rehydration medium, contains organic compounds possessing growth promoting properties, keeps the body cool. Lethal yellowing (LY) is the single most important plant disease affecting the coconut industry in Jamaica. It affects many palm species in Jamaica, Florida, and Guatemala. The disease-associated phytoplasma was reliably detected in immature tissues and trunk phloem at the onset of foliar symptoms in palms by PCR Myrie et al. (2006). Sharmila (2004) and Edwin (2007) reported phytoplasma associated with Kerala wilt disease in India. The symptoms of Kerala wilt disease (KWD) showed ribbing, unseasonable discolouration of leaves and generalized decline of palm growth. Phylogenetically, KWD phytoplasma is grouped in the new subgroup 16SrIV-C subsequent to the groups 16SrIV-A and 16SrIV-B for Mexican coconut lethal yellowing and Tanzanian coconut lethal decline, respectively. Martinez et al. (2008) reported Coconut lethal yellowing disease of phytoplasma on the southern coast of the Dominican Republic, Europe. The infected plants of coconut showed typical lethal yellowing symptoms. 16S rRNA gene sequence of Coconut phytoplama (DQ631639), indicated this phytoplasma was most similar (99·9%) to the strain associatedwith Yucatan coconut lethal decline (LDY) (U18753), a subgroup 16SrIV-B member (Lee et al., 1998), but belonging to a newly identified subgroup 16SrIV-E, while sharing only 98·3% identity with LY phytoplasma (AF498308, AF498309).

3.6. Phytoplasma Diseases in *Santalum album*

Santalum album sandal is a hemi-root parasitic tree, famous for its high-valued scented heartwood and oil. It commonly occurs in the dry regions of peninsular India, particularly in Karnataka and Tamil Nadu states. Sandal wood oil is useful in supporting the lymphatic, nervous and cardiovascular systems. It gives relief in itching, inflammation, nausea, vomiting, sunstroke and useful in healing wounds, scars and acne. Sandal spike is a major disease of sandal, attributed to phytoplasma aetiology, as shown by three independent groups at the same time. Khan et al. (2004) reported spike disease of sandal in India. The disease is characterised by witches'-broom symptoms consisting of small, narrow leaves which turn pale-green or yellow on branches acquiring a spike-like appearance. BLAST analysis revealed that *Santalum* phytoplasma (DQ0932357) is most similar (99%) to 'Candidatus Phytoplasma asteris'-related strains, previously classified as 16S rDNA RFLP subgroup 16SrI-B members. This is the first definitive identification of a subgroup 16SrI-B phytoplasma associated with sandal spike disease.

3.7. Phytoplasma Diseases in Rose

Rose essential oil is very valuable in fighting depression, anger and fear. It is skin friendly oil, which softens the skin and makes it glowing and charming. Rose essential oil also takes care of our heart and digestive system. Rose oil is very beneficial in curing eczema, stress and menstrual problems. It serves like a tonic for the liver, heart, stomach and uterus. For coping with emotional problems, rose essential oil is the best remedy. It is of great use in boosting the circulation of blood in the body. Rose rosette disease, also refereed as rose witches broom was first reported in Manitoba on wild rose species by Connors in 1941 and subsequently in other states of Canada and in the United States (Epstein and Hill, 1995).The disease is endemic in much of the south east, south-central and north-central United States (Hindal et al., 1988; Tipping and Sindermann, 2000). Similar symptoms known as rose dieback or rose wilt were recorded in garden rose by Cheo (1970) and Gumpf and Weathers (1974). In 1976, rose leaf curl (Slack et al., 1976a), which resembles rose wilt disease and rose spring dwarf were more fully described in the United States (Slack et al., 1976b). Due to the similarity in the mentioned diseases, Thomas (1981) named them rose degeneration syndrome. Chaturvedi et al. (2009a) reported little leaf disease on rose in India. The infected plants of rose showed yellowing, shortening of internodes and little leaf symptoms. Phylogenetic analysis of the rose phytoplasma (FJ429364) showed closest relationship with 16Sr RNA gene of several phytoplasma isolates of *Sesamum* phyllody (DQ431843), *Catharanthus roseus* (DQ097396), Sugarcane yellows (EU423900), Pigean pea little leaf (DQ343287), the members of '*Candidatus* phytoplasma asteris' 16SrI group. Therefore, the rose phytoplasma have been identified as an isolate of '*Ca.* P. asteris'.

3.8. Phytoplasma Diseases in *Catharanthus roseus*

Catharanthus roseus produce a class of secondary metabolites termed terpenoid indole alkaloids. Possible functions of these compounds include antimicrobial or antifungal activity, UV protection or nitrogen storage and transport. Their synthesis has mainly been studied for pharmaceutical interest. More than 100 alkaloids have been isolated from the different parts of the plant, many of them possessing remarkable pharmacological activity (Svoboda and Blake, 1975; Cordell, 1980). The root derived monomeric alkaloids '*ajmaciline*' and '*serpentine*' are used in treatment of cardiac and circular diseases, and the leaves derived dimeric alkaloids '*vincristine*' and '*vinblastine*' are potent anticancerous drugs. Detection of phytoplasmas in *Catharanthus roseus* has been reported all around the world (Ploaie et al., 1977; Shishlova and Andreeva, 1979; Mc Coy and Thomas, 1980; Dabek, 1982; Kar et al., 1983; Rao et al., 1983; Schmitt et al., 1983; Chen et al., 1984; Moreno et al. 1985; Grimaldi and Grasso , 1988; Musetti et al., 1992; 2000; 2002; Lepka et al., 1999; Musetti and Favali, 1999; Favali et al., 2008, Duduk et al., 2008). Many workers reported host-parasitic interaction and alterations due to phytoplasma infection in this species (Shepardson and Mc Crum, 1973). Periwinkle is the plant in which the majority of phytoplasma research was carried out, since it is the best host for maintaining phytoplasma strains in order to study their interaction with host. Okuda (1977) reported witches broom diseases of *C. roseus* in Japan. Chen and Hiruki (1978) reported the preservation of membranes of tubular bodies associated with phytoplasmas by tannic acid in *C. roseus* plants infected with aster yellows. Carling and

Millikan (1978) observed banded filaments associated with the aster yellows phytoplasmas in *C. roseus* in USA. Cousin and Abadie (1982) described the action of these pathogens on anthers of *C. roseus* with the help of light and electron microscopy. Lee and Davis (1983) separated sieve elements of *C. roseus* infected with phytoplasmas from other cell types by partial digestion of plant tissue with macerating enzymes in order to obtain enriched preparation for random cloning phytoplasma DNA (Davis et al., 1988). Petzold and Marwitz (1984) observed fluorescence in sieve tubes of *C. roseus* infected with after fixation with aldehydes. Shin and La (1984) used Dienes stain in detection of phytoplasma-associated diseases in *C. roseus* in Korea. Eastman et al. (1984) observed polymorphic phytoplasmas in mature sieve element of *C. roseus*. Kim et al. (1985) reported transmission of mulberry dwarf agent to *C. roseus* by the insect vector *Hishimonus sellatus* in Korea. Rocha et al. (1986) detected these prokaryotes in *C. roseus* by indirect immunofluorescence microscopy. Hiruki and Rocha (1986) observed phytoplasmas by DAPI staining of infected tissues. Schmitt et al. (1987) observed freeze-fracture electron microscopy (EM) of phytoplasmas in the phloem of *C. roseus*. Clark et al. (1989) developed serological discrimination among phytoplasmas using polyclonal and monoclonal antibodies developed from *C. roseus*. Yang (1989) reported dodder transmission red bird cactus witches' broom from *Pedilanthus tithymaloides* to *C. roseus* in Taiwan. Molecular cloning and detection of DNA of clover proliferation and little leaf disease in *C. roseus* were also carried out (Deng and Hiruki, 1990; Davis et al., 1990; 1992). Musetti et al. (2007) observed effects induced by fungal endophytes in *C. roseus* tissues infected by phytoplasma disease and Carginale et al. (2007) reported effect of pear decline phytoplasma on gene expression in *C. roseus* in Italy. Chaturvedi et al. (2009 b) reported little leaf and phyllody of *Catharanthus roseus* in India. The most characteristic symptoms of infected *C. roseus* plants were yellowing of the leaves, virescence, and proliferation, witche's broom, premature development of axillary buds, stunting of the entire plants, little leaf, phyllody and reduction of flower size. Phylogenetic analysis of *Catharanthus roseus* phytoplasma (EU694109) showed close relationship with the 16Sr RNA gene of Aster phytoplasma (AY265209, AF322645), *Scaphytopius* phytoplasma (AY180952, AY180943), *Nasturtium* phytoplama (AY665676), Periwinkle phytoplasma (EU727085), *Parthenium* phytoplasma (EU375485, EU375488). Therefore *Catharanthus roseus* phytoplasma is a member of 16SrI group of phytoplasma.

3.9. Phytoplasma Diseases in *Ziziphus jujuba*

Ziziphus jujuba known as Indian jujube or Ber is an important plant cultivated for its fleshy fruits rich in sugars and vitamins. In India, the ripe fruits are mostly consumed raw, but are sometimes stewed. The dried ripe fruit is a mild laxative; seeds are sedative and are taken to halt nausea, vomiting, and abdominal pains in pregnancy. Kusunoki et al. (2002) reported witches broom disease on *Ziziphus jujuba* in Japan. Wei et al. (2007) and Fan et al. (2008) reported Jujuba witch'es broom disease in China. Khan et al. (2009) reported little leaf and witche's broom disease on *Ziziphus jujuba* in India. Infected *Z. jujuba* plants showed severe rosetting, green little leaves and witches' broom symptoms. BLAST comparisons of both 16S rDNA sequences of *Ziziphus jujuba* phytoplasma (EU366162) shared 98% identity with those of members of the 16SrV elm yellows group, including accessions AB052875, AB052877 and AB052879. These accessions describe the new *Candidatus* Phytoplasma species,

'*Candidatus* Phytoplasma ziziphi', associated with jujube witches' broom in China, Japan and Korea (Jung et al, 2003). Therefore, phytoplasmas associated with witches' broom disease in *Z. jujuba* in India, are considered isolates of '*Ca.* Phytoplasma ziziphi'.

3.10. Phytoplasma Diseases in *Hibiscus rosa-sinensis*

Hibiscus rosa-sinensis L. is a sweet, astringent, cooling herb that checks bleeding, soothes irritated tissues and relaxes spasms (Bown, 1995). The flowers are aphrodisiac, demulcent, emmenagogue, emollient and refrigerant (Chopra et al., 1986). They are used internally in the treatment of excessive and painful menstruation, cystitis, venereal diseases, feverish illnesses, bronchial catarrh, coughs and to promote hair growth (Bown, 1995; Chopra et al., 1986). In Brazil, witches' broom disease of *Hibiscus* was first reported in São Paulo State in plants of *Hibiscus rosa-sinensis* L. The disease was characterized by symptoms of witches' broom, i.e. leaf yellowing and malformation, as well as by short internodes (Vicente et al., 1974).

Later, the disease was observed, in the State of Rio de Janeiro, in plants of the same species; they displayed similar symptoms and premature dropping of flowers (Kitajima et al., 1984; Kitajima, 1994; Davis, 1995). The disease has also been observed in naturally infected plants of *H. rosa-sinensis* in Brazil, Distrito Federal (P. S. T. Brioso, unpublished). In Australia, an unidentified phytoplasma has been reported to be associated with a witches' broom disease of *Hibiscus heterophyllus*, an Australian native species that is also grown commercially (Hiruki, 1987).

Many *Hibiscus* plants are affected by witches' broom disease in Brazil, which is characterized by excessive axillary branching, abnormally small leaves, and deformed flowers, symptoms that are characteristic of diseases attributed to phytoplasmas (Montano et al., 2001). Chaturvedi et al. (2010) reported yellows and little leaf disease on *Hibiscus* in India. The infected plants of *H. rosa-sinensis* showed symptoms of excessive yellowing, vein banding, little leaf, curling, puckering and stunting of the entire plant. Phylogenetic analysis of the *Hibiscus* phytoplasma (FJ939287, .FJ939288) showed close relationship with isolates of aster yellows '*Ca.* P. asteris' (16SrI group) i.e. rose phytoplasma (FJ429364) and aster yellows phytoplasma (AY549311) (Figure 2). Therefore, *Hibiscus* phytoplasma have been identified as isolates of '*Ca.* P. asteris.

3.11. Phytoplasma Diseases in *Bupleurum falcatum*

Bupleurum falcatum (Chai hu plants) is an important tonic herb for the liver and circulatory system of humans and can alleviate hepatitis. Chang et al. (2004) reported aster yellows phytoplasma associated with *Bupleurum falcatum* plant in Canada. Diseased plants showed rosetting, proliferation of auxiliary shoots at the nodes of the stem, witches'- broom, virescence and phyllody symptoms.

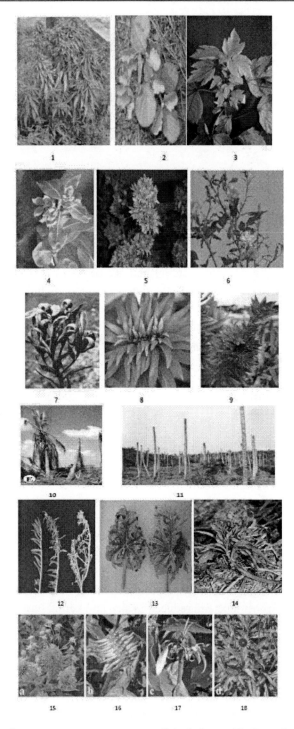

Figure 2. Phytoplasma disease symptoms on some medicinal plants :(1) *Cannabis* witche's –broom, (2) *Achyranthes* yellow leaf, (3) *Hibiscus* yellowing, (4) *Catharanthus roseus* plant showing phyllody symptom, (5) *Catharanthus* little leaf, (6) Discolouration in rose , (7) Flower virescence of lily, (8) Multiple meristem of lily, (9) Witches' broom disease of lily, (10) Advanced yellowing and loss of the entire crown of coconut, (11) Lethal yellowing of coconut, (12) *Portulaca* little leaf, (13) Yellowing, crinkling and tip necrosis of papaya, (14) Reddening and plant stunting of *Bupleurum falcatum,* (15,16,17) *Echinacea* floral malformation, (18) *Echinacea* leaf yellowing.

Alignment of the intergenic spacer region 16S-23S rDNA sequences of *Bupleurum falcatum* phytoplasma (AY394856) showed a high degree of homology with DNA sequences of Florida periwinkle virescence and western aster yellows phytoplasmas in parsley and Chinese aster.

Nucleotides 63, 67, 71, 96 and 197 represented the only sequential differences between these phytoplasmas and the chai hu phytoplasma. The results suggest that the *Bupleurum falcatum* phytoplasma belongs to the aster yellows subgroup I-A.

3.12. Phytoplasma Diseases in *Ocimum basilicum*

Ocimum plants are used in cold, cough fever, sore throat, hoarseness, earache, eye troubles, sinus, congestion, nemonia, respiratory disorder like bronchitis and asthama, acidity, flatulence and indigestion. Basil oil obtained from *Ocimum basilicum* is used in variety of medicine and perfumery. It has antibacterial activity against *Staphyllococcous aureus* and *Mycoplasma tuberculosis in vito* as well as other pathogens including fungi. Arocha et al. (2006 b) reported little leaf disease of *Ocimum basilicum* in Cuba. Diseased plants of *O. basilicum* showed typical little leaf and witches' broom symptoms. BLAST search analysis of 16S rRNA sequence of the *Ocimum* phytoplasma (DQ286577) showed 99% sequence similarities with the members of 16SrI group phytoplasma (Aster yellows; 'Candidatus phytoplasma asteris') affecting watercress (AY665676). Therefore, the *Ocimum* phytoplasma have been identified as an isolate of '*Ca*. P. asteris'.

3.13. Phytoplasma Diseases in *Areca catechu*

The areca nut palm (*Areca catechu* L.) is one of the most important commercial crops. The economic product is the fruit, called areca-nut, which is the most popular chewing substance in South East Asia. It is also used in socio-religious practices, in ayurvedic medicines against leucoderma, leprosy, cough, fits, worms anaemia and obesity. *Areca* tannins from areca nut are found to have inhibitory activities. Purushothama et al. (2007) observed yellow leaf disease of *Areca catechu* in India. The infected *A. catechu* plants showed yellowing of leaves, stems become spongy and friable, conducting strands get destroyed, rotting of the roots, nuts are reduced in size and kernel turns into black.

3.14. Phytoplasma Diseases in *Echinacea purpurea*

Echinacea pupurea is a medicinal plant.It has anti tumour property. *E. purpurea* can cut the chances of catching the cold by more than half and shorten the duration of cold by an average of 1.4 days. *E. purpurea* is popularly believed to be an immune stimulator, stimulating the bodie's non specific immune system and warding off infections. Radisek et al. (2008) identified a phytoplasma from the aster yellows group infecting purple coneflower (*Echinacea purpurea*) in Slovenia. Diseased plants showed symptoms of plant weakness, leaf yellowing, floral malformations, virescence and phyllody. A BLAST search revealed 100% sequence identity of *Echinacea* phytoplasma (EU416172) with poa stunt phytoplasma

(DQ640502) and clover phyllody phytoplasma strain CPh (AF222066) sequences, both belonging to the 16SrI-C subgroup of the aster yellows group (AY). Therefore *Echinacea* phytoplasma has been identified as a member of 16SrI-C subgroup.

3.15. Phytoplasma Diseases in *Tagetes* sp

The whole plant of *Tagetes* is anthelmintic, aromatic, digestive, diuretic, emmenagogue, sedative and stomachic (Bown, 1995). It is used internally in the treatment of indigestion, colic, severe constipation (Bown, 1995), coughs and dysentery. Externally, it is used to treat sores, ulcers, eczema, sore eyes and rheumatism.*Tagetes erecta* was found to be infected by witches'-broom Phytoplasma. Raj et al. (2008 b) worked out Marigold witches'-broom phytoplasma in Lucknow, India. The infected plants showed little leaf, yellowing, shortening of internodes and witches' broom symptoms. They cloned and sequenced the partial 16S ribosomal RNA gene of 1182 nt (Acc. EU516321). The BLAST search analysis of the *Tagetes* phytoplasma (EU516321) 16S rRNA sequence revealed 96% identities with respective sequence of several phytoplasma members of 16SrI group, 'Candidatus Phytoplasma asteris', Aster yellows phytoplasma strain (GQ365729), Mulberry yellow dwarf Phytoplasma (GQ249410), Mulberry dwarf Phytoplasma (FJ844439), Chinese Huanglongbing disease-associated Phytoplasma (EU544303), Bamboo witches'-broom Phytoplasma (FJ853161) and *'Amblyomma variegatum'* phytoplasma (FJ853155).

3.16. Phytoplasma Diseases in *Citrus aurantifolia*

Citrus aurantifolia provide world's most important, tasty and juicy fruit which are the richest source of vitamin C. Essential oil obtained from the leaves and fruit rind of *Citrus aurantifolia* used in medicine and perfumery. Arocha et al. (2006) reported die back disease of citrus in Ethiopia, Africa. Symptoms in *Citrus* include leaf interveinal chlorosis, mosaic or mottling, a reduction in the size and curling of leaves. The 16S rDNA phytoplasma sequences of a citrus phytoplasma (DQ286576) showed highest similarity (98%) with papaya yellow crinkle in Australia (Y10097), a member of the 16SrII group (*Candidatus* Phytoplasma aurantifolia). Alhudaib et al. (2009) detected Lime decline disease in Saudi Arabia. Symptoms of leaf yellowing, motling, little leaf, shortened internodes and necrosis were observed in the infected plants of *Citrus*. BLAST search analysis showed that the 16S rDNA sequences of *Citrus* phytoplasma (EU980537) was 98-99% identical to phytoplasma members of 16SrII, including the cactus witches' broom phytoplasma (EU099565) and the phytoplasma associated with the garden witches' broom disease in Iran in Yazd (DQ233656) and Fars (DQ233655). Therefore *Citrus* phytoplasma is identified as a member of 16SrII group.

3.17. Phytoplasma Diseases in *Datura inoxia*

Datura inoxia is an annual invasive weed grown in India, and used as a medicinal plant for therapeutic purposes. *Datura* leaves and flowers are the source of drug which is used in asthama. Raj et al. (2009) reported little leaf disease of *Datura inoxia* in India. The diseased plants exhibited proliferation of branches with shortened internodes and reduced-size leaves which give rise to the little leaf appearance. BLAST analysis of the 16S rRNA partial sequence of the phytoplasma identified in little leaf-affected *D. inoxia* revealed its highest identity (97%) with those of members of group 16SrVI, '*Candidatus* Phytoplasma trifolii'. Therefore *Datura* little leaf phytoplasma is identified as a member of '*Ca.* Phytoplasma trifolii'-related strain.

3.18. Phytoplasma Diseases in *Portulaca grandiflora*

Portulaca grandiflora commonly known as moss rose purslane, is a popular ornamental plant widely grown in temperate climates because it blooms all summer. *Portulaca* is also used for medicinal purposes since it is rich in vitamins A, B1, and C and has antimicrobial and cytotoxic activity. Ajayakumar et al. (2007) and Samad et al. (2008) reported little leaf disease of *Portulaca grandiflora* in India. Disease plants showed symptoms of a typical bud proliferation, curling, diminishing size of leaves, stunted growth and yellowing of the whole plant. Sequence analysis revealed the *Portulaca* little leaf phytoplasma (EF651786) to be most similar (98%) to Indian brinjal little leaf (EF186820) and '*Candidatus* Phytoplasma trifolii' (AY390261), two 16SrVI group phytoplasmas previously reported from India and Canada, respectively. *Portulaca* little leaf phytoplasma is identified as a member of 16SrVI group.

3.19. Phytoplasma Diseases in *Phoenix dactylifera*

Phoenix dactylifera (date palm) are used medicinally as a detersive (having cleansing power) and astringent in intestinal troubles. As an infusion, decoction, syrup, or paste, dates may be administered for sore throat, colds, bronchial catarrh, and taken to relieve fever and number of other complaints. One traditional belief is that it can counteract alcohol intoxication. The seed powder is also used in some traditional medicines. Alhudaib et al. (2008) reported lethal yellowing disease of *Phoenix dactylifera* in Saudi Arabia. The main symptoms of infected *P. dactylifera* plants were leaf stunting, yellow streaking and a marked reduction in fruit and stalk size, which progresses to no fruit production in the final stages. The 16S rDNA sequences of the phytoplasmas identified in date palm (DQ913090) was 100% identical and showed 98% homology to that of Aster yellows phytoplasma (AF322644) of 16SrI, *Candidatus* Phytoplasma asteris group.

3.20. Phytoplasma Diseases in *Lilium* sp

The bulb of *Lilium* plant is antiinflammatory, diuretic, emmenagogue, emollient and expectorant. They are used to relieve heart diseases, pain in the cardiac region and angina pectoris. They are used to treat coughs, sore throats, palpitations and boils. The flowers are carminative. They are used to strengthen the eye-lid muscles and are commended in the treatment of myopic astigmatism. It is not clear when aster yellows type disease was described for the first time in lilies. Probably the earliest description of aster yellows type disease in lilies was that of Ogilvie and Guterman in 1929 in the United States. They described a disease on *Lilium longiflorum* cultivars characterized by severe leaf chlorosis and malformation, stunted growth and flower distortion. In 1954, Brierley and Smith described symptoms of lily rosette on *L. longiflorum* 'Croft 'and 'Georgia'. The affected plants showed stunting and rosette-like symptoms. Bertaccini and Marani (1982) described flower and leaf malformation and discoloration in lily hybrid 'Pink Perfection' associated with multiple infection of lily mottle (LmoV) and lily symptomless (LSV) viruses and the presence of phytoplasmas in Italy. Similar symptoms were reported by Verhoeven and Horvat (1972) in lilies affected with LSV and *Cucumber mosaic virus* (CMV). Recently, on the basis of PCR amplification of 16SrDNA and RFLP analysis indicated that stunting and flower bud deficiency symptoms in hybrids 'Casablanca' were associated with infection with aster yellows phytoplasma and viruses (Kamińska et al., 1998, 2004a; Bertaccini et al., 2005). In 1997-2000 phytoplasma infection was reported in plants of several lily cultivars with different symptoms (Poncarová-Voracková et al., 1998; Kamińska and Korbin, 2000; Bertaccini et al., 2002). Cortés-Martínez et al. (2007) reported a new phytoplasma associated with a zig-zag line pattern in leaves of *Lilium* sp. in Mexico. Kamińska and Śliwa (2008) reported leaf scorch disease of lily plant in Poland. Symptoms of leaf malformation, necrosis and bud abscission were observed in diseased plants of lily. A BLAST search analysis of the sequence from lily phytoplasm (EF370450) revealed that it was most closely related to the phytoplasmas deposited in GenBank under accession numbers AY598319 and AJ542541, members of '*Ca.* Phytoplasma mali'. The lily phytoplasma is identified as a member of 16SrX group ('*Ca.* Phytoplasma mali').

3.21. Phytoplasma Diseases in *Tamarix chinensis*

The leaves of *Tamarix chinensis* are analgesic, antipyretic, antivinous, carminative, depurative, diuretic, febrifuge. It is also used in Aids, measles and rash surfacing. The wood is used in the treatment of anthrax-like sores. Zhao et al. (2009) reported witche's-broom disease of *Tamarix Chinensis* (Salt cedar tree) in China. Diseased salt cedar plants showed pronounced witches'-broom and little leaf symptoms. Phylogenetic analysis of the *Tamarix* phytoplasma 16S rRNA gene sequence indicated that *Tamarix* phytoplasma belonged to a subclade consisting of several mutually distinct '*Candidatus* Phytoplasma' species including '*Ca.* Phytoplasma prunorum', '*Ca.* Phytoplasma mali', '*Ca.* Phytoplasma pyri', and '*Ca.* Phytoplasma spartii'. Pairwise sequence identity scores calculated from an alignment of near-full-length 16S rRNA genes revealed that SCWB phytoplasma shared 96.6% or less sequence identity with each previously described or proposed '*Ca.* Phytoplasma' species, justifying the recognition of *Tamarix* phytoplasma as a novel taxon, '*Candidatus* Phytoplasma tamaricis'.

3.22. Phytoplasma Diseases in *Grindelia robusta*

Grindelia robusta is a perennial species native to California. The leaves and flowering tops of G. robusta are antiphlogistic, antispasmodic, balsamic, demulcent, expectorant, sedative, stomachic, vascular tonic and a blood purifier. The plant is applied externally as a compress on inflamed or irritated areas of the skin. Used internally, it slows down the heartbeat and reduces the stimulation of the nerve endings in the air passages that causes coughing - it is therefore extremely effective as a calming agent in the treatment of asthma. Bellardi (2009) reported virescence and phyllody disease on *Grindelia robusta* in Italy. The infected *G. robusta* plants showed virescence and phyllody symptoms. Phytoplasmas belonging to subgroup 16SrI-B (*Aster* yellows, *Candidatus* Phytoplasma asteris) were identified in *G. robusta* plants.

3.23. Phytoplasma Diseases in *Medicago sativa*

Medicago sativa is antiscorbutic, aperient, diuretic, oxytocic, haemostatic, nutritive, stimulant and tonic. Its expressed juice is emetic and is also anodyne in the treatment of gravel. The plant is taken internally for debility in convalescence or anaemia, haemorrhage, menopausal complaints, pre-menstrual tension, fibroids etc. A poultice of the heated leaves has been applied to the ear in the treatment of earache. The leaves can be used fresh or dried. The leaves are rich in vitamin K which is used medicinally to encourage the clotting of blood. This plant is valuable in the treatment of jaundice. Lee et al. (1993) reported Loofah witches'broom disease on *Medicago sativa* in Taiwan. Symptoms of witches' broom and little leaf were observed in infected plants of *M. sativa*. BLAST search analysis of 16Sr RNA sequences of *Medicago* phytoplasma (L33764) showed 100% identity with Loofah witches' broom phytoplasma strain China (AF086621) and 99% identity with Loofah withches' broom phytoplasmas strain Taiwn (AF353090, AF248956), member of 16SrVIII group. Therefore *Medicago* phytoplasma is identified as a member of 16SrVIII group.

3.24. Phytoplasma Diseases in *Rehmania glutinosa*

Rehmania glutinosa is used for loss of blood, yin deficiency, lower back pain with kidney deficiency from overwork (it replenishes the vital essence of the kidneys), lumbago, cough, hectic fever, diabetes, urinary incontinence, deafness, uterine bleeding, vertigo, tinnitus, and for regulating menstrual flow. *Rehmannia* has astringent properties that make it useful in stopping bleeding. It helps to protect and support the liver and adrenal glands. Pribylova et al. (2001) detected little leaf disease of *Rehmannia glutinosa* in Czech Republic, Europe. Infected plants of *R. glutinosa* showed severely proliferating shoots, leaves reduced in size with vein clearing and chlorosis, shortened internodes and virescent petals died in advanced stages of the disease.Restriction fragment length polymorphism (RFLP) analysis of phytoplasmal infected *Rehmania glutinosa* indicated the presence of aster yellows related phytoplasmas (16SrI-B). A comparison of the amplified sequence of *Rehmania* phytoplasma with 17 sequences available in the GenBank confirmed the classification of the phytoplasma in the subgroup 16SrI-B.

3.25. Phytoplasma Diseases in *Valerian* sp

Valerian is an effective stress reducer, and has benefit in cases of nervous tension, depression, irritability, hysteria, panic, anxiety, fear, stomach cramping, indigestion due to nervousness, delusions, exhaustion, and, of course, nervous sleeplessness. It also appears to have real benefits in cases of sciatica, multiple sclerosis, epilepsy, shingles, and peripheral neuropathy, including numbness, tingling, muscle weakness, and pain in the extremities. Testing has also revealed that it eases muscle cramping, rheumatic pain, migraines, uterine cramps, intestinal colic, and stress-related heart problems and hypertension. Khadhair et al. (2008) reported phytoplasmal disease on *Valerian* sp. in Canada. Diseased plants of *Valerian* sp. showed typical aster yellows symptoms. Restriction fragment length polymorphism (RFLP) was used to analyse the partial 16Sr DNA sequences (1.2 kb) of *Valerian* phytoplasma DNA samples after restriction with four endonucleases (AluI, HhaI, MseI and RsaI). The restriction patterns of these strains were found to be identical with the RFLP pattern of the AY phytoplasma reference control (AY-27 strain). Based on the RFLP data, the *Valerian* phytoplasma is identified as a member of subgroup A of the AY 16SrI group.

3.26. Phytoplasma Diseases in *Vernonia cineria*

Vernonia cineria is sweet, cold, tonic, stomachic, astringent and cures consumption, asthma, bronchitis and fevers it is one of the best remedies for the treatment of typhoid. In case of female diseases, particularly in Leucorrhoea, its juice is used and it is given to the patients with gud (jaggery). The juice of *Vernonia cineria* is good remedy for intestinal worms also. Brown et al. (2008) observed typical lethal yellowing symptoms in *Vernonia cineria* in Jamaica. Blast analysis determined *Vernonia phytoplasma* sequence (EU057983) to be most similar (99%) to that of CLY phytoplasma in Jamaica (AF49807) and Florida (AF498309), member of 16SrIV group. Therefore *Vernonia* phytoplasma is identified as a member of 16SrIV group.

3.27. Phytoplasma Diseases in *Polygala* sp

Livingston et al. (2006) reported 16SrII group in *Polygala mascatense* plant associated with *Polygala* witche's-broom phytoplasma in Oman. Arocha et al. (2008) observed phyllody disease of *Polygala paniculata* in Cuba. The infected plants of *Polygala* sp. showed typical witches' broom and phyllody symptoms. BLAST search analysis of 16Sr RNA sequence of *Polygala* phytoplasma (AY787140) showed 99% identity with Papaya bunchy top phytoplasma (DQ868533), *Euphorbia heterophylla* phytoplasma (DQ286952), *Malvastrum* phytoplasma (DQ286951) and *Crotolaria* phytoplasma (GU113154), member of 16SrII group. Therefore, *Polygala* phytoplasma is identified as a member of 16SrII group.

Table 1. Worldwide Distribution of Phytoplasma on Medicinal plants

S. No.	Medicinal Plants Host Species	Diseases	Country (s) of origin	References
1.	*Medicago sativa* (Fabaceae)	Loofah, witches' broom (LfWB)	Taiwan	Lee et al. (1993)
2.	*Ocimum basilicum* (Lamiaceae)	Basil little leaf	Cuba	Arocha et al. (2006b)
3.	*Cannabis sativa* (Cannabinaceae)	Witches' broom	India	Raj et al. (2008a); Mall. (2009)
4.	*Achyranthes aspera* (Amaranthaceae)	Yellows disease	India	Raj et al.(2008c)
5.	*Catharanthus roseus* (Apocynaceae)	Periwinkle little leaf Maryland aster yellows American aster yellows Periwinkle virescence Yellows Periwinkle witches broom Yellows disease of periwinkle *Vinca* proliferation Phyllody disease of periwinkle Little leaf disease of periwinkle Virescence and phyllody Periwinkle phyllody Stunting of periwinkle Little leaf disease of periwinkle Yellows and phyllody Mexican periwinkle virescence Virescence, witches' broom and proliferation Little leaf and phyllody disease	Connecticut USA Maryland USA Florida USA California USA Brazil USA Japan Romania Jamaica India USA China Italy USA Russia Mexico Colombia India	Davis et al. (1990) Lee and Davis (1992) Seemüller et al. (1994) Lee et al. (1991); Shaw et al. (1991) Kitajima and Costa (1979) Mc Coy and Thomas (1980) Okuda (1977) Ploaie et al. (1977) Dabek (1982) Rao et al. (1983) Eastman et al. (1984) Chen et al. (1984) Grimaldi and Grasso (1988) Davis et al. (1990) Shishlova and Andreeva (1979) Gundersen et al. (1994) Duduk et al. (2008) Chaturvedi et al. (2009b)

Table 1. Worldwide Distribution of Phytoplasma on Medicinal plants (Continued)

S. No.	Medicinal Plants Host Species	Diseases	Country (s) of origin	References
6.	*Portulaca grandiflora* (Portulacaceae)	Little leaf disease	India	Ajayakumar et al. (2007); Samad et al. (2008)
7.	*Rosa alba* (Rosaceae)	Little leaf disease	India	Chaturvedi et al. (2009a)
8.	*Hibiscus rosa-sinensis* (Malvaceae)	*Hibiscus* witches' broom	Brazil	Montano et al. (2001)
		Yellows and little leaf disease	India	Chaturvedi et al. (2010)
9.	*Ziziphus jujuba* (Rhamnaceae)	Jujuba witches' broom disease-DL	China	Wei et al. (2007); Fan et al. (2008)
		Witches' broom	Japan	Kusunoki et al. (2002)
		little leaves and witches' broom	India	Khan et al. (2008)
		Jujube witches' broom disease	South Korea	Han and Cha (2002)
10.	*Cocos nucifera* (Arecaceae)	Coconut lethal yellowing	Jamaica	Myrie et al.(2007)
		Coconut yellow decline	Malaysia	Nejat et al. (2009)
		Kerala wilt disease	India	Sharmila (2004); Edwin (2007)
		Coconut lethal yellowing	Dominican Republic, Europe	Martinez et al. (2008)
11.	*Santalum album* (Santalaceae)	Spike disease	India	Khan et al. (2006b)
12.	*Carica papaya* (Caricaceae)	Papaya bunchy top	Cuba	Arocha et al. (2003, 2007, 2009)
		Die back disease	Cuba	Arocha et al. (2006a)
		Papaya bunchy top	Ethiopia, Africa	Arocha et al.(2008)
			Australia	White et al. (1998)
		Dieback, yellow crinkle and mosaic		
13.	*Citrus aurantifolia* (Rutaceae)	Die back disease Lime decline disease	East Shewa, Africa Saudi Arabia	Arocha et al. (2006) Alhudaib et al. (2009)
14.	*Echinacea purpurea* (Asteraceae)	Yellowing, virescence and phyllody Phyllody	Slovenia, Europe Maryland USA	Radisek et al. (2009) Lee et al. (2008)

Table 1. Worldwide Distribution of Phytoplasma on Medicinal Plants (Continued)

S. No.	Medicinal Plants Host Species	Diseases	Country (s) of origin	References
15.	*Withania somnifera* (Solanaceae)	Witches' broom Little leaf	India India	Samad et al. (2006a) Khan et al. (2006)
16.	*Rehmania glutinosa* (Scrophulariaceae)	Little leaf	Czech Republic, Europe	Pribylova et al. (2001)
17.	*Phoneix dactylifera* (Arecaceae)	Lethal yellowing	Saudi Arabia	Alhudaib et al. (2008)
18.	*Tamarix chinensis* (Tamaricaceae)	Witches' broom disease	China	Zhao et al., 2009
19.	*Areca catechu* (Arecaceae)	Yellow leaf disease	India	Purushothama et al. (2007)
20.	*Polygala mascatense* (Polygalaceae)	Polygala Witches' broom	Oman	Livingston et al. (2006)
21.	*Valerian* sp. (Valerianaceae)	Aster yellows disease	Canada	Khadhair et al. (2008)
22.	*Bupleurum falcatum* (Apiaceae)	virescence and Witches' broom	Canada	Chang et al. (2004)
23.	*Datura inoxia* (Solanaceae)	Little leaf	India	Raj et al. (2009)
24.	*Tagetes erecta* (Asteraceae)	Witches' broom	India	Raj et al. (2008b)
25.	*Grindelia robusta* (Asteraceae)	virescence and phyllody	Italy	Bellardi (2009)
26.	*Lilium* sp. (Liliaceae)	Zig-Zag line pattern in leaves Leaf scorch or leaf burn	Mexico Poland	Cortés-Martínez et al. (2007) Kamińska and Śliwa (2008b)
27.	*Vernonia cinerea* (Asteraceae)	Lethal Yellowing disease	Jamaica	Brown et al. (2008)

4. Phytoplasma Distribution in Medicinal Plants

Phytoplasma cause diseases in several medicinal plants and resulted in serious threat as a source of alternative natural host for the spread of these pathogens to other economically important plant species and thereby chances of causing severe yield and/or quality losses are maximum. So far, 20 phytoplasmas belonging to 14 groups have been identified on different medicinal plants (Tables 1 and 2).

Table 2. Symptoms of Phytoplasma Diseases Occurring on Medicinal Plants

S. No.	Medicinal Plants Host Species	Diseases	Symptoms	References
1.	*Medicago sativa* (Fabaceae)	Loofah witches' broom (LfWB)	Witches' broom	Lee et al. (1993)
2.	*Ocimum basilicum* (Lamiaceae)	Basil little leaf	Little leaf	Arocha et al. (2006b)
3.	*Cannabis sativa* (Cannabinaceae)	Witches' broom disease	Excessive green, Tiny,narrow shortened leaves,Shortening of internodes,Little leaf and latly witches' broom	Raj et al. (2008a) Mall (2009)
4.	*Achyranthes aspera* (Amaranthaceae)	Yellowing disease	yellowing	Raj et al. (2008c)
5.	*Carica papaya* (Caricaceae)	Papaya bunchy top	Mosaic, yellow, crinkle	Arocha et al. (2003)
		Papaya bunchy top	Stunting, shortening of internodes, leaf chlorosis, deformation, necrosis, crinkling and yellowing	Arocha et al. (2007, 2009)
		Die back disease	Bright yellowing of upper young leaves, mosaic, crinkling leaf tip Necrosis	Arocha et al. (2006a; 2008)
		Dieback, yellow crinkle and mosaic	Dieback, yellow crinkle and mosaic	White et al. (1998)
6.	*Citrus aurantifolia* (Rutaceae)	Die back disease	Leaf interveinal Chlorosis, mosaic, mottling , mottling, reduction in size, curling of leaves, Twig drying and dieback	Arocha et al. (2006)
		Lime decline disease	Leaf yellowing, motling, little leaf and yellowing of the foliage. Internodes get shorter and branches decline until they become completely dried and necroyic in the final stage, with no leaves and no fruit production	Alhudaib et al. (2009)
7.	*Portulaca grandiflora* (Portulacaceae)	Little leaf disease Little leaf disease	Bud proliferation, Downward curling diminishing size of leaves, stunted growth	Ajayakumar et al. (2007) Samad et al. (2008)
8.	*Echinacea purpurea* (Asteraceae)	Yellowing, virescence and phyllody phyllody	Plant weakness, leaf yellowing, floral malformation, virescence phyllody	Radisek et al. (2009) Lee et al. (2008)

Table 2. Symptoms of Phytoplasma Diseases Occurring on Medicinal Plants (Continued)

S. No.	Medicinal Plants Host Species	Diseases	Symptoms	References
9.	*Withania somnifera* (Solanaceae)	Witches' broom	Phyllody, little leaf, dense clusters of highly proliferating branches, shortened internodes	Samad et al. (2006)
		Little leaf	Little leaf	Khan et al. (2006a)
10.	*Ziziphus jujuba* (Rhamnaceae)	Jujuba witches' broom disease-DL	Witches' broom	Wei et al.(2007); Fan et al. (2008)
		Witches' broom	Witches' broom, Severe decline	Kusunoki et al. (2002)
		little leaves and witches' broom	severe rosetting, green little leaves and witches' broom	Khan et al. (2008)
		Jujube witches' broom disease	witches' broom	Han and Cha (2002)
11.	*Cocos nucifera* (Arecaceae)	Coconut lethal yellowing	lethal yellowing	Myrie et al. (2007)
		Coconut yellow decline		
		Kerala wilt disease	yellow decline	Nejat et al. (2009)
		Coconut lethal yellowing	discolouration of leaves and generalized decline of palm growth, lethal yellowing and wilting	Sharmila (2004); Edwin (2007)
			lethal yellowing	Martinez et al. (2008)
12.	*Santalum album* (Santalaceae)	Spike disease	Witches' broom small, narrow leaves, pale green branches	Khan et al. (2006b)
13.	*Phoneix dactylifera* (Arecaceae)	Lethal yellowing	Leaf stunting, yellow steaking, mask reduction in fruit and stalk size	Alhudaib et al. (2008)
14.	*Tamarix chinensis* (Tamaricaceae)	Witches' broom disease	Witches' broom	Zhao et al. (2009)
15.	*Areca catechu* (Arecaceae)	Yellow leaf disease	Yellowing of leaves in inner whorl	Purushothama et al. (2007)
16.	*Polygala mascatense* (Polygalaceae)	Polygala Witches' broom	Witches' broom	Livingston et al. (2006)
17.	*Rehmania glutinosa* (Scrophulariaceae)	Little leaf and chlorosis	Proliferating shoots, clearing, chlorosis, shortened internodes, virescent petals	Pribylova et al. (2001)

No.	Plant	Disease name	Symptoms	Reference
18.	*Catharanthus roseus* (Apocynaceae)	Periwinkle little leaf	Little leaf	Davis et al. (1990)
		Maryland aster yellows in periwinke	Yellowing	Lee and Davis (1992)
		American aster yellows in periwinkle	Yellowing	Seemüller et al. (1994)
		Periwinkle virescence	Virescence	Lee et al. (1991);Shaw et al. (1991)
		Mexican periwinkle virescence	Virescence	Gundersen et al. (1994)
		Periwinkle yellows	Yellowing	Kitajima and Costa (1979)
		Periwinkle witches' broom	Yellowing	Mc Coy. and Thomas (1980)
		Yellows disease of periwinkle	Virescence,phyllody,proliferation and dwarfing Yellowing	Okuda (1977)
		Vinca proliferation	proliferation	Ploaie et al. (1977)
		Phyllody disease of periwinkle	Phyllody	Dabek (1982)
		Little leaf disease of periwinkle Virescence and phyllody	Little leaf and phyllody	Rao et al. (1983)
			Virescence, phyllody, shortening of internodes, branching of leaves with Phyllody	Eastman et al. (1984)
		Periwinkle phyllody		Chen et al. (1984)
		Periwinkle stunting	Small pale green leaves, shortened internodes and stunting	Grimaldi and Grasso (1988)
		Little leaf disease of periwinkle	Little leaf	Davis et al. (1990)
			Yellows and phyllody	
			Little leaf	
		Periwinkle yellow and phyllody	Yellows and phyllody	Shishlova and Andreeva (1979)
		Litle leaf and phyllody disease	Litle leaf and phyllody	Chaturvedi et al. (2009b)
19.	*Rosa alba* (Rosaceae) *Rosa sp.* (Rosaceae)	Little leaf disease	Little leaf disease	Chaturvedi et al. (2009a)
		Dieback, rose rosette,witches' broom and bud proliferation	Dieback, rose rosette, witches' broom and bud proliferation	Kamińska and Sliwa (2004)

Table 2. Symptoms of Phytoplasma Diseases Occurring on Medicinal Plants (Continued)

S. No.	Medicinal Plants Host Species	Diseases	Symptoms	References
20.	*Hibiscus rosa-sinensis* (Malvaceae)	*Hibiscus* witches' broom Yellows and little leaf disease	Witches' broom Leaf yellowing Yellowing and little leaf	Montano et al. (2001) Chaturvedi et al. (2010)
21.	Valerian sp. (Valerianaceae)	Aster yellows disease	typical aster yellows symptoms	Khadhair et al. (2008)
22.	*Bupleurum falcatum* (Apiaceae)	virescence and witches'- brooms	reddish-yellow discoloration, followed by stunting, virescence and witches' brooms	Chang et al. (2004)
23.	*Datura inoxia* (Solanaceae)	Little leaf	proliferation of branches with shortened internodes and little leaf	Raj et al. (2009)
24.	*Tagetes erecta* (Asteraceae)	Witches' broom	Witches' broom	Raj et al. (2008b)
25.	*Grindelia robusta* (Asteraceae)	virescence and phyllody	virescence and phyllody	Bellardi (2009)
26.	*Lilium* sp. (Liliaceae)	*Lilium* virescence Zig-Zag line pattern in leaves of *Lilium* Leaf scorch or leaf burn of *Lilium*	Virescence and alteration of reproductive structure Zig-zag lines between midribs of leaves, dwarfism Leaf malformation and necrosis and flower bud abscission	Bertaccini and Marani (1982) Cortés-Martínez et al. (2007) Kamínska and Śliwa (2008b)
27.	*Vernonia cinerea* (Asteraceae)	Lethal Yellowing disease	Lethal yellowing	Brown et al. (2008)

Table 3. Classification of Phytoplasmas Detected on Medicinal Plants Worldwide

S. No.	Medicinal Plants Host Species	Strain	Phytoplasma Group	Accession Nos. (16Sr)/ (rp)	Primes used	References
1.	*Medicago sativa* (Fabaceae)	Loofah witches' broom (LfWB),(ArAWB),Alfalfa witches' broom	16SrVIII,16SrVI I,16SrI	L33764/L27027	P1/P7andR16F2n/R16R 2	Lee et al. (1993)
2.	*Ocimum basilicum* (Lamiaceae)	'*Ca*. P. asteris'	16SrI	--	--	Arocha et al. (2006b)
3.	*Achyranthes aspera* (Amaranthaceae)	'*Ca*. P. asteris'	16SrI	EU573926	P1/P6 and R16F2n/R16R2	Raj et al. (2008c)
4.	*Catharanthus roseus* (Apocynaceae)	Periwinkle little leaf (CN1)	16SrI	--	P1/P6 and R16F2n/R16R2	Davis et al. (1990)
		Maryland aster yellows (AY1) American aster yellows (AAY)	16SrI	L33767	--	Lee and Davis (1992)
		Periwinkle virescence (VR, BLTVA)	16SrI	X68373	--	Semüller et al. (1994)
		Mexican periwinkle virescence (MPV) '*Ca*. P. asteris'	16SrVI	--	--	Lee et al. (1991); Shaw et al. (1991)
			16SrXIII 16SrI	EU694109	P1/P6 and R16F2n/R16R2	Gundersen et al. (1994) Chaturvedi et al. (2009b)
5.	*Rosa canina* (Rosaceae)	--	16SrX,16SrV	--	P1/P6 and R16F2n/R16R2	Jarausch et al. (2001)
	Rosa alba (Rosaceae)	'*Ca*. P. asteris'	16SrI	FJ429364	P1/P6 and R16F2n/R16R2	Chaturvedi et al. (2009a)
	Rosa sp.(Rosaceae)	--	16SrI,16SrX-A	--	--	Kaminska et al. (2004a)
6.	*Echinacea purpurea* (Asteraceae)	'*Ca*. P. asteris'	16SrI	--	P1/P7 and R16F2n/R16R2	Lee et al. (2008)
		'*Ca*. P. asteris'	16SrI	EU416172	P1/P7, Fu5/Ru3 and R16F2n/R16R2	Radisek et al. (2009)

Table 3. Classification of Phytoplasmas Detected on Medicinal Plants Worldwide (Continued)

S. No.	Medicinal Plants Host Species	Strain	Phytoplasma Group	Accession Nos. (16Sr)/ (rp)	Primes used	References
7.	*Hibiscus rosa-sinensis* (Malvaceae)	'Ca. P. brasiliense'	16SrXV	AF147708	P1/P4 and P4/P7	Montano et al. (2001)
		'Ca. P. asteris' (GKP-1)	16SrI	FJ939287	P1/P4 and P4/P7	Chaturvedi et al. (2010)
		'Ca. P. asteris' (GKP-2)	16SrI	FJ939288	P1/P4 and P4/P7	Chaturvedi et al. (2010)
8.	*Ziziphus jujba* (Rhamnaceae)	'Ca. P. ziziphi' -related strain	16SrV	EF661852	P1/P7	Wei et al. (2007)
		'Ca. P. ziziphae'	16Sr V	--	--	Fan et al. (2008)
		--	16Sr V	--	--	Kusunoki et al. (2002)
		'Ca. P. ziziphi'	16SrV	EU366162	P1/P6 and	Khan et al. (2008); Deng & Hiruki (1991); Gundersen & Lee (1996)
		'Ca. P. ziziphi'	16SrV	AY072722	R16F2n/R16R2n --	Han and Cha (2002)
9.	*Santalum album* (Santalaceae)	'Ca. P. asteris'-related strains	16SrI	DQ0932357	P1/P7 and R16mF2/R16mR1	Khan et al. (2004), (2006b)
10.	*Carica Papaya* (Caricaceae)	--	16SrXVII	AY725234	PBTF1/PBTR1	Arocha et al. (2003)
		'Ca. P. aurantifolia'	16SrII	DQ285659	P1/P7 , R16F2n/R16R2 and PBTF1/PBTR1	Arocha et al. (2006a); Davis et al (1998)
		'Ca. P. aurantifolia'	16SrII	--	P1/P7 and R16F2n/R16R2	Arocha et al. (2007) Gundersen and Lee (1996);
		'Ca. P. aurantifolia'	16SrII	--	R16mF2/R1 and fU5/rU3	Lorenz et al. (1995); Arocha et al. (2009)
11.	*Portulaca grandiflora* (Portulacaceae)	--	--	--	P1/P6 and R16F2n/R16R2	Deng and Hiruki (1991);Lee et al.(1993); Ajaya kumar et al.(2007)
		--	16SrVI	EF651786	P1/P6 and R16F2n/R16R2	Samad et al.(2008)

No.	Plant species (Family)	Phytoplasma name	16Sr group	GenBank accession	Primers	Reference
12.	*Polygala mascatense* (Polygalaceae)	Polygala witches' broom (PWB)	16SrII	--	--	Livingston et al. (2006)
	Polygala paniculata (Polygalaceae)	--	16SrII	AY787140	--	Arocha et al. (2008)
13.	*Cannabis sativa* (Cannabinaceae)	'*Ca.* P. asteris'	16SrI	EU439257	P1/P6 and R16F2n/R16R2	Raj et al. (2008a)
		'*Ca.* P. asteris'	16SrI	FJ227937	P1/P6 and R16F2n/R16R2	Mall (2009)
14.	*Withania somnifera* (Solanaceae)	--	16SrVI	--	P1/P6 and R16F2n/R16R2	Samad et al. (2006a)
15.	*Citrus aurantifolia* (Rutaceae)	--	16SrII	DQ286576	P1/P7 and R16F2n/R16R2	Arocha et al. (2006)
		'*Ca.* P. aurantifolia'	16SrII	EU980537	R16F2n/R16R2	Alhudaib et al. (2009)
16.	*Rehmania glutinosa* (Scrophulariaceae)	'*Ca.* P. asteris'	16SrI	--	R16F2n/R16R2	Pribylova et al. (2001)
17.	*Phoenix dactylofera* (Arecaceae)	--	16SrI	DQ913090	P1/P7 and R16F2n/R16R2	Alhudaib et al. (2008)
18.	*Tamarix chinensis* (Tamaricaceae)	'*Ca.* P. tamaricis'	16SrXXX	--	--	Zhao et al. (2009)
19.	*Areca catechu* (Arecaceae)	--	--	--	P1/P7 and R16F2n/R16R2	Purushothama et al. (2007)
20.	*Cocos nucifera* (Arecaceae)	'*Ca.* P. cynodontis'	16SrXIV	EU328159	P1/P7 and R16F2/R16R2 or fU5/rU3	Nejat et al. (2009)
		--	16SrIV	AY158660	P4/P7	Sharmila (2004); Edwin (2007
					P1/P7 and	Martinez et al. (2008)
		--	16SrIV	DQ631639	LY16Sf/LY16Sr	
21.	*Valerian* sp. (Valerianaceae)	'*Ca.* P. asteris'	16SrI	--	P1 / P7 , R16F2n / R2 and P3 / P7	Khadhair et al. (2008)
22.	*Bupleurum falcatum* (Apiaceae)	--	16SrI	AY394856	R16F2 /R16R2	Chang et al. (2004)
23.	*Datura inoxia* (Solanaceae)	'*Ca.* P.trifolii'	16SrVI	EU573925	P1/P6 and R16F2n/R16R2	Deng & Hiruki (1991); Gundersen & Lee (1996); Raj et al. (2009)

Table 3. Classification of Phytoplasmas Detected on Medicinal Plants Worldwide (Continued)

S. No.	Medicinal Plants Host Species	Strain	Phytoplasma Group	Accession Nos. (16SrI)/ (rp)	Primes used	References
24.	*Tagetes erecta* (Asteraceae)	'*Ca. P.* asteris'	16SrI	EU516321	--	Raj et al. (2008b)
25.	*Grindelia robusta* (Asteraceae)	'*Ca. P.* asteris'	16SrI	--	--	Bellardi (2009)
26.	*Lilum* sp. (Liliaceae)	--	16SrI and or16SrX	--	--	Kaminska et al.(2004a)
		--	16SrI	AY839617	R16F2n/R2	Bertaccini et al.(2005)
		'*Ca. P.* asteris'	--	--	--	Cortés-Martínez et al.(2007)
		--	16SrXII	AY169309	P1/P6 and R16F1/R1-S P1/P7, fA/rA, R16F2n/R16R2, R16(I)F1/R16(I)R1 and fAT/rAS	Deng and Hiruki (1991); Lee et al.(1998); Chung (2008) Kaminska and Śliwa (2008b)
		'*Ca* P. mali'	16SrX	EF370450		
27.	*Vernonia cinerea* (Asteraceae)	--	16Sr IV	EU057983	P1/P7 and LY16Sf/LY16-23Sr	Deng and Hiruki (1991); Smart et al. (1996); Brown et al. (2008)

Table 4. Sequence similarity (in %) of 16S rRNA gene of different phytoplasmas identified in medicinal plants worldwide based on the Genomatix DiAlign Program

S. No.	Phytoplasmas	Acc. No.	2	3	4	5	6	7	8	9	10	11	12	13	14	15	16	17	18	19	20	21	22	23	24	25	26	27	28	29	30	31	32	33	34	35
1	Echinacea	EU016172	88	89	86	90	83	86	98	86	96	89	91	88	89	85	79	99	88	94	98	98	98	93	7	89	95	99	97	88	98	86	98	87	84	98	87
2	Zizphus JWB-KO	AY072722		99	87	80	87	84	87	91	85	96	89	92	91	84	77	87	84	88	88	88	87	9	87	87	88	85	93	88	85	87	94	83	88	92
3	Zizphus JWB	AY197661			87	81	87	85	87	91	88	97	81	93	93	82	77	88	85	89	89	80	88	9	87	87	89	86	93	89	85	88	94	82	89	93
4	Hibiscus Brazil	AF147708				78	82	96	85	84	83	85	93	88	88	93	77	85	86	85	86	86	85	7	95	85	85	85	85	86	93	84	85	92	86	84
5	Phoenix	DQ913090					85	87	98	80	90	88	83	83	82	76	88	90	94	97	97	97	96	14	86	96	99	98	85	97	84	90	85	78	99	85
6	Pernonia	EU057983						86	87	89	84	93	79	93	92	80	88	85	86	86	88	88	85	16	87	85	88	81	92	87	86	85	91	81	88	89
7	Ingawe Pratnagar	EU362651							85	91	83	85	85	86	92	85	24	86	85	87	87	87	85	10	98	85	87	97	85	87	97	87	83	95	85	82
8	Cannabis GKP	FJ227937								84	96	87	91	89	89	84	35	98	92	98	98	98	98	31	98	94	98	98	86	98	85	98	86	84	98	85
9	Medicago	L33764									85	90	82	90	90	82	76	84	83	85	85	86	84	6	85	83	83	83	89	85	84	83	90	82	85	89
10	Carthaomus Maryland	L33767										86	89	87	87	83	79	95	91	96	96	96	96	7	86	93	96	94	85	96	84	93	85	82	95	82
11	Zizphus Lucknow	EU366161											82	94	94	85	38	89	85	88	88	88	87	7	85	88	88	87	91	96	86	88	93	82	88	91
12	Carica Cuba	AY725234												83	83	80	74	92	96	92	92	91	91	5	88	88	92	88	85	92	84	92	85	80	91	81
13	Cocos LYF-C5	AF498308													99	86	79	88	87	87	89	89	88	5	88	87	89	85	94	88	87	88	92	86	89	90
14	Cocos LYF-C3	AF498309														86	78	89	87	87	89	89	88	5	88	86	89	85	94	88	86	88	92	86	89	90
15	Carica Ethiopia	DQ385659															72	85	83	83	84	84	84	8	95	84	85	83	84	84	95	84	81	98	85	82
16	Lilium Siberia	EF370450																74	34	34	53	53	52	16	51	47	47	71	52	41	51	69	51	71	47	47
17	Lilium Czech Republic	AY339617																	94	94	99	98	98	24	89	95	99	98	88	98	86	99	87	84	99	86
18	Lilium Ph-lily	AY169309																		99	94	94	93	5	87	90	94	94	84	93	86	94	84	83	93	83
19	Rosa	FJ439364																			99	99	98	5	87	95	99	99	87	99	86	99	87	84	99	86
20	Carthaomus Lucknow	DQ097396																				98	98	5	89	96	99	99	87	99	86	99	87	84	99	86
21	Hibiscus GKP1	FJ939287																					98	5	88	95	99	98	87	99	86	98	87	85	99	86
22	Hibiscus GKP2	FJ939288																						5	87	95	98	97	87	98	86	98	86	85	98	85
23	Cocos Kerala	AY158660																							5	5	5	10	5	5	5	7	4	6	5	4
24	Citrus Al-Hassan	EU980537																								86	88	88	87	88	96	88	85	95	88	84
25	Ingawe Lucknow	EU516321																									96	95	85	93	84	96	85	84	95	83

Table 4. Sequence similarity (in %) of 16S rRNA gene of different phytoplasmas identified in medicinal plants worldwide based on the Genomatix DiAlign Program (Continued)

#	Name	Accession									
26	Achyranthe s	EU573926	98		96	86	99	87	85	99	86
27	Catharanth us AAY	X68373		87	99	86	99	87	83	98	84
28	Cocos Malaysia	EU358159			87	86	87	92	84	87	91
29	Catharanth us GKP	EU604109			87	96	86	99	87	84	96	84
30	Polygala	AY787140				86		85	95	85	85
31	Catharanth us China	EU375834						87	84	99	86
32	Portulaca	EF651786							81	86	95
33	Citrus Ethiopia	DQ286576								85	81
34	Cannabis Lucknow	EU439257									85
35	Datura	EU573925									

5. Phytoplasma Detection and Identification

Most of the phytoplasmas infecting medicinal plants were characterized on the basis of symptoms, DAPI staining, electron microscopy, PCR/RFLP analysis and phylogenetic relatedness.

5.1. Symptoms

Plants infected by phytoplasmas exhibit variety of symptoms that suggests profound disturbances in the normal balance of growth regulators (Lee and Davis, 1992). The most characteristic symptoms caused by phytoplasmas in medicinal plants are virescence/phyllody (development of green leaf like structures instead of flowers), sterility of flowers, proliferation of axillary buds resulting in witches broom behaviour, abnormal internodes elongation and generalized stunting, yellows, little leaf, phloem necrosis, chlorosis, crinkling, shoot proliferation, leaf burn and death of the plant (McCoy et al., 1989). Samad et al. (2006) observed typical disease symptoms on *Withania somnifera* which include phyllody, little leaf, dense clusters of highly proliferating branches with shortened internodes, and witches'-broom. Khan et al. (2006 b) reported witches'-broom symptoms, consisting of small, narrow leaves which turn pale-green or yellow on branches on *Santalum album*. Favali et al. (2008) reported the most characteristic symptoms on *C. roseus* plants are yellowing of the leaves, virescence, phyllody and proliferation, witches' broom induced by the premature development of axillary buds, inhibition of root growth. A different range of symptoms produced by phytoplasma on different medicinal plant species are listed in Table 2.

Phytoplasma disease symptoms on different medicinal plants:- *Cannabis* witches' – broom, *Achyranthes* yellow leaf, *Hibiscus* yellowing, *Catharanthus roseus* plant showing phyllody symptom, *Catharanthus* little leaf, discolouration in rose , flower virescence of lily, multiple meristem of lily, witches' broom disease of lily, advanced yellowing and loss of the entire crown of coconut, lethal yellowing of coconut, *Portulaca* little leaf, yellowing, crinkling and tip necrosis of papaya, reddening and plant stunting of *Bupleurum falcatum*, Echinacea floral malformation and leaf yellowing are shown in Figure 2.

5.2. Microscopy and Staining Technique

In earlier days the phytoplasmas were detected on the basis of DAPI staining and electron microscopy observations. Microscopic methods including TEM and light microscopy have been used to detect phytoplasmas, but most sensitive is the DAPI (DNA-specific-6-diaminido-2-phenylindole) fluorescence microscopy technique. Shin and La (1984) use Dienes' stain and Hiruki and Rocha (1986) use DAPI stain in the detection of mycoplasma like organisms-associated diseases of *C. roseus* plant. Detection of phytoplasma by electron microscopy was carried out *C. roseus* (Cousin and Abadie, 1982). Pribylova et al. (2001) detected numerous polymorphic bodies in phloem tissue of leaf midribs and petioles of *Rehmannia glutinosa* plant through electron microscopy examination in Czech Republic, Europe. Recently bio-imaging methods requiring sensitive, specific and non-toxic fluorescent dyes and the use of confocal or multiphoton microscopy have allowed identification of phytoplasmas in living tissues. Among these, microscopic methods do not attain pathogen identification, and all of them are not always sufficiently sensitive to detect phytoplasma infections in low-titer hosts.

5.3. PCR/RFLP Assays and Phylogenetic Relationships

The identification of phytoplasmas in diseased plants relied longtime on symptomatology; however some times absence of peculiar symptoms in infected plants occurs and makes it difficult to clearly identify all phytoplasma-associated diseases. For this purpose identification methodology is required for quick and reliable detection of phytoplasmas at early infection stages.

Molecular detection methods include dot and Southern blot hybridization and PCR technology. Dot and Southern blot hybridization assays were used in phytoplasma detection for some years; however, both are currently completely replaced by PCR assays. PCR assays using universal primers are most useful for preliminary detection of phytoplasma diseases. Several universal and many phytoplasma group-specific primers have been designed for detection of phytoplasmas (Clark and Davies, 1984; Deng and Hiruki, 1991; Lee et al., 1993, 1995, 2000; Lorenz et al., 1995; Smart et al., 1996; Gundersen and Lee, 1996; Khadhair et al., 1998; Berges et al., 2000). Nested PCR assay, designed to increase both sensitivity and specificity, was performed by using a group-specific primers. Therefore, nested-PCR is capable of detection of dual or multiple phytoplasmas present in the infected tissues in case of mixed infection (Lee et al., 1994, 1995). Application of PCR to the detection of phytoplasma-associated with medicinl plant diseases has greatly facilitated the identification of a wide array of phytoplasmas in medicinal plants (Marcone and Rao, 2008; Favali et al., 2008; Raj et al., 2008 a, b). Nested-PCR assay increases both sensitivity and specificity and is a valuable technique in the amplification of phytoplasmas from samples in which unusually low titers are present, or substantial inhibitors that may interfere with the PCR efficacy are present (Marwitz, 1990; Lee et al., 1995; Heinrich et al., 2001). For amplification of phytoplasma ribosomal DNA (rDNA) by PCR assays, the universal phytoplasma primer pairs P1/P7, P4/P7 (Schneider et al., 1995), and P1/P6 (Deng and Hiruki, 1991) are among those most used to amplify 16S ribosomal region of phytoplasmas plus spacer region; among primers amplifying only 16S ribosomal region the R16F2n/R16R2 (Gundersen and Lee, 1996) are those most employed since RFLP profiles necessary for preliminary phytoplasma identification are widely available (Lee et al., 1995, 1998). PCR amplified products could also be sequenced directly from amplicons or cloned and finally submitted to GenBank. These sequences are used to determine the genetic relatedness of the phytoplasmas. The taxonomic and molecular classification of phytoplasmas detected on medicinal plants throughout the world is listed in Table 3.

6. Phytoplasma Transmission

Phytoplasma transmission occurs through sap-sucking insect vectors mainly belonging to the family Cicadellidea (leafhoppers), Fulgoridea (planthoppers). Phytoplasmas can also be spread via vegetative propagation such as the grafting of a piece of infected plant onto a healthy plant, cutting, micropropagation or other ways to propagate plant germplasm avoiding sexual reproduction are also propagating the phytoplasmas.

A number of insect vectors were responsible for transmission of phytoplasma on medicinal plants (Arocha et al., 2005; Favali et al., 2008; Harrison and Oropeza, 2008). Phytoplasma disease that occurs on *C. roseus* plants in nature is periwinkle yellows, transmitted by the leafhopper *Macrosteles quadripunctulatus* (Bosco et al., 1997). Natural infections of perinkle are reported in gardens, in different Italin regions.The artificial transmission of phytoplasma to periwinkle by insects, was largely used to study the transmission characteristics and the spread of these pathogens (Carraro et al., 1991). Artificial transmission of phytoplasmas, from host plants to *C. roseus* and back to host plants, can be obtained by grafting and by dodder (Marwitz et al., 1974; Carraro et al., 1988, 1991, 1992, 2004). In particular, it has been also demonstrated that dodder transmits different phytoplasmas to periwinkle with different efficiency, may be due to their pathogenic effects on the vector plant (Carraro et al., 1991; Musetti et al., 1992).

Survey of insect populations in Florida established that *Myndus crudus* was by far the most abundant potential vector on coconut palms and the populations of this planthopper species were as much as 40 time higher in areas of high Coconut Lethal yellowing incidence than in disease free areas (Howard, 1980).

Ponnamma et al. (1991) identified a vector responsible for spread of yellow leaf disease of *Areca catechu* from infected to healthy plant is *Proutista moesta* in India.

Aster yellows phytoplasma is transmitted to chai hu plants from other infected plants in Alberta by aster leafhoppers (*Macrosteles* sp.). These insects were commonly found associated with various economical crops in Alberta (Khadhair et al., 1997c). They are naturally capable of feeding on a wide range of plants and are highly mobile (Chang et al., 2004).

Leafhopper vectors of phytoplasmas infecting papaya are unknown; a species of *Orosius* has been identified as a candidate for transmission studies of papaya diseases in Australia (Padovan and Gibb, 2001). The leafhopper *Empoasca papayae* has been reported to be a natural vector of papaya bunchy top disease (Davis et al., 1998).

Jujube witches' broom (JWB) phytoplasma was transferred to the host plant, *Zizipus jujuba*, by the leafhopper *Hovenia tomentella* (Kusunoki et al., 2002).

7. Genetic Diversity

Medicinal plants phytoplasmas show wide geographical distribution (Table 1). The 'Ca. P. asteris' belonging to 16SrI group is the major group associated with medicinal plants worldwide (Table 3). So far more than 27 medicinal plant species were reported as phytoplasma infected. Based on the sequences retrieved from Genbank identified phytoplasmas mainly belong to 16SrI, 16SrII, 16SrIV, 16SrV, 16SrVI, 16SrVII, 16SrVIII, 16SrX, 16SrXII, 16SrXIII, 16SrXIV, 16SrXV, 16SrXVII and 16SrXXX (Fig. 2).

Phytoplasma of the 16SrX apple proliferation group were found associated with Papaya bunchy top symptomatic papaya plants from Havana and V. Clara provinces, with 93% infection rate (Arocha et al., 2003), but the disease is wide spread to other provinces throughout the country as well in contrast to the situation in sugarcane, no latent infection had previously been reported from Australia (Gibb et al., 1996; 1998; White et al., 1998; Padovan and Gibb, 2001), but recent studies in Cuba have found that 10.6% of symptomless papaya plants analysed countained phytoplasmas (Arocha et al., 2005d). The intergenic sequence (AF257547) of the phytoplasma identified in Cuban papaya plantation showed 98% homology with that of apricot chlorotic leaf roll phytoplasma of Italy from the 16SrX goup (Arocha et al., 2003). Phylogenetic analysis indicated that this phytoplasma is more closely related to the phytoplasma associated with papaya dieback (Stolbur, 16SrXII group) than the other phytoplasma associated with papaya diseases in Australia which belong to the 16SrII, peanut witche's broom group (mosaic and yellow crinkle).

Rose proliferation and stunting as well as rose leaf curl and shoot dieback symptoms in rose cultivars were associated with aster yellows phytoplasmas (AY, 16SrI-B). It was also found, that two rose cultivars, with shoot proliferation or flower proliferation symptoms were infected by phytoplasma classified to apple proliferation group (16SrX-A) (Kamińska and Śliwa, 2004). Jarausch et al. (2001) reported the occurrence of European stone fruit yellows phytoplasma (16SrX-B), 'Candidatus phytoplasma prunorum' and rubus stunt (16SrV-E), in asymptomatic Rosa canina plants surrounding peach orchards.

Thirteen medicinal plant species Cannabis sativa, Achyranthes aspera, Santalum album, Withania somnifera, Portulaca grandiflora,Areca catechu, Ziziphus jujuba, Cocos nucifera, Datura inoxia, Tagetes erecta, Rosa alba, Catharanthus roseus and Hibiscus rosa-sinensis were reported to be associated with phytoplasma in India; phytoplasmas identified mainly belong to 16SrI, 16SrIV, 16SrV and 16SrVI groups as shown in Fig. 2. Phytoplasmas from Cannabis sativa (Raj et al., 2008a; Mall et al., 2009), Achyranthes aspera (Raj et al., 2008c), Santalum album (Khan et al., 2006b), Withania somnifera (Samad et al., 2006; Khan et al., 2006a) and Portulaca grandiflora (Ajayakumar et al. 2007; Samad et al.,2008), Areca catechu (Purushothama et al., 2007), Ziziphus jujuba (Khan et al., 2008), Cocos nucifera (Sharmila, 2004; Edwin, 2007), Datura inoxia (Raj et al., 2009), Tagetes erecta (Raj et al., 2008b), C. roseus, Rosa alba and Hibiscus rosa-sinensis (Chaturvedi et al., 2009 a,b; 2010) are molecularly characterized by sequencing of the 16S ribosomal gene.

Cannabis phytoplasma (EU439257; FJ227937), Achyranthes phytoplasma (EU573926), Santalum phytoplasma (DQ0932357) and Tagetes phytoplasma strain Lucknow (EU516321) shared highest 99% similarity with the 16Sr RNA gene of several phytoplasmas belonging to 16SrI group. Hibiscus rosa-sinensis phytoplasmas strains GKP1 (FJ939287) and GKP 2 (FJ939289) showed 98% homology between them however, separately each of them showed highest identity (99%) with several phytoplasmas of 16SrI group. Portulaca phytoplasma (EF651786), Datura phytoplasma (EU573925) and Withania phytoplasma showed highest identity (99%) with several phytoplasmas of 16SrVI group. Tagetes phytoplasma strain Pantnagar (EU362631), Ziziphus phytoplasma (EU366162), Cocos phytoplasma (AY158660) showed 99% identity with the 16S rRNA gene of several phytoplasmas belonging to 16SrII, 16SrV and 16SrIV group respectively. Sequence homology results revealed that C. roseus phytoplasma (EU694109) and rose phytoplasma (FJ429364) shared 99% sequence similarity with the 16Sr RNA gene of aster yellows phytoplasmas from *C. roseus* or from other medicinal plants or woody species always detected in infected plants from India,. Therefore both phytoplasmas were identified as strains in the 16SrI group (Figure 3). Sequence similarity of 16Sr DNA among different phytoplasma strain identified in medicinal plants in all over the world is shown in table 4.

8. Management Approaches

Control of epidemic outbreak of phytoplasma diseases can be carried out theoretically either by controlling the vector or by eliminating the pathogen from the infected plants by meristem tip culture, antibiotics or other chemicals (Bertaccini, 2007).

At the present, insect vector control using pesticides is the tool of choice for limiting outbreaks of phytoplasma diseases; however, removal of sources of inoculum is efficient in the case of mollicute diseases spread by monophagous vector feeding on the affected plant. The vector control is difficult to achieve when wild reservoir plants are sources of contaminations for polyphagous leafhoppers. Similarly, it is easier to control monophagous insects reproducing on the affected crop than insect making their life cycle on wild plants.

Phytoplasmas can be eliminated from their plant hosts, as they are generally thermo-labile and are not present in the shoot meristem (Lee and Davis, 1992). Furthermore they are sensitive to some antibiotics such as tetracycline (Ishiie et al., 1967; Heintz, 1989). Several methods have been applied to clean plant material for phytoplasmas; these include *in vitro* tissue culture such as shoot tip (Dale and Cheyne, 1993) or micropropagation (Davies and Clark, 1994) sometimes in combination with heat or antibiotic treatment.

Preventative or therapeutic antibiotic treatments using oxytetracycline-HCL (OTC) administered by trunk injection to palms (Hunt et al., 1974; McCoy, 1982) is an effective method for control of Lethal Yellowing in coconut and other susceptible palm species.Used proactively in mandatory inoculation zones as part of an integrated management program in Collier Country , southwestern Florida, OTC treatments have been largely successful in suppressing local spread of Lethal Yellowing thereby protecting most of the country's local population of about 80,000 vulnerable Atlatic tall coconuts for the last 30 years (Fedelem, 2000).

Symptoms of periwinkle little leaf disease of *C. roseus* caused by phytoplasmas were reduced by treatment with gibberellic acid or tetracycline (Kar et al., 1983). Phytoplasma could be eliminated in shoot-tip cultures of *C. roseus* employing oxytetracycline. Rose plants treated with tetracycline showed no remission of symptoms (Epstein and Hill, 1995).

Ajayakumar et al. (2007) demonstrated temporarily amelioration of phytoplasma symptoms by treatment with tetracycline antibiotic in *Portulaca grandiflora* plants infected by *Candidatus* Phytoplasma. During the study a set of infected *P. grandiflora* plants displaying symptoms were treated with one of two antibiotics. Each set of 20 plants was treated for 6 weeks by foliar spray with tetracycline hydrochloride or penicillin at 250, 500 and 1000 μg/mL concentration at weekly intervals. Plants sprayed with distilled water served as controls. The antibiotic was dissolved in sterile water and applied on the infected plants by hand sprayer in the evening under glasshouse conditions. All infected plants showed signs of recovery from the disease symptoms 4 weeks after treatment with tetracycline hydrochloride and appeared healthy after 6 weeks. However, by 6 weeks after ceasing the antibiotic treatment, the characteristic symptoms of the disease reappeared on newly emerged leaves and branches. On the contrary, symptoms of the disease became more severe following penicillin or distilled water treatment.

Foliar spray of oxytetracycline, tetracycline hydrochloride or penicillin and or dipping of cuttings of infected plants in indole-3-acetic acid (IAA) or indole-3-butyric acid (IBA) have been attempted by various workers in India and abroad for remission of Phytoplasma in various plants or their control to some extent.

Therefore, a real way to control phytoplasma infection is to prevent the outbreaks by producing clean material or by finding phytoplasma resistant varieties. Knowledge about the mechanisms of plant host resistance to phytoplasmas is little, but the paucity of effective disease management strategies for these diseases lends a high priority to these questions. Efforts continue to identify germplasm encoding natural resistance to Mollicutes, and to incorporate such genes via selection and breeding programs may involve resistance to either the pathogen itself or to the insect vector. Plant defense related proteins, known to be active in host responses to invasion by other types of pathogens, might occur in responses to mollicute infection; confirmation of this hypothesis would require demonstration that the compound is in the right place at the right time, and is present in effective concentrations (Garnier et al., 2001).

Conclusion

Medicinal plants constitute a group of industrially important plant which is of great value for domestic use and for export. Plant based drugs are being increasingly preffered in medicinal science. Phytoplasma cause diseases in several medicinal plant causing serious economic losses. Therefore, phytoplasma diseases are the major constraints in profitable cultivation of medicinal plants and lower its quantum and quality and gaining international importance because of unspecific symptoms, various losses and diverse epidemiology throughout the world. Epidemics of these diseases have compelled withdrawal of many medicinal plant varieties from cultivation.

Knowledge of the diversity of phytoplasmas has been expanded by recent studies and the availability of molecular tools for pathogen identification. The diversity of the potential reservoir of disease has been increased with the discovery of new phytoplasmas hosts. The potential reservoir of phytoplasmas in on medicinal plants may be even larger than already reported one. There is already evidence available, for host plants other than medicinal plants, that phytoplasmas can be detected in plant species before symptoms appearance, that phytoplasmas are not always detectable in every part of a plant, and that the location of phytoplasma in a plant can vary over time. New disease outbreaks occur from time to time in various geographic regions. Numerous new phytoplasma strains have been identified in the last few years and a preliminary classification of known and new phytoplasma strains has revealed that phytoplasmas are more diverse than previously thought .Hence, it would be, of prime importance to study the diverse nature of phytoplasma and their taxonomy affecting different plant species inworldwide.

Future Prospects

Molecular tools such as monoclonal antibodies, DNA-based probes, and PCR-based sensitive detection procedures have largely replaced traditional procedures based on biological properties, greatly advancing phytoplasmal disease diagnotics and facilitating phytoplasma characterization. It is axiomatic that evolutionary speciation is driven by genes other than those, such as 16SrRNA and ribosomal protein genes, that are commonly used for phylogenetic analysis, classification and delineation and description of '*Candidatus* phytoplasma' species. While conserved genes are useful in phytoplasma strain classification and species delineation, their utility is due to sequence variability that is correlated with, but not determinant of, species evolution. Thus, it is sequence drift in niche–isolated or niche-unique strain populations that results in conserved gene sequence variability. This implies that some closely related species may not be resolved by analysis of conserved genes and that incipient species tend to remain unrecognized. For these reasons and for practicality, it is important at this stage of phytoplasmas taxonomy to link phenotypic or biological characteristic with molecular criteria in definition and description of phytoplasma taxa, especially at species level. Ultimately, as more is learned about factors involved in host-pathogen interactions and nucleotide sequences controlling these interactions, it should be possible to bridge molecular criteria and biological properties through judicious choices of suites of nucleotide sequences applicable for distinguishing and describing phytoplasma species. In our view, use of multigene sequences with varying degrees of variability will eventually afford definitions of phytoplasmas at strain, species or higher level consistent with phylogenies theoretically based on complete genome sequences. This outlook engenders the concept that formal genus phytoplasma taxonomy will become a reality, in spite of inability to isolate these intriguing microbes in artificial cultures, and will one day be based entirely upon gene information. Phytoplasma associated diseases are molecularly distinguishable in most of the cases at the 16Sr DNA level. Therefore, epidemiological studies can be carried out in order to eliminate infected plants to prevent further epidemic spreading. The main limitation to the real application of these procedures that can be very successful in eliminating or reducing the impact of phytoplasma diseases is that agricultural-related problems are not under consideration in many countries worldwide for opposite reasons (over production or not qualified production) people working in this field are not always aware of the risk connected with the trading or the maintenance in field of phytoplasma infected plants. It is presumed that phytoplasma infected natural plants may act as a reservoir and insect vectors feeding on them may carry the destructive pathogen to the agricultural crops. Therefore, the current developed practices in identification and characterization of phytoplasmas should be updated and more concised which would be quite helpful in phytoplasmas taxonomy and a sound practical management approach could be planned accordingly.

References

Ajaykumar, P.V., Samad, A., Shasany, A.K., Gupta, M.K., Alam, M. and Rastogi, S. (2007). First record of a '*Candidatus* phytoplasma' associated with little leaf disease of *Portulaca grandiflora*. *Australian Plant Disease Notes*, 2: 67-69.

Alhudaib, K. , Arocha, Y. , Wilson, M. and Jones, P. (2008). First report of a 16SrI, *Candidatus* Phytoplasma asteris group phytoplasma associated with a date palm disease in Saudi Arabia. *Plant Pathology* 57: 366.

Alhudaib, K., Arocha, Y., Wilson, M. and Jones, P. (2009). Molecular identification, potential vectors and alternative hosts of the phytoplasma associated with a lime decline disease in Saudi Arabia. *Crop Protection*, 28: 13-18.

Alma, A., Bosco, D., Danielli, A., Bertaccini, A., Vibio, M., and Arzone, A. (1997). Identification of phytoplasmas in eggs, nymphs and adults of *Scaphoideus titanus* Ball reared on healthy plants. *Insect Molecular Biology*, 6: 115-121.

Al-Saady, N.A. and Khan, A.J. (2006). Phytoplasmas that can infect diverse plant species worldwide. *Physiol. Mol. Biol. Plant,* 12: 263-281.

Anonymous (2004). IRPCM Phytoplasma/Spiroplasma Working Team Phytoplasma taxonomy group, '*Candidatus* Phytoplasma', a taxon for the wall-less, non-helical prokaryotes that colonize plant phloem and insects. *Int. J. Syst. Evol. Microbiol,* 54: 1243-1255.

Arocha, Y., Horta, D., Peralta, E. and Jones, P. (2003). First report on molecular detection of phytoplasmas in papaya in Cuba. *Plant Disease,* 87: 1148.

Arocha, Y., Horta, D., Pinol, B., Palenzuela, I., Picornell, S., Almeida, R. and Jones, P. (2005). First report of Phytoplasma associated with Bermuda grass white leaf disease in Cuba. *Plant Pathol.*, 54: 233.

Arocha ,Y., Pinol, B., Picornell, B., Almeida ,R. and Jones, P. (2006a) first report of the 16SrII ('*Candidatus* phytoplasma aurantifolia') Group associated with a bunchy top disease of papaya in Cuba. *Plant Pathology*, 55:821.

Arocha, Y., Pinol., B., Picornell, B., Almeida, R., Jones, P. and Boa, E. (2006b). Basil little leaf: a new disease associated with a phytoplasma of the 16SrI (Aster Yellows) group in Cuba. *Plant Pathol.*, 55: 82.

Arocha, Y., Pinol, B., Lopez, M., Miranda, I., Almeida, R., Wilson, M. and Jones, P. (2007). Bunchy top symptom' of papaya in Cuba: new insights, *Bulletin of Insectology,* 60: 393-394.

Arocha, Y., Almeida, R., Vigheri, N., Florent, N., Betts, P., Monger, W.A., Harju, V., Mumford, R.A., Bekele, B., Tadesse, D. and Jones, P. (2008). Unveiling the aetiology of papaya diseases in Cuba, Democratic Republic of Congo (DRC) and Ethiopia. *Rev. Protección Veg.,* 23: 21-25.

Arocha, Y., Pinol, B., Acosta, K., Almeida, R., Devonshire, J., Van de Meene, A., Boa, E. and Lucas, J. (2009). Detection of phytoplasma and potyvirus pathogens in papaya (*Carica papaya* L.) affected with 'Bunchy Top Symptom' (BTS) in eastern Cuba. *Crop Protection*, 28: 640-646.

Bellardi, M.G., Contaldo, N., Benni, A., Curini, M., Epifano, F., Genovese, S. and Bertaccini, A. (2009). Effects of phytoplasma infection on the quality of Grindelia robusta essential oil. *Plant Pathology*, 91: 240.

Berges, R., Rott, M. and Seemüller, E. (2000). Range of phytoplasma concentrations in various host plants as determined by competitive polymerase chain reaction. *Phytopathology*, 90: 1145-1152.

Bertaccini, A. and Marani, F. (1982). Electron microscopy of two viruses and mycoplasma-like organism in lilies with deformed flowers. *Phytopathologia Mediterranea*, 21: 8-14.

Bertaccini, A., Kamińska, M., Botti, S. and Martini, M. (2002). Molecular evidence for mixed phytoplasma infection in lily plants. *Acta Horticulturae*, 568: 35-41.

Bertaccini, A., Franova, J., Botti, S. and Tabanelli, D. (2005). Molecular characterization of phytoplasmas in lilies with fasciation in the Czech Republic. *FEMS Microbiology Letters*, 249: 79-85.

Bertaccini, A. (2007). Phytoplasmas: diversity, taxonomy, and epidemiology. *Frontieres in Bioscience*, 12: 673-689.

Bertaccini, A., Calari, A. and Felker, P. (2007). Developing a method for phytoplasma identification in cactus pear samples from California. *Bulletin of Insectology*, 60: 257-258.

Bertaccini, A. and Maini, S. (2007). *Bulletin of Insectology*. Vol. 60(2), A. Bertaccini, S. Maini)(eds.) pp. 99-407. Department of Agroenvironmental Sciences and technologies, Alma Mater Studiorum University of Bologna.

Bosco, D., Minucci, C., Boccardo, G. and Conti, M. (1997). Differential acquisition of chrysanthemum yellows phytoplasma by three leafhopper species. *Entomologia Experimentalis et Applicata,* 83: 219-224.

Bové, J.M. (1984). Wall-less prokaryotes of plants. *Annual Revue of Phytopathology*, 22: 361-396.

Bown, D. (1995). Encyclopedia of herbs and their uses. Dorling Kindersley, London.

Brown, S.E. (2008). First Report of Lethal Yellowing Group (16Sr IV) of Phytoplasmas in *Vernonia cinerea* in Jamaica. *Plant disease*, 92: 1132.

Brown, S.E., Been, B.O. and McLaughlin, W.A. (2008). First report of the presence of the leathal yellowing group (16Sr IV) of phytoplasma in the weeds *Emelia fosbergii* and *Synedella nodiflora* in Jamaica. *Plant Pathology* : http: // www.bspp.org.uk / ndr / jan 2008/2007 - 75. asp.

Carginale, V., Luca, V.D., Capasso, C., Baldi, M.R., Maria, G., Pastore, M., Bertaccini, A., Carraro, L. and Capasso, A. (2007). Effect of pear decline phytoplasma on gene expression in *Catharanthus roseus*. *Bulletin of Insectology*, 60: 213-214.

Carling, D.E. and Millikan, D.F. (1978). Banded filaments associated with the aster yellows MLO in *Vinca rosea*. *Canadian Journal of Microbiology*, 24: 1417-1418.

Carraro, L., Osler, R., Refatti, E. and Poggi-Pollini, C. (1988). Transmission of the possible agent of apple proliferation to *Vinca rosea* by dodder. *Rivista di Patologia Vegetale*, 24: 43-52.

Carraro, L., Osler, R., Loi, N. and Favali, M.A. (1991). Transmission characteristics of the clover phyllody agent by dodder. *Journal of Phytopathology*, 133: 15-22.

Carraro, L., Osler, R., Refatti, E. and Favali, M.A. (1992). Natural diffusion and experimental transmission of plum leptonecrosis. *Acta Horticulturae,* 309: 285-290.

Carraro, L., Ermacora, P., Loi, N. and Osler, R. (2004). The recovery phenomenon in apple proliferation-infected apple trees. *Journal of Plant Pathology,* 86: 141-146.

Chang, K.F., Hwang, S.F., Khadhair, A.H., Kawchuk, L.M., Howard, R.J. and Blade, S.F. (2004). Aster yellows phytoplasma associated with chai hu plants in Canada. *Journal of Plant Diseases and Protection*, 111: 218–224.

Chaturvedi, Y., Singh, M., Rao, G.P., Snehi, S.K. and Raj, S.K. (2009a). First report of association of 'Candidatus phytoplasma asteris' (16SrI group) with little leaf disease of rose (*Rosa alba*) in India. *Plant Pathology*, 58: 788.

Chaturvedi, Y., Tewari, A.K., Upadhyaya, P.P., Prabhuji, S.K. and Rao, G.P. (2009b). Association of 'Candidatus phytoplasma asteris' with little leaf and phyllody disease of Catharanthus roseus in Eastern Uttar Pradesh, India. Medicinal Plants, 1: 103-108.

Chaturvedi, Y., Singh, M., Snehi, S.K., Raj , S.K. and Rao, G.P. (2010). First report of 'Candidatus Phytoplasma asteris' (16Sr I group) associated with yellows and little leaf diseases of Hibiscus rosa-sinensis in India. Plant Pathology, 59:796.

Chen, M. H. and Hiruki, C. (1978). The preservation of membranes of tubular bodies associated with mycoplasma like organisms by tannic acid. Canadian Journal of Botany, 56: 2878-2882.

Chen, Z.Y., Shen, J.Y., Peng, B.Z., Zheng, G.B. and Chen, M.Y. (1984). Mycoplasma associated with periwinkle phyllody disease. Acta Phytopathologica Sinica, 14: 233-234.

Cheo, P. (1970). Rose wilt or dieback-a new virus disease attacks rose in California. Lasca Leaves, 20: 88-89.

Chopra, R.N., Nayar, S.L. and Chopra, I.C. (1986). Glossary of Indian medicinal plants (Including the supplement). Council of Scientific and Industrial Research, New Delhi.

Christensen, N.M., Axelsen, K. B., Nicolaisen, M. and Schulz, A. (2004). Phytoplasmas and their interactions with hosts. Trends in Plant Science, 11: 526-535.

Chung, B. N. (2008). Phytoplasma detection in Chrysanthemum and Lily. In: Characterization, Diagnosis and Management of Phytoplasmas. N. A.Harrison, G. P. Rao and C. Marcone (eds.) pp. 175-194. Studium Press LLC, Texas, USA.

Clark, M.F. and Davies, D.L. (1984). Mycoplasma detection and characterization. In Report East Malling Research Station, 108-109 pp.

Clark, M.F., Davies, D.L., Buss, S.L. and Morton, A. (1989). Serological discrimination among mycoplasma-like organisms using polyclonal and monoclonal antibodies. Acta Horticulturae, 234: 107-113.

Connors, I. L. (1941). 20th Annual Report of the Canadian Plant Disease Survey, 1940. pp. 1-7.

Cordell, G.A. (1980). The botanical chemical biosynthesis and pharmacological aspects Catharanthus roseus (L.) G. Don.(Apocynaceae). In: Recent Advances in Natural Product Research. W. S. Woo and B. H. Han (eds:) pp. 65-72. Seoul National University Press, Seoul.

Cortés-Martínez, N.E., Moctezuma, E.V., Molina, L.X.Z. and Aguilar-Rios, J. (2007). A new phytoplasma associated with a zigzag line pattern in leaves of Lilum spp. In Mexico. Bulletin of Insectology, 60: 283-284.

Cousin, M-T. and Abadie, M. (1982). Action of mycoplasmas on the anther. Light and electron microscope study. Station de Pathologie Vegetale, 5: 41-57.

Dabek, A.J. (1982). Transmission experiments on coconut lethal yellowing disease with Deltocephalus flavicosta Stal, a leafhopper vector of periwinkle phyllody in Jamaica. Phytopathology Z., 103: 109-119.

Dale, P.J. and Cheyne, V.A. (1993). The elimination of clover diseases by shoot tip culture. Annals of Applied Biology, 123: 25-32.

Davies, D.L. and Clark, M.F. (1994). Maintenance of mycoplasmalike organisms occurring in Pyrus species by micropropagation and their elimination by tetracycline therapy. Plant Pathology, 43: 819-823.Davis, R.E., Lee, I.M., Dally, E.L., Delwitt, N. and Douglas, S.M. (1988). Cloned nucleic acid hybridization probes in detection and classification of mycoplasma like organisms (MLOs). Acta Horticulturae, 234: 115-122.

Davis, R.E., Lee, I.M., Douglas, S.M. and Dally, E.L. (1990). Molecular cloning and detection of chromosomal and extrachromosomal DNA of the mycoplasma like organism associated with little leaf disease in periwinkle (*Catharanthus roseus*). *Phytopathology*, 80: 789-793.

Davis, R.E., Dally, E.L., Bertaccini, A., Credi, R., Osler, R., Carraro, L., Lee, I.M. and Barba, M. (1992). Cloned DNA probes for specific detection of Italian periwinkle virescence mycoplasmalike organism (MLO) and investigation of genetic relatedness with other MLO. *Phytopathologia Mediterranea*, 31: 5-12.

Davis, R.E. and Sinclair, W.A. (1998). Phytoplasma identity and disease etiology. *Phytopathology*, 88: 1372-1376.

Deng, S.J. and Hiruki, C. (1990). Molecular cloning and detection of DNA of the mycoplasma like organism associated with clover proliferation. *Canadian Journal of Plant Pathology*, 12: 383-388.

Deng, S. and Hiruki, C. (1991). Amplification of 16S rRNA genes from culturable and non-culturable mollicutes. *Journal of Microbiological Methods,* 14: 53-61.

Doi, Y., Teranaka, M., Yora, K. and Asuyama, H. (1967). Mycoplasma or PLT group-like micro-organisms found in the phloem elements of plants infected with mulberry dwarf, potato witches, broom, aster yellow or *Paulownia* witches' broom. *Annals of Phytopathological Society of Japan,* 33: 259-266.

Duduk, B., Mejia, J.F., Calari, A. and Bertaccini, A. (2008). Identification of 16SrIX group phytoplasmas infecting Colombian periwinkles and molecular characterization on several genes. IOM 17th International Congress, Tienjin, China: 112: 83.

Eastman, C.E., Schultz, G.A., Fletcher, J., Hemmanti, K. and Oldfield, G.N. (1984). Virescence of horseradish in Illinois. *Plant Disease*, 68: 968-971.

Edwin, B.T. and Mohankumar, C. (2007). Kerala wilt disease phytoplasma: Phylogenetic analysis and identification of a vector, Proutista moesta. *Physiological and Molecular Plant Pathology* 71: 41-47.

Epstein, A.H. and Hill, J. (1995). The biology of rose rosette disease: a mite-associated disease of uncertain etiology. *Journal of Phytopathology*, 143: 353-360.

Fan, X.P. , Wang, X., Tian, J.B. , Paltrinieri, S., Bertaccini, A. , Petriccione, M. and Pastore. M. (2008). Molecular Detection of *Candidatus* Phytoplasma *Ziziphae jujube* Cultivars. *Phytopathology,* 156: 326 - 331

Favali, M.A., Fossati, F., Toppi, L.S.D. and Musetti, R. (2008). *Catharanthus roseus* phytoplasmas. In: *Characterization, Diagnosis and Management of phytoplasmas*. N. A. Harrison, G. P. Rao, C. Marcone (eds:) pp. 195-218. Studium Press LLC, Texas, USA.

Garnier, M., Foissac, X., Gaurivaud, P., Laigret, F., Renaudin, J., Saillard, C. and Bové J.M. (2001). Mycoplasmas, plants, insect vectors: a matrimonial triangle. *C. R. Acad. Sci.*, 324: 923–928.

Gibb, K., Persley D., Schneider, B. and Thomas, J. (1996).Phytoplasma associated with *Papaya* disease in australia.-*Plant Disease*, 80:174-178.

Gibb, K.S., Schneider, B. and Padovan, A.C. (1998). Differential detection and relatedness of phytoplasmas in papaya. *Pl. Pathol.,* 47 : 325-332.

Girach, R.D. and Khan, A.S.A. (1992). Ethananomedicinal uses of *Achyranthes apera* leaves in Orissa (India). *International Journal of Pharmacognosy,* 30: 113-115.

Grimaldi, V. and Grasso, S. (1988). Mycoplasma disease of *Dimophotheca sinuata* and *Catharanthus roseus* in Sicily. *Acta Horticulturae*, 234: 137-143.

Gumpf, D.J. and Weathers, L.G. (1974). Detection of a new infectious disease of roses in California. *Acta Horticulturae*, 36: 53-57.

Gundersen, D.E., Lee, I.M., Rehner, S.A., Davis, R.E. and Kingsbury, D.T. (1994). Phylogeny of mycoplasmalike organisms (phytoplasmas): a basis for their classification. *Journal of Bacteriology*, 176: 5244-5254.

Gundersen, D. E. and Lee, I-M. (1996). Ultrasensitive detection of phytoplasmas by nested-PCR assays using two universal primer pairs. *Phytopathologia Mediterranea*, 35: 144-151.

Han, S. and Cha, B. (2002). Genetic Similarity Between Jujube Witches' Broom and Mulberry Dwarf Phytoplasmas Transmitted by *Hishimonus sellatus* Uhler. *Plant Pathol. J.,* 18: 98-101.

Hanboonsong, Y., Choosai, C., Panyim, S., and Damak, S. (2002). Transovarial transmission of sugarcane white leaf phytoplasma in the insect vector *Matsumuratettix hiroglyphicus* (Matsumura). *Insect Molecular Biology*, 11: 97-103.

Harrison, N.A. and Oropeza, C. (2008a). Coconut Lethal Yellowing, In:*Characterization, Diagnosis and Management of Phytoplasmas* .N.A. Harrison, G.P. Rao and C. Marcone.(eds). pp.219-248. Plant Pathogens Series -5. Studium Press LLC, U.S.A.

Harrison, N.A., Rao, G.P. and Marcone, C. (2008b). *Characterization, Diagnosis and Management of Phytoplasmas*. N.A. Harrison, G.P. Rao, C. Marcone (eds.) pp. 1-399. Studium Press LLC, U.S.A.

Heinrich, M., Botti, S., Caprara, L., Arthofer, W., Strommer, S., Hanzer, V., Katinger, H., Laimer da Câmara Machado, M. and Bertaccini, A. (2001). Improved detection methods for fruit tree phytoplasmas. *Plant Molecular Biology Reporter*, 19: 169-179.

Heintz, W. (1989). Transmission of a new mycoplasma-like organism (MLO) from *Cuscuta odorata* (Ruiz et Pav.) to herbaceous plants and attempts to its elimination in the vector. *Journal of Phytopathology,* 125: 171-186.

Hindal, D.F., Amrine, J.W., Williams, R.L. and Stasny, T.A. (1988). Rose rosette disease on multiflora rose (*Rosa multiflora*) in Indian and Kentucky. *Weed Technology*, 2: 442-444.

Hiruki, C. and Rocha, A.D.A. (1986). Hystochemical diagnosis of mycoplasma infections in *Catharanthus roseus* by means of a fluorescent DNA-binding agent, 4'-6'-diamidino-2-phenylindole-2 HC1 (DAPI). *Canadian Journal of Plant Pathology*, 8: 185-188.

Hiruki, C. (1987). Witches' broom of *Hibiscus heterophyllus*, a mycoplasma disease occurring in Australia. *Ann. Phytopathol. Soc. Japan*, 53: 1-6.

Howard, F.W. (1980). Population densities of Myndus crudus Van Duzee (Homoptera: Cixiidae) in relation to coconut lethal yellowing distribution in Florida. *Principes*, 24: 174-178.

Ishiie, T., Doi, Y., Yora, K. and Asuyama H. (1967). Suppressive effects of antibiotics of tetracycline group on symptom development of mulberry dwarf disease. *Annals of Phytopathological Society of Japan*, 33: 267-275.

Jarausch, W., Jarausch-Wehrheim, B., Danet, J.L., Broquaire, J.M., Dosba, F., Saillard, C. and Garnier, M. (2001). Detection and identification of European stone fruit yellows and other phytoplasmas in the surroundings of apricot chlorotic leaf roll-affected orchards in southern France. *European Journal of Plant Pathology*, 107: 209-217.

Jung, H.Y., Sawayanagi, T., Wongkaew, P., Kakizawa, S., Nishigawa, H., Wei, W., Oshima, K., Miyata, S.I., Ugaki, M., Hibi., T. and Namba, S. (2003). '*Candidatus* Phytoplasma oryzae', a novel phytoplasma taxon associated with rice yellow dwarf disease. *Int. J. Syst. Evol. Microbiol.,* 53: 1925-1929.

Kaminska, M., Korbin, M., Komorowska, B. and Pulawska , J. (1998). Stunting and flower buds deficiency of *Lilium* sp.: a new phytoplasma associated disease. *Acta Physiol. Plant.,* 20: 49-53.

Kamińska, M. and Korbin, M. (2000). Phytoplasma infection in *Lilium* sp. plants. *Phytopathol. Pol.,* 20: 45-57.

Kaminska, M., Sliwa, H. and Rudzinska-Langwald, A. (2004). Phytoplasma diseases of ornamental crops. *Progress in plant protection,* 44: 776-779.

Kamińska M. and Śliwa H. (2004). First report of phytoplasma belonging to apple proliferation group in roses in Poland. *Plant Disease,* 88: 1283.

Kamińska, M. and Śliwa, H. (2008a). Mixed infection of dahlia in Poland with apple proliferation and aster yellows phytoplasmas. *Plant Pathology,* 57: 363.

Kamińska, M. and Śliwa, H. (2008b). First report of '*Candidatus* Phytoplasma mali' in oriental lilies and its association with leaf scorch in Poland. *Plant Pathology,* 57: 363.

Kar, R.K., Kabi, T. and Pattnaik, H. (1983). Chemotherapy of periwinkle little leaf disease. *Current Science,* 52: 496-497.

Kawakita, H., Saiki, T., Wei, W., Mitsuhasi, W., Watanabe, K., and Sato, M. (2000). Identification of mulberry dwarf phytoplasmas in genital organs and eggs of the leafhopper *Hishimonoides sellatiformis. Phytopathology,* 90: 909-914.

Khadhair, A.H., Hiruki, C. and Hwang , S.F. (1997). Molecular detection of alfalfa witches'-broom phytoplasma in four leafhopper species associated with infected alfalfa plants. *Microbiol. Res.,* 152: 269–275.

Khadhair, A.H., Kawchuk, L.M., Taillon, R.C. and Botar, G. (1998). Detection and molecular characterization of an aster yellows phytoplasma in parsley. *Canadian Journal of Botany,* 20: 55-61.

Khadhair, A.H., Hiruki, C. and Deyholos, M. (2008). Molecular Characterization of Aster Yellows Phytoplasma Associated with Valerian and Sowthistle Plants by PCR–RFLP Analyses. *Phytopathology,* 156: 326 – 331.

Khan, J.A., Srivastava, P. and Singh, S.K. (2004). Efficacy of nested-PCR for the detection of phytoplasma causing spike disease of sandal. *Current Science,* 86: 1530-1533.

Khan, J.A., Srivastava, P. and Singh, S.K. (2006a). Sensitive detection of a phytoplasma associated with little leaf symptoms in *Withania somnifera. European Journal of Plant Pathology,* 115: 401-408.

Khan, J.A., Srivastava, P. and Singh S.K. (2006b). Identification of a '*Candidatus* Phytoplasma asteris'-related strain associated with spike disease of sandal (*Santalum album*) in India. *Plant Pathology,* 55: 572.

Khan, M.S , Raj, S.K. and Snehi, S.K. 2008. Natural occurrence of '*Candidatus* Phytoplasma ziziphi' isolates in two species of jujube trees (*Ziziphus* spp.) in India. *Plant Pathology,* 57: 1173.

Kim, Y.H., La, J. and Kim, Y.T. (1985). Transmission and hystochemical detection of mulberry dwarf mycoplasma in several herbaceous plants. *Korean Journal of Plant Pathology,* 1: 184-189.

Kitajima, E.W. and Costa, A.S. (1979). Mycoplasma-like organisms associated with yellow-type diseases in cultivated plants and ornamentals in Săo Paulo state and the Federal district. *Fitopatologia Brasileira,* 4: 317-327.

Kusunoki, M., Shiomi, T., Kobayashi, M., Okudaira, T., Ohashi, A. and Nohira, T. (2002). A Leafhopper (*Hishimonus sellatus*) Transmits Phylogenetically Distant Phytoplasmas: Rhus Yellows and Hovenia Witches' Broom Phytoplasma. *General Plant Pathology,* 68: 147-154.

Lee, I.M. and Davis, R.E. (1983). Phloem-limited prokaryotes in sieve elements isolated by enzyme treatment of diseased plant tissues. *Phytopathology*, 73: 1540-1543.

Lee, I.M., Davis, R.E. and Hiruki, C. (1991). Genetic relatedness among clover proliferation mycoplasmalike organisms (MLOs) and other MLOs investigated by nucleic acid hybridization and restriction fragment length polymorphism analyses. *Applied Environmental Microbiology,* 57: 3565-3569.

Lee, I.M. and Davis, R.E. (1992). Mycoplasmas which infect plants and insects. In: *Mycoplasmas: Molecular Biology and Pathogenesis*. J. Maniloff, R. N. McElhaney, L. R. Finch and J. B. Baseman, (eds.) pp 379-390. American Society for Microbiology, Washington, DC, USA.

Lee, I.M., Hammond, R.W., Davis, R.E. and Gundersen, D.E. (1993). Universal amplification and analysis of pathogen 16S rDNA for classification and identification of mycoplasmas like organisms. *Phytopathology*, 83: 834-842.

Lee, I.M., Gundersen, D.E., Hammond, R.W. and Davis, R.E. (1994). Use of mycoplasma like organism (MLO) group-specific oligonucleotide primers for nested-PCR assays to detect mixed-MLO infections in a single host plant. *Phytopathology*, 84: 559-566.

Lee, I.M., Bertaccini, A., Vibio, M. and Gundersen, D.E. (1995). Detection of multiple phytoplasmas in perennial fruit trees with decline symptoms in Italy. *Phytopathology*, 85: 728-735.

Lee, I.M., Gundersen-Rindal, D.E., Davis, R.E. and Bartoszyk, M. (1998). Revised classification scheme of phytoplasmas based on RFLP analyses of 16S rRNA and ribosomal protein gene sequences. *Intl. J. Syst. Bacteriol,* 48: 1153-1169.

Lee, I.M., Davis, R.E. and Gundersen-Rindal, D.E. (2000). Phytoplasma: phytopathogenic mollicutes. *Annual Revue of Microbiology*, 54: 221-255.

Lee, I.M., Bottner, K.D., Dally, E.L. and Davis, R.E. (2008). First report of Purple Coneflower phyllody associated with a 16SrI-B phytoplasma in Maryland. *Plant Disease*, 92: 654.

Lepka, P., Stitt, M., Moll, E. and Seemüller, E. (1999). Effect of phytoplasmal infection on concentration and translocation of carbohydrates and aminoacids in periwinkle and tobacco. *Physiology and Molecular Plant Pathology*, 55: 59-68.

Livingston, S., Al-Azri, M.O., Al-Saady, N.A., Al-Subhi, A.M. and Khan, A.J. (2006). First report of 16Sr DNA II group phytoplasma on *Polygala mascatense*, a weed in Oman. *Plant Disease*, 90: 248.

Lorenz, K.H., Schneider, B., Ahrens, U. and Seemüller, E. (1995). Detection of the apple proliferation and pear decline phytoplasmas by PCR amplification of ribosomal and nonribosomal DNA. *Phytopathology*, 85: 771-776.

Mall, S., Rao, G.P. and Upadhyaya, P.P. (2010). Molecular characterization of Aster yellows (16SrI) group phytoplasma infecting *Cannabis sativa* in Eastern Uttar Pradesh. *Indian Phytopathology*, (accepted).

Marcone, C. and Rao, G.P. (2008). 'Candidatus Phytoplasma cynodontis': The causal agent of Bermuda Grass White Leaf Disease. In: *Characterization, Diagnosis and Managemen of Phytoplasma.* N. A. Harrison, G. P. Rao and C. Marcone (eds.) pp 353-364. Studium Press LLC,U.S.A.

Martinez, R.T., Narvaez, M., Fabre, S., Harrison, N., Oropeza, C., Dollet, M. and Hichez, E. (2008). Coconut lethal yellowing on the southern coast of the Dominican Republic is associated with a new 16SrIV group phytoplasma. *Plant Pathology,* 57: 366.

Marwitz, R., Petzold, H. and Ozel, M. (1974). Studies on the transfer of the possible causal agent of apple proliferation to a herbaceous host. *Phytopathology*, 81: 85-91.

Marwitz, R. (1990). Diversity of yellows disease agents in plant infections. *Zentralblatt fur Baktenologie, Suppl.*, 20: 431-434.

Mc Coy, R.E. and Thomas, D.L. (1980). Periwinkle witches' broom on South Florida. *Proceedings of the Florida State Horticultural Society*, 93: 179-181.

McCoy, R.E., Caudwell, A., Chang, C.J., Chen, T.A., Chiykowski, L.N., Cousin, M.T., Dale, J.L., deLeeuw, G.T.N., Golino, D.A., Hackettt, K.J., Kirkpatrick, B.C., Marwitz, R., Petzold, H., Sinha, R.C., Suguira, M., Whitcomb, R.F., Yang, I.L., Zhu, B.M. and Seemuller, E. (1989). Plant diseases associated with mycoplasma-like organisms. In: The Mycoplasmas, R. F. Whitcomb and J. G. Tully (eds.) pp. 545-640. Academic Press, San Diego, USA.

Mikuriya, T.H. (1969). Historical aspects of *Cannabis sativa* in Western Medicine. *New Physician* ,18: 902-08.

Montano, H.G., Davis, R.E., Dally, E.L., Hogenhout, S., Pimentel, J. P. and Brioso, P. S. (2001). 'Candidatus Phytoplasma brasiliense', a new phytoplasma taxon associated with hibiscus witches' broom disease. *International Journal of Systematic and Evolutionary Microbiology*, 51: 1109-1118.

Moreno, P., Llacer, G. and Medina, V. (1985). Description and comparison of several yellow disease on *Vinca rosea. Agricola*, 28 (suppl.): 287-310.

Musetti, R., Favali, M.A., Carraro, L. and Osler, R. (1992). An attempt to differentiate by microscopic methods two plant mycoplasma-like organisms. *Cytobios*, 72: 71-82.

Musetti, R. and Favali, M.A. (1999). Histological and ultrastructural comparative study between *Prunus* varieties of different susceptibility to plum leptonecrosis. *Cytobios*, 99: 73-82.

Musetti, R., Favali, M. and Pressacco, L. (2000). Histopathology and polyphenol content in plants infected by phytoplasmas. *Cytobios*, 102: 133-147.

Musetti, R., Loi, N., Carraro, L. and Ermacora, P. (2002). Application of immunoelectron microscopy techniques in the diagnosis of phytoplasma diseases. *Microscopy and Research Teqhnique*, 56: 462-464.

Musetti, R., Olizzotto, R., Grisan, S., Martini, M., Borselli, S., Carraro, L. and Osler, R. (2007). Effects induced by fungal endophytes in *Catharanthus roseus* tissues infected by phytoplasmas. *Bulletin of Insectology*, 60: 293-294.

Myrie ,W., Paulraj ,L., Dollet, M., Wray ,D., Been, B.O.and McLauglin ,W. (2007). First report of lethal yellowing disease of coconut palms caused by phytoplasma on Nevis Island. *Plant Disease*, 90: 834.

Nejat, N., Sijam, K., Abdullah, S.N.A., Vadamalai, G. and Dickinson, M. (2009). Phytoplasmas associated with disease of coconut in Malaysia: phylogenetic groups and host plant species. *Plant Pathology*, 58: 1152-1160.

Okuda, S. (1977). Studies on the causal agents of yellows or witches' broom diseases of plants. *Special Bulletin of the College of Agriculture Utsunomiya University*, 32: 70.

Padovan, A. and Gibb, K. (2001). Epidemiology of Phytoplasma disease in Papaya in Northern Australia. *Journal of Phytopathology*, 149: 649-658.

Petzold, H. and Marwitz, R. (1984). Fluorescence in sieve tubes of mycoplasma infected plants after fixation with aldehydes. *German Federal Republic*, 91: 286-293.

Ploaie, P.G., Petre, Z. and Ionica, M. (1977). Identification of some plant diseases with symptoms of proliferation, chlorosis and dwarfing associated with mycoplasma in Romania. *Analele Institutulve de Cercetari pentree Protectia Plantelor*, 12: 17-25.

Poncarová-Vorácková Z., Fránová J., Válová P., Mertelik J., Navrátil M. and Nebesárová J. (1998). Identification of phytoplasma infecting *Lilium martagon* in the Czech Republic. *Journal of Phytopathology*, 146: 609-612.

Ponnamma, K.N., Rajeev, G. and Solomon, J.J. (1991). Detection of mycoplasma-like organisms in *Proutista moesta* (Westwood) a putative vector of yellow leaf disease of arecanut. *Journal of Plants Crops*, 19: 63-65.

Pribylova, J., Spak, J., Fránová, J. and Petrzik, K. (2001). Association of aster yellows subgroup 16SrI-B phytoplasmas with a disease of *Rehmannia glutinosa* var. *purpurea*. *Plant Pathology, 50: (DOI:* 10.1046/j.1365-3059.2001.00638.x).

Purushothama, C.R.A., Ramanayaka, J.G., Sanos, T., Casati, P. and Blanco, P.A. (2007). Are phytoplasmas the etiological agent of yellow leaf disease of *Areca catechu* in India? *Bulletin of Insectology*, 60: 161-162.

Radisek, S., Ferant, N., Jakse, J. and Javornik, B. (2009). Identification of a phytoplasma from the aster yellows group infecting purple coneflower (*Echinacea purpurea*) in Slovenia. *Plant Pathology*, 58: 392.

Raj, S.K., Snehi, S.K., Khan, M.S. and Kumar, S. (2008a). 'Candidatus Phytoplasma asteris' (group 16SrI) associated with a witches '-broom disease of *Cannabis sativa* in India. *Plant Pathology*, 57: 1173.

Raj, S.K., Khan,M.S., Snehi,S.K. and Kumar,S. (2008b). Marigold witches'-broom phytoplasma isolate Lucknow 16S ribosomal RNA gene, partial sequence. (unpublished).

Raj, S.K., Snehi, S.K., Kumar, S. Pratap, D. and Khan, M.S. (2008c). Association of 'Candidatus Phytoplasma asteris' (16SrI group) with yellows of *Achyranthes aspera* in India. *Plant Pathology*, (accepted)

Raj, S.K., Snehi, S.K., Kumar, S., Khan, S. (2009). First finding of 'Candidatus Phytoplasma trifolii' (16SrVI group) associated with little leaf disease of *Datura inoxia* in India. *Plant Pathology* , 18 (http://www.bspp.org.uk/publications/new-disease-reports/volumes.php/).

Rao, B.L.S., Husain, A. and Manohar, S.K. (1983). Association of mycoplasma like bodies with little leaf disease of Periwinkle (*Catharanthus roseus* G.) in India. *Indian Journal of Plant Pathology*, 1: 122-124.

Rocha, A.D.A., Okhi, S.T. and Hiruki, C. (1986). Detection of mycoplasma like organisms in situ by indirect immunofluorescence microscopy. *Phytopathology*, 76: 864-868.

Samad, A., Shasany ,A.K., Gupta, S., Ajayakuar, P.V., Darokar, M.P. and Khanuja, S.P.S. (2006). First Report of a 16SrVI Group Phytoplasma Associated with Witches'-Broom Disease on *Withania somnifera*. *Plant Disease*, 90: 248.

Samad, A., Ajaykumar, P.V., Shasany, A.K., Gupta, M.K., Alam, M. and Rastogi, S. (2008). Occurrence of a clover proliferation (16Sr VI) group phytoplasma associated with little leaf disease of *Portulaca grandiflora* in India. *Plant Disease*, 92: 832.

Schmitt, U., Peterzold, H. and Marwitz, R. (1983). On the pleomorphism of MLO in *Catharanthus roseus* (*Vinca rosea*). *Phytopathology Z.*, 108: 314-326.

Schmitt, U., Peterzold, H. and Martwitz, R. (1987). Bud like structure of mycoplasma-like organisms (MLO) demonstrated by freeze-fracturing. *Naturwissenschaften,* 74: 396-397.

Schneider, B., Seemüller, E., Smart, C.D. and Kirkpatrick, B.C. (1995). Phylogenetic classification of plant pathogenic mycoplasma-like organisms or phytoplasmas, In: *Molecular and Diagnostic Procedures in Mycoplasmology, Vol. I. Molecular Characterization* (R.S., Tully (eds) pp. 369-380. Academic Press Inc., San Diego, California, USA.

Seemüller, E., Schneider, B., Maureer, R., Ahrens, U., Daire, X., Kison, H., Lorenz, K.H., Firrao, G., Avinent, L., Sears, B.B. and Stackebrandt, E. (1994). Phylogenetic classification of phytopathogenic mollicutes by sequence analysis of 16SrDNA. *International Journal of Systematic Bacteriology,* 44: 440-446.

Sharmilaa, L.B., Bhaskerb, S., Thellyc, M.T., Edwina B.T. and Mohankumara, C. (2004). Cloning and Sequencing of Phytoplasma Ribosomal DNA (rDNA) Associated with Kerala Wilt Disease of Coconut Palms. *J. Plant Biochemistry & Biotechnology,* 13: 01-05.

Shaw, M.E., Kirkpatrick, B.C. and Golino, D.A. (1991). Causal agent of tomato big bud disease in California is the beet leaf hopper transmitted virescence agent. *Phytopathlogy,* 81: 1210.

Shepardson, S., and Mc Crum, R.C. (1973). Effect of gibberellic acid on mycoplasma like organism-infected and healthy periwinkle. *Plant Disease Reporter,* 63: 865-869.

Shin, H.D. and La, Y.L. (1984). Use of Dienes' stain in diagnosis of plant mycoplasmal diseases and modification of diagnostic procedure. *Korean Journal of Plant Protection,* 23: 215-220.

Shishlova, Z.H.N. and Andreeva, L.G. (1979). Some biological features and diseases of *Catharanthus roseus* in geographic investigations in the Rostov botanic garden. *Referativnyi Zhurnal,* 3: 108-110.

Slack, S.A., Traylor, J.A., Williams, H.E. and Nyland, G. (1976 a). Rose leaf curl, a distinct component of a disease complex which resembles rose wilt. *Plant Disease Reporter,* 60: 178-182.

Slack, S.A., Traylor, J.A., Nyland, G. and Williams, H.E. (1976 b). Symptoms, indexing and transmission of rose spring dwarf disease. *Plant Disease Reporter,* 60: 183-187.

Smart, C.D., Schneider, B., Blomquist, C. L., Guerra, L.J., Harrison, N.A., Ahrens, U., Lorenz, K.H., Seemüller, E. and Kirkpatrick, B.C. (1996). Phytoplasma-specific PCR primers based on sequences of the 16S-23S rRNA spacer region. *Applied Environmental Microbiology,* 62: 2988-2993.

Svoboba, G.H. and Blake, D.A. (1975). The phytochemistry and Pharmacology of *Catharanthus roseus* (L.) G. Don. In: *The Catharanthus alkaloids,* W.I. Taylor and N.R .Fornsworth (eds.) pp.45-83. Marcel Dekker Inc., New York.

Tamura, K., Dudley, J., Nei, M. and Kumar, S. (2007). MEGA4: Molecular Evolutionary Genetics Analysis (MEGA) software version 4.0. *Molecular Biology and Evolution,* 24: 1596–1599.

Tedeschi, R., Ferrato, V., Rossi, J. and Alma, A. (2006). Possible phytoplasma transovarial transmission in the psyllids *Cacopsylla melanoneura* and *Cacopsylla pruni. Plant Pathology,* 55: 18–24

Thomas, B.J. (1981). Some degeneration and dieback diseases of the rose. Ann. Rep. Glasshouse Crops Res. Inst.: 178-190.

Thompson, J.D., Higgins, D.G. and Gibson, T.J. (1994). CLUSTAL W: improving the sensitivity of progressive multiple sequence alignment through sequence weighting, position-specific gap penalties and weight matrix choice. *Nucleic Acids Res.* 22: 4673-4680.

Tipping, P.W. and Sindermann, A.B. (2000). Natural and augmented spread of rose rosette disease of multiflora rose in Maryland. *Plant Disease*, 12: 1344.

Verhoeven, M. and Horvat, F. (1972). La deformation des fleurs du lis: une grave maladie provoquee par un compexe de virus: methods d' identification. *Ann. Phytopathol.*, 4: 311-323.

Vicente, M., Caner, J. and July, J.R. (1974). Corpusculos do tipo micoplasma em *Hibiscus rosa-sinensis*. Arq. Inst. Biol. Saho Paulo, 41: 53-58.

Wei, W. (2007). Molecular Identification of a New Phytoplasma Strain Associated with the First Observation of Jujube Witches'-Broom Disease in Northeastern China Plant disease. *Plant Disease*, 91: 1364.

White, D.T., Blackhall, L.L., Scott, P.T. and Waldh, K.V. (1998). Phylogenetic positions of phytoplasma associated with dieback, yellow crinkle and mosaic diseases of papaya and their proposed inclusion in 'Candidatus phytoplasma australiensce' and a new taxon, 'Candidatus phytoplasma australasia'. *International Journal of Systematic and Evolutionary Microbiology*, 48: 941-951.

Yang, I.L. (1989). Dodder transmission and microscopic observations of red-bird cactus witches' broom disease. (1989). *J. Agric. Res. China*, 38: 463-467.

Zhao, Y., Sun, Q., Davis, R.E., Lee, I. and Liu, Q. (2007). First report of witches'-broom disease in a *Cannabis* species and its association with a phytoplasma of Elm yellows group (16SrV). *Plant Disease*, 91: 227.

Zhao, Y., Sun, Q., Wei, W., Davis, R. E., Wu, W. and Liu, Q. (2009). 'Candidatus Phytoplasma tamaricis', a novel taxon discovered in witches'-broom-diseased salt cedar (*Tamarix chinensis* Lour.) *International Journal of Systematic and Evolutionary Microbiology*, 59:2496.

In: Medicinal Plants and Sustainable Development
Editor: Chandra Prakash Kala

ISBN 978-1-61761-942-7
© 2011 Nova Science Publishers, Inc.

Chapter 10

Morphological Marker for Characterization of Two Important Endangered Himalayan Medicinal Plants: *Swertia chirayita* and *Swertia angustifolia*

Arvind Bhatt[*1] and *A. K. Bisht*[2]

[1]School of Biological Sciences, Universiti Sains Malaysia, 11800 Penang, Malaysia
[2]Department of Botany, Govt. Degree College, Narayan Nagar,
Didihat, Pithoragarh, Uttarakhand, India

Abstract

Many species of genus *Swertia* growing in the Himalayan region are used as medicine, especially for curing of fever. The present study deals with two endangered and medicinally important Swertia species of the Himalayan region - *S. chirayita* and *S. angustifolia*. Attempts were made to characterize these species by morphological markers.

Morphologically, seeds of *S. chirayita* and *S. angustifolia* differ in their external features i.e., colour, weight, length, width shape index and size index. These distinguishing characteristics features can be utilized for proper identification and reduce the chance of adulteration.

Keywords: Medicinal plants, adulteration, morphology, *Swertia chirayita* and *S. angustifolia*.

[*] Tel: 604-653-3828, Fax: 604-656-5125. E-mail: arvin_bhatt@rediffmail.com

Introduction

According to the estimates of WHO, over 80% of people in developing countries depend upon traditional medicine for their primary health care. The possible reason behind this may the perception of using medicinal plants having lesser side effects (Kamboj, 2000).

Unfortunately, the increase in demand has also increased the threat of depletion from the wild. Adulteration is one of the important issues pertaining to trade and marketing of medicinal plants.

Since the quality considerations are important for promoting medicinal plant products, therefore, it is essential to standardize methodologies. *S. chirayita* (Roxb. ex Fleming) Karsten, a critically rare plant species (Samant et al., 1998), distributed throughout temperate Himalaya (Kashmir to Bhutan and Khasia hills) between 1200-3000 m asl (Garg, 1987).

The whole plant is intensely bitter (Nadkarni, 1998) and used in various treatments i.e. blood purifier, skin disease, bitter tonic for fever, indigestion, laxative, anthelmentic, antidiarrhoetic, antiperiodic and bronchial asthma (Mukherjee, 1953; Dastur, 1956; Anonymous, 1976; Dey, 1980; Kirtikar and Basu, 1984). In ayurveda *S. chirayita* is used as kafpit samak, bransodhan, diban, aam pachan, pitsarak, anuloman, krimighan, raktasodhak, sothhar, dahahar and katu postik (Kapoor, 2000). Chirayita has great demand due to various uses in pharmaceutical industry. Every year about 600-1000 Qtl of Chirayita is imported into India and sold in Market @75/kg (Chauhan, 1999). Task Force Report on conservation and sustainable use of medicinal plants in India indicates that over 272 Quintal Chirayita (value over Rs 23 Lakhs) was imported from Nepal in 1997-98. This scenario affects the extent and magnitude of demand of Chirayita in the country.

Reckless exploitation with ever increasing popularity of this species owes largely the responsibility of the present state of true Chirayita have become a rare item in commerce. This has diverted focus to other available species of *Swertia*, particularly *S. angustifolia* which is morphological similar to the *S. chirayita* (Garg, 1987). This morphological similarity might be one of the causes of adulteration. The present investigations were carried out salient morphological seeds characterization of *S. chirayita* and *S. angustifolia*. Reliable and fast identification/ characterization of seeds have great importance and economical value particularly in medicinal plants sectors where adulteration is a common problem.

Identification of propagules (such as seeds) on the basis of external morphological characters can serve a simple and quick method of species identification. Species identification is an important step towards establishing standards for characterization based on morphological variations, particularly, the species which are used as an adulterants in pharmaceutical industry. *S. angustifolia* is most commonly used adulterant of *S. chirayita*.

Therefore, it is important to identify simple morphological markers for characterization of *S. chirayita* and *S. angustifolia*. The increasing demand leads to the overexploitation of species from the wild. As such, *S. chirayita* and *S. angustifolia* are classified as critically rare and endangered respectively (Samant et al., 1998).

Materials and Methods

Mature seeds were collected from all of the five distantly located populations of *S. chirayita* and *S. angustifolia* from west Himalaya (Table 1). Seeds obtained from different individuals were pooled for each population. The morphology of seed was studied by recording seed length, seed width, size index and shape index in three replicates of ten seeds each from each population (Sharma et al., 2000).

Seed length and width were measured using compound microscope (Hund Wetzlar, Japan). The length and width of the seed was calculated by multiplying the measurement of one ocular unit to the number of ocular units occupied by the length and width of the seed.

Weight of 50 seeds in three replicates was determined from each population of both the species with the help of electronic balance (Afcoset, ER-182A, India). Product of seed length and seed width (length x width) gave the size index and seed length divided by width gave the shape index of the seeds (Sharma et al., 2000).

Table 1. Morphological markers of seed (*Swertia chirayita* and *Swertia angustifolia*)

Code	Seed weight (mg/ 50 seeds)*	Seed length (μm)	Seed width (μm)	Size Index	Shape Index
Swertia chirayita					
Kanchula (Sc_1)	9.9 ± 0.52	842.17	619.04	521336.92	1.36
Kalaseer (Sc_2)	10.2 ± 0.32	808.13	598.66	483795.11	1.35
Pullag (Sc_3)	9.5 ± 0.70	825.84	618.93	511137.15	1.33
Dora (Sc_4)	10.4 ± 0.50	827.23	612.24	506463.29	1.35
Dugalbitha (Sc_5)	10.1 ± 0.95	808.13	619.04	500264.79	1.31
S. angustifolia					
Jalana (Sa_1)	0.86 ± 0.05	482.99	315.64	152450.96	1.53
Majkhali (Sa_2)	0.83 ± 0.15	477.55	292.51	139688.15	1.63
Katarmal (Sa_3)	0.86 ± 0.20	476.16	318.36	151590.29	1.50
Killburry (Sa_4)	0.76 ± 0.15	459.86	285.71	131386.60	1.61
Deenapani (Sa_5)	0.96 ± 0.20	404.44	314.28	127107.40	1.29

Results and Discussion

Seeds of both the species are easily identifiable on the basis of external morphological characters such as seed shape, colour and other features. Seeds differ in their colour, which varies from reddish brown (*S. chirayita*) to brown (*S. angustifolia*). However, both the species have globose seeds. There was considerable variation in seed weight of both the species. The seed weight of *S. angustifolia* was lesser and ranged between 0.76 mg / 50 seeds (Sa_4) to 0.96 mg (Sa_5) as compared to *S. chirayita* seeds [9.5 (Sc_3) to 10.4 mg / 50 seeds (Sc_4)]. Similarly other parameters showed higher values for *S. chirayita* as compared to *S. angustifolia* i.e., average seed length (808.13-842.17 μm - *S. chirayita* and 404.44-482.99 μm - *S. angustifolia*), seed width (598.66-619.04 μm - *S. chirayita* and 285.71-318.36 μm - *S.*

angustifolia) and size index (483795.11-521336.92- *S. chirayita* and 127107.40152450.96- *S. angustifolia*) (Table 1).

On the basis of distinguishing seed morphological characters of *S. chirayita* and *S. angustifolia*, a key has been developed for quick and correct identification of these species (Table 2). *S. chirayita* has two fimbriate glands on each petal while *S. angustifolia* have one gland on each petal.

Table 2. Identification key based on seed morphology for *S. chirayita* and *S. angustifolia*

Species	Seed weight (mg/50 Seeds)	Seed length (µm)	Seed width (µm)	Size Index	Shape Index
S. chirayita	9.5-10.4	808.13-842.17	598.66-619.04	483795.11-52133692	1.31-1.36
S. angustifolia	0.76-0.96	404.44-482.99	285.71-318.36	127107.40-152450.96	1.29-1.63

Present study revealed that the size of seeds is larger in *S. chirayita* as compared to *S. angustifolia*. Such difference in morphology of seeds between the two species of the same genera is often attributed to the differences in their genetic makeup besides the heterogeneity of the environment (Jazen, 1977). Substantial variation in seed size has been documented both among and within species in different sets of condition (Michael et al., 1988; Westoby et al., 1992). In present case, the variation in seed mass was observed among the populations of both the species. These differences in seed mass distribution among populations can be attributed to difference in genotype or environmental /habitat conditions. Variations in seed mass can also occur due to different position of seeds on mother plant, resulting in the variation in seed filling (Gutterman, 1992). Further, in a population where mother plant is subjected to differing environmental conditions (temperature, availability of soil water and nutrients etc.) such variation in seed mass between the populations can occur (Milberg et al., 1996). Under present investigation, substantial variation in seed size was observed between the target species. This has been previously reported for other species (Harper et al., 1970; Leishmann et al., 1995) and evolutionary causes are found responsible for such variation (Silvertown and Charlesworth, 2001). This study indicates the possibility of using seed morphology, such as, seed weight, colour, shape etc., for easy segregation of species, which can finally reduce the chances of adulteration. Previous study also reports that the morphological variation in *S. chirayita* and *S. angustifolia*, which can be utilize for the species identification in nature (Table 3). These characteristics of plant can serve as the tool to identify the two species of *Swertia* (Karan et al., 1997). Species identification on the basis of seed morphology can reduce unnecessary uprooting of the plant for the sake of identification. Moreover, it can help in checking large-scale adulteration.

Table 3. Morphological characteristics of target species

Characteristics	S. chirtayita*	S. angustifolia
The Plant	80-110 cm long, stout, branching towards the top	30-70 cm long, trichotomously branched
Stem	Robust, round, angular near the top, green	Purplish green, quadrangular
Leaf	70-90x35-40 mm sessile, elliptic, acute, 7-nerved	2.5-7x0.8-2 cm subsessile, narrowly lanceolate, acute, 3-5 nerved
Flower	Tetramerous, dia 10-12 mm	Tetramerous, 0.6-1.2 cm across
Calyx	4, gamosepalous, smaller than corolla, oblong, tip acute, green, 1- nerved, 5-6 mm	4, partite, shorter or longer than corolla
Corolla	4, gamosepalous, greenish petals which are violet in the centre, two glands on each petal, each gland is a depression which is bright green inside. Margin of the depression is covered by long purple hair which converge to form a summit 6x4 mm	4, ovate-lanceolate, one solitary gland at base of each petal which is covered by glaborous scale. Pits margin fimbriate.
Androecium	4, versatile, filament and anthers purple in colour, filament base slightly dilated	4, filamentous, linear anthers oblong

*- Karan et al (1997).

Conclusion

The present study could be helpful for the characterization / identification of *S. chirayita* and *S. angutifolia*. The possibility of using seed morphology such as, seed weight, colour, shape size index and shape Index, can be used for species identification even at the preliminary stage in order to reduce the chances of adulteration.

The seed morphological characters of species can be used as a taxonomic trait, but should be combined with other traits for the diagnostic determination of species.

Acknowledgments

The authors thank Dr. U. Dhar, Dr R.S. Rawal and Dr. I. D. Bhatt for their help and support during the course of this study.

References

Anonymous (1976). *The Wealth of India*. CSIR Publication, New Delhi. Vol. X: 77-81.
Bewley, J.D. and Black, M. (1994). *Seeds*. Physiology of Development and Germination. Plenum Press, New York, London.
Bhattacharjee, S.K. (2001). *Handbook of Medicinal Plants*. Pointer Publishers, Jaipur.
Chauhan, N.S. (1999). *Medicinal and Aromatic Plants of Himachal Pradesh*. Indus Publishing Company, New Delhi.

Dastur, J.F. (1956). *Medicinal Plants of the India and Pakistan.* D.B. Taraporewala Sons and Co. Ltd., Bombay.

Datta, S.C. (1965). Germination of seeds of two arid zone species. *Bull. Bot. Soc. Beng.,* 19: 51-53.

Dey, A.C. (1980). *Indian Medicinal Plants Used in Ayurvedic Preparation.* Bishen Singh Mahendra Pal Singh, Dehradun. India.

Garg, S. (1987). *Gentianaceae of the North West Himalaya (a revision).* International Bioscience Monograph 17, Today and Tomorrow's Publication Co, New Delhi.

Gutterman, Y. (1992). Maternal effect on seeds during development. In: *Seeds: The Ecology of Regeneration in Plant Communities.* Fenner, M. (Ed.). pp. 27- 59.Wallingford, UK, Cab International.Hammett, K.R.W., Murray, B.G., Matkham, K.R., Hallett, I.C. and Osterloh, I. (1996). New interspecifichybrid in *Lathyrus* (Leguminosae): *Lathyrus annuus x L. hieroslymitanus. Bot. J. Linn. Soc.,* 122: 89-101.

Harper, J.L., Lovell, P.H. and Moore, K.G. (1970). The shapes and size of seeds. *Ann. Rev. Ecol. Syst.,* 1: 327-356.

Janzen, D.H. (1977). Variation in seed size within a crop of a Costa Rican *Mucuna andreana* (Leguminosae). *Am J of Bot.,* 64: 347-349.

Kamboj, V.P. 2000. Herbal medicine. *Current Science,* 95: 57-65.

Kapoor, L. D. *(2000). Handbook of Ayurvedic Medicinal Plants.* CRC Press, Boca Raton, USA.

Karan, M., Vasisht, K., Handa, S.S. (1997). Morphological and chromatographic comparison of certain Indian species of *Swertia. J. Med. Aromat.. Plant. Sci.,* 19: 955-963.

Kirtikar, K.R. and Basu, B.D. (1984). *Indian Medicinal Plants* - Volume III, Bishen Singh Mahendra Pal Singh, Dehradun, India.

Leishman, M.R., Westoby, M. and Jurado, E. (1995). Correlates of seed size variation: a comparison among fire temperate floras. *J Ecol.,* 83: 517-529.

Michaels, H.J., Benner, B., Hartgerink, A.P., Lee, T.D. and Rice S. (1988). Seed size variation: magnitude, distribution and ecological correlates. *Evolutionary Ecology,* 2: 157-166.

Milberg, P., Anderson, L., Elfverson, C. and Regner, S. (1996). Germination characteristics of seeds differing in mass. *Seed Science Res.,* 6: 191-197.

Mukherjee, B. (1953). *The Indian Pharmaceutical Codex.* Vol. 1, C.S.I.R., New Delhi.

Nadkarni, K.M. (1998). *(Reprint), Indian Plants and Drugs with their Medicinal Properties and Uses.* Asiatic Publishing House Delhi.

Samant, S. S., Dhar, U. and Palni, L. M. S. (1998). *Medicinal Plants of Indian Himalaya: Diversity, Distribution potential Values.* Gyanodaya Prakashan, Nainital.

Sharma, K.D., Singh, B.M., Sharma, T.N., Katoch, M . and Guleria, S. (2000). Molecular analysis of variability in *Podophyllum hexandrum* Royle- an endangered medicinal herb of north western Himalaya. *Plant Gen. Res. Newsletter,* 124: 57-61.

Silvertown, J. and Charlesworth, D. (2001). *Introduction to Plant Population Biology.* 4th ed. Blackwell Science.

Westoby, M., Jurado, E. and Leishman, M. (1992). Comparative evolutionary ecology of seed size. *Trends Ecol. and Evol.,* 7: 368-372.

In: Medicinal Plants and Sustainable Development
Editor: Chandra Prakash Kala

ISBN 978-1-61761-942-7
© 2011 Nova Science Publishers, Inc.

Chapter 11

Aconitum naviculare:
A Threatened and Endemic Medicinal Plant of the Himalaya

Bharat Babu Shrestha[1]* and Stephano Dall'Acqua[2]
[1]Central Department of Botany, Tribhuvan University, Kathmandu, Nepal
[2]Department of Pharmaceutical Sciences, University of Padova,
Padova, Italy

Abstract

Aconitum naviculare, a Himalayan endemic, is an endangered medicinal herb of the alpine region. With recorded distribution from west Nepal to Bhutan, including Tibet, *A. naviculare* is highly prioritized ethnomedicinal plant. The whole plant is medicinally used. Most commonly, aqueous extract of this plant has been used against various kinds of fever. The plant is perennial with biennial tuberous root and annual aerial parts. Phytochemical analyses have led to the isolation of 11 alkaloids, 3 flavonoid glycosides and 4 phenol glycosides. In a preliminary bioassay, two alkaloids (navirine B and chellespontine) showed some cytotoxic activities against tumor cell lines [colon (LoVo) and ovarian (2008) cell lines]. Due to narrow distribution range and habitat degradation, the natural population of this plant is highly fragmented and declining. Some attempts have been made to domesticate this plant in Manang and Mustang districts of Nepal. Given the high value of *A. naviculare* in ethnomedicine of remote mountains, natural rarity, and dwindling population, we recommend to develop and implement conservation management plan for this plant at regional level which would include monitoring natural population, protection of habitats, and development of agro-technology for domestication.

Keywords: conservation, ethnomedicinal uses, phytochemistry, threat.

* E-mail: bhabashre@yahoo.com

Introduction

The Himalayan region is rich in medicinal plants and the traditional knowledge of their uses. Given the low access to modern health care systems, high mountain people of the Himalaya have been traditionally using >50 % of locally available plant species for their health care (Kunwar and Bussmann, 2008). Due to renewed interest on ethnomedicinal plants as source of potential bioactive natural products (Cordell, 2000; Ji et al., 2009), several research groups worldwide have been working on phytochemisty and bioactivity of the Himalayan medicinal plants (e.g. Taylor et al., 1995; Tomimori, 2000; Rajbhandari et al., 2007). Therefore, the number of references on phytochemistry and bioactivity of the Himalayan medicinal plants is rapidly increasing in recent time. However, the biological/ecological studies of the medicinal plants of the Himalaya are lagging behind, and it is available only for a few high profile species (Dhar et al., 2000; Ghimire, 2008).

Aconitum species, well known for the presence of bioactive compounds (Pelletier and Mody, 1981; Pelletier et al., 1983), are important components of ethnomedicine (Baral and Kurmi, 2006) and trade of medicinal plants in Nepal (Olsen and Larsen, 2003). Most of the medicinally important *Aconitum* species have been categorized as critically endangered in their natural habitats (CAMP, 1998). Out of 34 species of *Aconitum* reported from Nepal, fifteen species are endemic to Nepal and twenty two to the Himalaya (Press et al., 2000). Among these Himalayan endemic species, *Aconitum naviculare* is naturally rare and highly valued ethnomedicinal plant which is found in trans-Himalayan alpine regions from western Nepal to Bhutan including Tibet. Recently, some phytochemical and biological studies of *A. naviculare* have been undertaken. In this review, we have summarized ethnomedicinal uses, phytochemistry and biological information available for this species. These information will be important in research and development (R and D) effort for this valuable medicinal plant in future.

Species Identification

Aconitum naviculare (Figure 1) is a perennial herb with fusiform white tuberous root; stems ascending, 10-30 cm; leaves mostly congested in proximal part of stems, petiolate, blade orbicular-cordate, deeply 3-5 lobed, lobes obovate, further shallowly 2- or 3- lobuled, lobules dentate, teeth obtuse, leaves of distal part of stem 1 or 2, much smaller than proximal one, sub sessile, deeply 3 lobed; flowers in loose raceme; sepals tinged dull reddish purple/violet blue, with dark purple veinlets, lower surface pubescent, persistent in fruits, helmet navicular; petals clawed, head 3-4 mm; fruit of 5 follicles, sparsely pubescent (Ohba et al., 2008).

Life History

Aconitum naviculare is a perennial herb with biennial tuberous root and annual aerial parts. The plant reproduces sexually by seeds. The tuberous root with apical dormant bud functions as perennating organs.

Seeds germinate and winter buds sprout during June when the soil surface is exposed after snow melt. In *in vitro* experiment, the seed germination was 49% after ten weeks of cold storage, and it declined with storage period (Shrestha, 2010).

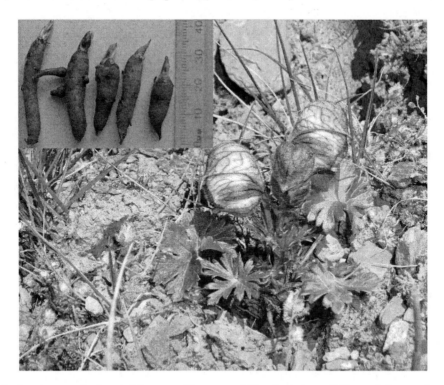

Figure 1. *Aconitum naviculare* in Manang valley, central Nepal, at about 4300 m asl. Inset: tuberous root.

Germination was epigeal, in which the elongating hypocotyle carries the cotyledons above the substrate surface, which expand and become green to be active photosynthetically. Flowering occurs from mid September to early October, and fruiting during October. The persistent sepals cover the developing fruit.

In average a plant bears three flowers, and a fruit (with five follicles) contains 55 seeds (Shrestha, 2010). Seeds are small (mass: 0.47 µg/seed) with a lamellate (gill like structures) seed coat.

In addition to gravity dispersal, seeds are dispersed by strong continental wind. Seeds remain dormant until next growing season.

Ethnomedicinal Uses

Aconitum naviculare is an important ethnomedicinal plant of the trans-Himalayan region including Tibet. *Amchis* (traditional herbal healer trained in Tibetan medicine) as well as individual local people use this plant for traditional healthcare.

It is the most prioritized species in term effectiveness and frequency of use among the medicinal plants used by local people of Manang, central Nepal (Bhattarai et al., 2007;

Shrestha et al., 2007). *A. naviculare* has been used in a wide range of internal disorders. In Dolpa (western Nepal), the plant is used against poisoning, fever due to poisoning, and bile fever (Lama et al., 2001). In Mustang (central Nepal), the plant is used in disorders of gall bladder in Mustang, central Nepal (Chetri et al., 2006).

In Manang (central Nepal), it is used against fever, headache, jaundice, high blood pressure and cold (Bhattarai et al., 2006; Shrestha et al., 2007). In Tibet, the plant is used as sedative, analgesic and febrifuge (Gao et al., 2004) as well as for the treatment of gastricism, hepatitis and nephritis (Cao et al., 2008). This plant has been included in the list of medicinal plants of Bhutan (Nawang, 1996) and flora of Sikkim (Shrivastava, 1998), but we could not find references on ethmomedicinal use of this plant in these areas.

The whole plant body is medicinally important. *Amchis* prefer to use tuberous root because this part is considered more effective than other parts. However, local people in Manang often collect aerial parts when the plant is in bloom (Shrestha et al., 2007).

In absence of flower, *A. naviculare* is often confused with associated species of *Geranium* and *Delphinium*. Shepherds are the main collectors of this plant for use in individual households. They bring the plant material down to the village and share with relatives and privileged people in the society. Sometimes, they send dry material of *A. naviculare* to their relatives in Kathmandu, the capital city of Nepal.

The collected plant material is air dried in shade by hanging inside the house (Figure 2). In some households, the dried plant material is crushed and stored in airtight bottles.

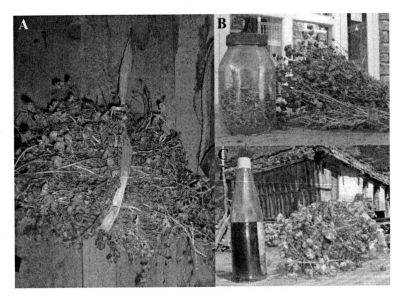

Figure 2. Traditional use of *Aconitum naviculare* in Manang, central Nepal. A) Arial part of flowering *A. naviculare* hanged on the wall inside the home for air drying, B) Storage of crushed *A. naviculare* in plastic bottle, and C) Aqueous extract of the plant prepared for immediate use by a shepherd.

During administration, about one gram of dried plant material is boiled with two glasses of water for about half an hour and the black, bitter decoction is drunk twice a day (Shrestha et al., 2007).

The bitter decoction makes the patient weak, probably due to presence of antibiotics in the plant material. To restore vigor the decoction is often taken along with *ghee* (butter).

Phytochemistry

Although the chemical constituents of plants of the genus *Aconitum* have been extensively studied, mainly due to the presence of toxic and bioactive alkaloids, there are only few works regarding the phytochemical composition of *A. naviculare*.

Eleven alkaloids, three flavonoid glycosides and four phenol glycosides have been reported from this plant.

Among them five alkaloids and three flavonoid glycosides are known only from this plant while the rests are also reported from other plants. Gao et al. (2004) isolated and characterized six alkaloids (Figure 3); they are navirine (compound 1), isoatisine (2), hordenine (3), atisine (4), hetisinone (5) and delfissinol (6). Among them navirine (1) was reported as a new diterpenoid alkaloid while other five alkaloids are known in other plants too. Cao et al. (2008) reported two new C-20 alkaloids: naviculine A (7) and B (8). Other terpenoid alkaloids were reported by our research group (Dall'Acqua et al. 2008); they are navirine B (9), navirine C (10) and chellespontine (11). This latter one was previously isolated from aerial part of *Consolida hellespontica* (Desai et al., 1993).

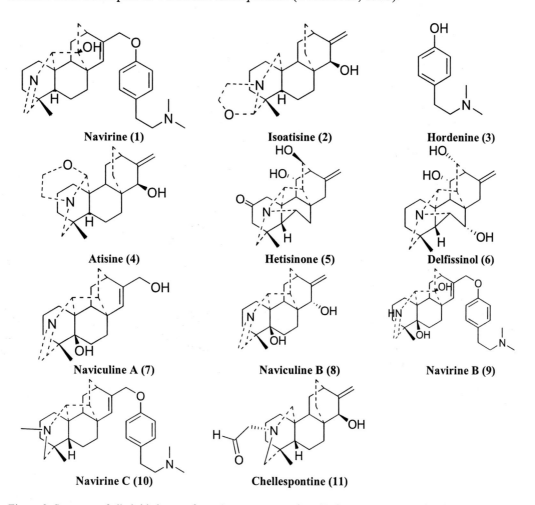

Figure 3. Structure of alkaloids known from *Aconitum naviculare* (References, compound 1-6: Gao et al. 2004; 7-8: Cao et al., 2008; and 9-11: Dall'Acqua et al., 2008).

Bioactivity of the diterpenoid alkaloids from *A. naviculare* has been assessed in a few instances.

In an attempt to evaluate cytotoxic activity against tumor cell lines, the navirine B (9) was found active against colon and ovarian cell lines (LoVo and 2008, respectively) while chellespontine (11) was active only against LoVo cells (Dall'Acqua et al., 2008).

Further biological studies are needed for scientific validation of traditional uses of this plant and to understand potential mechanism of action as well as potential toxic effects.

Flavonoid and phenolic glycoside are other classes of phytoconstituents commonly found in the plants of genus *Aconitum*. Three new glycoside derivatives of flavonoid (compounds 12-14) were reported by Shrestha et al. (2006) as quercetin and kaempferol glycosides with two to five sugar units (Figure 4).

Four glycoside derivatives of phenol (Figure 5) have been also reported from *Aconitum naviculare*; they are kaempferol glycosides (15 and 16) and phenylpropanoids glycosides (17 and 18) (Dall'Acqua et al., 2008). Such types of glycoside derivatives of phenol are relatively common in several plant species.

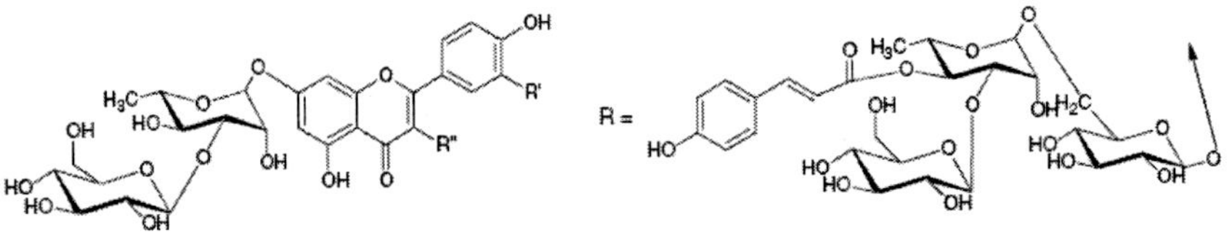

(12): R′=H; R″=R (13): R′=OH; R″=R (14): R′= R″=OH

Figure 4. Structure of flavonoid glycosides isolated from *Aconitum naviculare* (Shrestha et al., 2006).

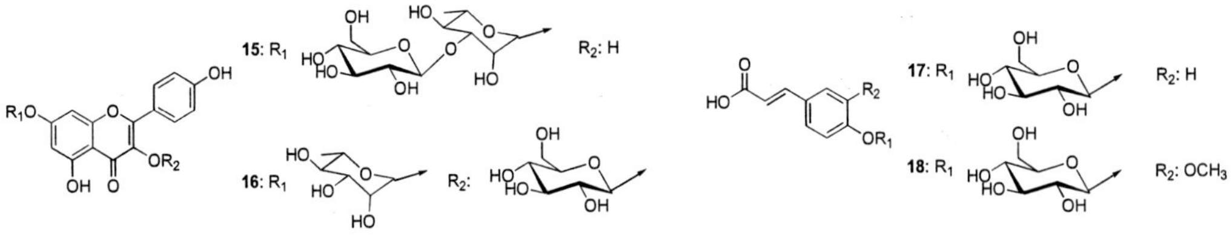

Figure 5. Structure of phenol derivatives isolated from *Aconitum naviculare* (Dall'Acqua et al., 2008).

Distribution and Abundance

Aconitum naviculare is endemic to the Himalaya (Stainton, 1997) with recorded distribution from Bhutan to western Nepal including Tibet. In Bhutan, the species is mainly found in northern districts (Upper Mangde Chu, Upper Bumthang Chu, Upper Kuru Chu and Upper Kulong Chu districts) between 3960 and 4570 m asl (Grierson and Long, 1984).

In Sikkim, it has been reported from Thangu-Giagong between 4600 and 4900 m asl (Shrivastava, 1998). In Nepal, the plant is found in trans-Himalayan regions of Solukhumbu, Manang, Mustang and Dolpa districts. From Solukhumbu district (eastern Nepal), *A. naviculare* has been collected at 4000 m asl along Benikharka-Yurigolcha route (pers. obs. by BBS of the specimen (no. 61658) collected by Dr K.R. Rajbhandy in 1985 and deposited in National Herbarium of Nepal, Kathmandu, KATH). In Manang district, *A. naviculare* is mainly found in Manang valley from 4090 to 4650 m asl (Shrestha and Jha, 2009). In Mustang, specimen of this plant has been collected from Chabarbu (4010 m asl), Ghemi-Jhaite (4350 m asl), Thanti (4520 m asl) and Kungale (4771 m asl) (Ohba et al. 2008). Specimens of *A. naviculare* has been also collected form Dho-Tarap (4200 m asl), Tsharka (4230 m asl) and Mukut Himal camp (elevation not mentioned) area of Dolpa district (Ghimire et al. 2008). In Tibet, the plant is found in southern part between 3200 and 5000 m asl (Liangqian and Kodata, 2001). Gao et al. (2004) collected specimens of this plant from National Forest Park of Huzhubei Mountain, Qinghai province, Tibet.

A. naviculare grows in alpine regions. The common habitats are meadow, grassy slope, rocky slope, cliff edge and juniper scrub. In Manang (central Nepal), the plant is found exclusively on sunny southern slope (aspect: 108° SE to 240° SW), often in association with sclerophyllous and thorny plant species such as *Juniperus squamata*, *Ephedra gerardiana*, *Cotoneaster microphyllus*, *Caragana gerardiana* and *Berberis* spp. (Shrestha and Jha 2009). These thorny species appear to be important for the persistence of local population of this species because of the protective role played by them against livestock damage and human collection (Shrestha, 2010).

A. naviculare is naturally rare with restricted distribution. Quantitative data on abundance of this species is mostly lacking. However, it has been reported as 'rare' in Dolpa, westen Nepal (Lama et al., 2001) and Bhutan (Nawang, 2006). In Manang valley, central Nepal, the estimated area of occupancy of this plant was about 50 ha with average density of 7 plants/m^2 within the area of occupancy (Shrestha, 2010).

Threat Status and Conservation

Shrestha (2010) evaluated threat status of *Aconitum naviculare* against IUCN Redlist threat categories and found that the species is qualified for 'endagered' category in Nepal based on geographic range size and population fragmentation (criteria: B2ab (iii)). Similar regional assessment of this species in Sikkim, Bhutan and Tibet is not available.

Being endemic to alpine region of the Himalaya, *A. naviculare* belongs to a group of plants with 'nowhere to go' in the context of global warming. Such species are of grave conservation concern (Hawkins et al., 2008). In addition to this, *A. naviculare* is naturally rare and habitat specialist. The population and habitat of this plant are under high anthropogenic pressure. In Dolpa, western Nepal, harvesting of whole plant for medicine is a major anthropogenic threat to this plant (Lama et al., 2001).

In Manang valley, central Nepal, the aerial part of the plant is collected before seed set (Shrestha et al., 2007). In this valley the habitats of *A. naviculare* coincides with the areas with high livestock pressure. In five of the six sites examined in Manang valley, this plant is mainly confined in the bushes of sclerophyllous and thorny species (Shrestha and Jha, 2009). In such bushes, collection by human and damage by livestock trampling are relatively low.

There is no recorded trade of *A. naviculare* in Nepal and elsewhere. Due to lack of trade value, this plant has been overlooked by policy makers and researchers. Because the plant is Himalayan endemic with 'nowhere to go' and highly prioritized in traditional medicine, *A. naviculare* deserve conservation management with legal status.

The abundance of this naturally rare plant appears to be declining due to human collection for traditional uses, and habitat degradation (Shrestha, 2010). Himalayan Amchi Association (HAA) and a private herbal farm (Khamso Nature Product) have initiated to domesticate this plant in Mustang and Manang, respectively, in small scale (per. obs. of BBS).

Given the high value of *A. naviculare* in ethnomedicine of remote mountains, natural rarity, and dwindling population, we recommend to develop and implement conservation management plan for this plant at regional level which would include monitoring natural population, protection of habitats, and development of agro-technology for domestication.

Conclusion

Aconitum naviculare is biologically and phytochemically less studied medicinal plant of the alpine Himalaya, with recorded distribution from Bhutan to west Nepal.

Phytochemical analysis done so far has led to the isolation of eleven alkaloids, three flavonoid glycosides, and four phenol glycosides. Though the plant has been most preferred for the treatment of common diseases, such as, fever and headache, there was no commercial collection from the wild.

However, naturally rare and fragmented population, habitat degradation due to high grazing pressure, and collection of the plant before seed set warrant for the need of conservation of this important plant species.

Acknowledgments

We are grateful to Prof. Mohan Bikarma Gewali, Central Department of Chemistry, Tribhuvan University, and Prof. Pramod Kumar Jha, Central Department of Botany, Tribhuvan University, Kathmandu, for their comments on the first draft of this manuscript.

References

Baral, S.R. and Kurmi, P.P. (2006). *A Compendium of Medicinal Plants in Nepal*. R. Sharma, Kathmandu.

Bhattarai, S., Chaudhary, R.P., and Taylor, R.S.L. (2006). Ethnomedicinal plants used by the people of Manang district, central Nepal. *Journal of Ethnobiology and Ethnomedicine*, 2:41 doi: 10.1186/1746-4269-2-41. http://www.ethnobiomed.com/content/2/1/41.

Bhattarai, S., Chaudhary, R.P., and Taylor, R.S.L. (2007). Prioritization and trade of ethnomedicinal plants by the people of Manang district, central Nepal. In: *Local Effects of Global Changes in the Himalayas: Manang, Nepal*. Chaudhary, R.P., Aase, T.H., Vetaas, O.R. and Subedi, B.P. (eds.). pp. 151–169. Tribhuvan University, Nepal and University of Bergen, Norway.

C.A.M.P. (1998). *Selected medicinal plants of northern, northeastern and central India: conservation assessment and management plans (CAMP)*. Forest Department of Uattar Pradesh, Lucknow.

Cao, J.-X., Li, L.-B., Ren, J., Jiang, S.-P., Tian, R.-R., Chen, X.-L., Peng, S.-L., Zhang, J. and Zhu, H.-J. (2008). Two new C20-diterpernoid alkaloids from the Tibetan medicinal plant *Aconitum naviculare* Stapf. *Helvetica Chimica Acta,* 91:1954–1960.

Chetri, M., Chapagain, N.R. and Neupane, B.D. (2006). *Flowers of Mustang: A Pictorial Guide Book.* National Trust for Nature Conservation, Annapurna Conservation Area Project, Upper Mustang Biodiversity Conservation Project, Kathmandu, Nepal.

Cordell, G.A. (2000). Biodiversity and drug discovery – a symbiotic relationship. *Phytochemistry,* 55: 463–480.

Dall'Acqua, S., Shrestha, B.B., Gewali, M.B., Jha, P.K., Carrara, M. and Innocenti, G. (2008). Diterpenoid alkaloids and phenolic glycosides from *Aconitum naviculare* (Brühl) Stapf. *Natural Product Communication,* 3: 1985–1989.

Desai, H.K., Joshi, B.S., Pelletier, S.W., Sener, B., Bingol, F. and Baykal, T. (1993). New alkaloids from *Consolida hellespontica. Heterocycles,* 36: 1081–1089.

Dhar, U., Rawal, R.S. and Upreti, J. (2000). Setting priorities for conservation of medicinal plants – a case study in the Indian Himalaya. *Biological Conservation*, 95: 57–65.

Gao, L., Wei, X. and Yang, L. (2004). A New diterpenoid alkaloid from a Tibetan medicinal herb *Aconitum naviculare* Stapf. *Journal of Chemical Research,* 4: 307–308.

Ghimire, S.K., Samkota, I.B., Oli, B.R. and Parajuli, R.R. (2008). *Non-Timber Forest Products of Nepal Himalaya*. WWF Nepal, Kathmandu.

Ghimire S.K. (2008). Medicinal plants in the Nepal Himalaya: current issue, sustainable harvesting, knowledge gaps and research priorities. In: *Medicinal Plants in Nepal: An Anthology of Contemporary Research*. Jha, P.K., Karmacharya, S.B., Chettri, M.K. Thapa, C.B. and Shrestha, B.B. (eds.). pp. 25–42. Ecological Society (ECOS), Kathmandu.

Grierson, A.J.C. and Long, D.G. (1984). *Flora of Bhutan*. Vol 1, Part 2. pp. 188–462. Royal Botanical Garden, Edinburgh.

Hawkins, B., Sharrock, S. and Havens, K. (2008). *Plants and Climate Change: Which Future*? Botanic Gardens Conservation International, Richmond (UK).

Ji, H.-F., Li, X.-J. and Zhang, H.-Y. (2009). Natural products and drug discovery. *EMBO Reports*, 10: 194–200.

Kunwar, R., and Bussmann, R.W. 2008. Ethnobotany in the Nepal Himalaya. *Journal of Ethnobiology and Ethnomedicine*, 4: 24 doi:10.1186/1746–4269–4–24

Lama Y.C., Ghimire, S.K. and Aumeeruddy-Thomas, Y. (2001). *Medicinal Plants of Dolpo: Amchis' Knowledge and Conservation*. WWF Nepal Program, Kathmandu.

Liangqian, L. and Kodata, Y. (2001). *Aconitum* L. In: *Flora of China*, vol. 6, *Caryophyllaceae through Lardizabalaceae.* Zhengyi, W., Raven, P.H. and Deyuan, H. (eds.). pp. 149–222. Science Press, Beijing, and Missouri Botanical Garden Press, St. Louis.

Nawang, R. (1996). Medicinal Plants. In: *FAO Non-Wood Forest Products of Bhutan*. Food and Agriculture Organization (FAO) of United Nations, Bangkok, Thailand. URL: http://www.fao.org/docrep/X5335E/X5335E00. htm (accessed on Dec 19, 2008)

Ohba, H., Iokawa, Y. and Sharma, L.R. eds. (2008). *Flora of Mustang, Nepal.* Kodansha Scientific Ltd, Tokyo.

Olsen, C.S., and Larsen, H.O. (2003). Alpine medicinal plant trade and Himalayan mountain livelihood strategies. *The Geographical Journal,* 169: 243–254.

Pelletier, S.W. and Mody, N.V. (1981). Diterpenoid alkaloids. In: The Alkaloids, Vol. 17. R.H.F. Manske (ed.). pp. 1–103. Academic Press. New York.

Pelletier, S.W., Mody, N.V., Joshi, B.S. and Schramm, L.C. (1983). 13C and proton NMR shift assignments and physical constants of C19- diterpenoid alkaloids. In: *Alkaloids: Chemical and Biological Perspectives*, Vol. 2. S.W. Pelletier (ed.). pp. 206–462. John Wiley Sons, New York.

Press, J.R., Shrestha, K.K. and Sutton, D.A. (2000). *Annotated Checklist of the Flowering Plants of Nepal.* The Natural History Museum, London.

Rajbhandari, M., Mentel, R., Jha, P.K., Chaudhary, R.P., Bhattarai, S., Gewali, M.B., Karmacharya, N., Hipper, M. and Lindequist, U. (2007). Antiviral activity of some plants used in Nepalese traditional medicine. eCAM, doi:10.1093/ecam/nem156.

Shrestha, B.B. (2010). *Ecology and Phytochemisty of Selected Medicinal Plants in Central Nepal.* Ph D dissertation, Central Department of Botany, Tribhuvan University, Kathmandu.

Shrestha, B.B. and Jha, P.K. (2009). Habitat range of two alpine medicinal plants in a trans-Himalayan dry valley, central Nepal. *Journal of Mountain Science*, 6: 66–77.

Shrestha B.B., Jha, P.K. and Gewali, M.B. (2007). Ethomedicinal use and distribution of *Aconitum naviculare* (Bruhl) Stapf in upper Manang central Nepal. In: *Local Effects of Global Changes in the Himalayas: Manang, Nepal*. Chaudhary, R.P., Aase, T.H., Vetaas, O.R. and Subedi, B.P. (eds.). pp 171–181. Tribhuvan University, Nepal and University of Bergen, Norway.

Shrestha B.B., Dall'Acqua, S., Gewali, M.B., Jha, P.K. and Innocenti, G. (2006). New flavonoid glycosides from *Aconitum naviculare* (Bruhl) Stapf, a medicinal herb from the trans-Himalayan region of Nepal. *Carbohydrate Research,* 341: 2161–2165.

Shrivastava, R.C. (1998). *Flora of Sikkim (Ranunculaceae – Moringaceae).* Oriental Enterprises, Dehradun, India.

Stainton, A. (1997). *Flowers of the Himalayas: A Supplement.* Oxford University Press, New Delhi.

Taylor, R.S.L., Manandhar, N.P. and Towers, G.H.N. (1995). Screening of selected medicinal plants of Nepal for antimicrobial activities. *Journal of Ethnopharmacology,* 46:153–159.

Tomimori, T. (2000). On the constituents and biological activities of some Nepalese medicinal plants [Article in Japanese] [Abstract]. *Yakugaku Zasshi,* 120: 591–606.

C. Indigenous Knowledge on Medicinal Plants

In: Medicinal Plants and Sustainable Development
Editor: Chandra Prakash Kala

ISBN 978-1-61761-942-7
© 2011 Nova Science Publishers, Inc.

Chapter 12

Do Animals Eat What We Do? Observations on Medicinal Plants Used By Humans and Animals of Mundanthurai Range, Tamil Nadu

Jayanti Ray Mukherjee [1,4*], *V. Chelladurai* [2], *J. Ronald*,
G. S. Rawat [1], *J.P. Mani* [2] *and M. A. Huffman* [3]

[1] Wildlife Institute of India, Chandrabani, Dehradun, Uttarakhand, India
[2] Survey of Medicinal Plant Unit, Siddha, Palayamkottai, Tamil Nadu, India
[3] Primate Research Institute, Kyoto University, Inuyama Aichi 484 Japan.

Abstract

Though humans are known to have learnt the use of medicinal plants by observing animals, rarely have studies compared their use. Using published literature, interviews, and personal observations, we compared the medicinal plant used by the Kani tribals, to those ingested by wild animals in Kalakad-Mundanthurai Tiger reserve in southern India. By dividing Mundathurai range into four zones according to vegetation types, we recorded plant species, estimated their conservation status, and noted animal use of these medicinal plants. Within our study area, the highest number of medicinal plants occurred in the dry forests, followed by the wet-evergreen patches, and the moist deciduous forests. We documented 260 plant species of medicinal importance that are used by Kani tribals for 45 different ailments, 44% of which are also used by wild animals. Interestingly, the highest numbers of plant species consumed by wild animals are known to have therapeutic properties against skin disorders and infections, followed by those for fever and as general health tonics. We also found that approximately 7.7% of the medicinal plants used by Kani tribals are endemic, among which 10 species fall under rare and endemic IUCN category. Our study provides baseline information on medicinal

---

[*] E-mail: jayanti.rm@gmail.com; Phone number: 011-435-8818674. Current address: Dept of Wildland Resources, Utah State University, Logan, Utah 84321, USA.

plants used by Kani tribals and wild animals that might be crucial for future assessment of the status of these species within the Tiger reserve.

Keywords: conservation status of medicinal plants, ethnobotany, Kalakad-Mundanthurai Tiger reserve, medicinal plants used by Kani tribals, rare and endemic medicinal species.

Introduction

The interdependence of plants and human beings dates back to prehistory. It was Harshberger, who first described "ethnobotany" as the science of "the use of plants by aboriginal people" (Jain and Mudgal, 1999). Since then, ethnobotany has dealt with the natural relationship of humans and plants. It is said that humans have acquired much of this knowledge from nature by observing animals treating their own ailments and then testing these crude drugs themselves to evaluate their curative, tonic or hallucinogenic powers (e.g. Huffman, 2003; Pope, 1969). In fact, animals have a quite high probability to teach us something about the medicinal use of plants and 'zoopharmacognosy' is a branch of science to describe the process by which an animal selects plants or plant parts to cure themselves (Rodriquez and Wrangham, 1993). Since most of the wild plants exhibit several healing properties, it is believed that the wild animals that feed on a variety of food plants get enough nutrients and therapeutic elements to keep themselves healthy. This was first suggested by Janzen (1978), who argued that if animals can avoid feeding on leaves with toxic compounds, they may very well consume plants with medicinal properties that would help keep themselves in good health.

Virtually, quite a few species of wild plants, which have anthelmentic properties, are known to be consumed by wild animals as a part of their diet. Elephants are known to go for selected species of plants when they suffer from diarrhoea (VC and JRM, personal observation), while cases of wild African elephants thought to ease difficult labour by feeding on wild plants have also been reported (Huffman, 2003). Several studies have documented the use of medicinal plants by the primates, particularly chimpanzees, baboons, and gorillas across equatorial Africa, swallowing leaves to purge themselves of some intestinal parasites (Rodriguez and Wrangham, 1993; Wrangham, 1995; Huffman, 1997; Huffman and Caton, 2001). Chimpanzees are also reported to chew the bitter pith of plants, which brings a change in their health and stamina and reduce parasite load within 24 hours after ingestion (Huffman and Seifu, 1989; Huffman et al., 1993). A study (Carrai et al., 2003) documented in lemurs (*Propithecus verreauxi*) show that there is a significant increase in the ingestion of tannins in pregnant females and lactating mothers, which was proposed to be ingested for their astringent, anti-abortive and anti-hemorrhagic properties. The diet of gorillas contains a wide range of known human medicinal plants with various activities of potential value to these apes (Cousins and Huffman, 2002). But, most of the above mentioned studies emphasize on the chemical components of the diet in few species. In addition to chemical analysis of a single medicinal plant species, it is important to understand the dependency of humans and animals on plants and their overlap in using them.

Mundanthurai range (224.69 sq. km; 77^0 5' to 77^0 40' E long and 8^0 50' to 8^0 55' N lat) (referred to as Mundanthurai from now), within Kalakad-Mundanthurai Tiger reserve, lies at the southern fringe of the Western Ghats mountain range in the Indian Peninsula. This region falls in one of the 12 mega-biodiversity 'hotspots' of the world (Myers et al., 2001). Apart from its high species richness, this subcontinent is particularly known for its rich natural resources, aesthetic and cultural values, and rich wealth of medicinal plants (Anonymous, 1976). Saint Agastyar, who resided in these hills, is believed to be the founder of the modern 'Siddha' cult of medicine. The local tribe of this region, 'Kani', who are also the endemic tribe of southern Western Ghats, is believed to have inherited these treatises on medicine and traditional use of rich ethno-botanical lore of wild medicinal plants growing in their surroundings (Pate, 1917).

Owing to its rich biodiversity and vicinity to human settlements, this region is constantly under the threat of over exploitation of its valuable natural resources (Ali and Pai, 2001). Besides supporting rich forests types like tropical wet evergreen, semi evergreen, tropical moist deciduous, tropical dry deciduous (Champion and Seth, 1968), scrub lands along with different kinds of plantations, these hill ranges serves as an important catchment for several perennial rivers, which forms the lifeline for millions in the adjoining eastern plains. It is estimated that the Mundanthurai range contains *ca*. 1000 species of angiosperms belonging to 80 families (Ray and Rawat, 2002) and 77 species of mammals (Johnsingh, 2001). This area harbours several endemic and rare plant species, many of which are of medicinal importance. The residing Kani tribals are distributed in five settlements within the study area, harbouring a population of about more than 600, within the reserve.

In this observational study, our primary objective was; 1) to relate plants of known medicinal values that are utilized by Kani tribals to those consumed by wild animals and 2) to document distribution status of these plant species, in order to identify the current threats, if any, to these species. Although, this study is not a surrogate for detailed observations on animal behaviour and their diet or analysis of plant chemical constituents, to our knowledge, this is a first attempt to understand the overlap in medicinal plants consumed by humans and animals.

Materials and Methods

The field observations were made as a part of a study on the flora and vegetation at Mundanthurai. Data were collected on the distribution of various medicinal plant species throughout Mundanthurai range by regular perambulation of the study area. The entire area was divided into 2' x 2' (3.6 x 3.6 km) grids on 1:25,000 scale Survey of India topographic maps of Tirunelveli District. Each of these grids was subdivided into four 1' x 1' (1.8 x 1.8 km) segments. We randomly selected four of these sub grids based on their vegetation types (Champion and Seth, 1968, Ramesh, 1996), dry deciduous forest (elevation 200-300 m), moist deciduous forest (300-500 m), savannah woodlands (500-650 m), and wet evergreen (650-1000 m) forests.

Within each sub grid, an approximate diagonal line transect (Mueller-Dombois and Ellenberg, 1974) of 2 km was laid. Along each transect, vegetation sample plots were laid at every 150 m interval, making it 14 plots in each grid and each vegetation type. For trees and woody climbers, square plots of 30m x 30m were used to record number of tree and climber species, (Mueller-Dombois and Ellenberg, 1974; Kent and Coker, 1994). Concentric to the larger plot nested plots of one 8 x 8 m was laid for shrubs and five concentric plots (four corners and one centre) for herbs and grasses. Along both side of the line transect within the same sub grids, animals were recorded and identified and information was collected on plant-species diet of these animals and plant parts used. In addition, each sub grid was also extensively perambulated for information on plant-species diet of animals. These results were consolidated with published literature (Johnsingh and Sankar, 1994; Krishnamani and Kumar, 2000; Sundarraj and Johnsingh, 1996) on the food habits of wild herbivores from this area. The distribution of plants and animals were calculated based on these data (detailed analytical results beyond the scope of this study), and was confirmed with the available data base on these plants.

For ethnobotanical information, one of the authors (VC), who is also a Siddha medicine doctor, conducted frequent interviews (n = 60 individuals) with simple questionnaires conducted with the Kani tribals. These questionnaires revealed information on plant species used, ailment or purpose of use and plant parts used for each ailment. The medicinal uses of the known therapeutic plants by the Kani tribals aided to assess the range and possibility of bioactive supplementation potentially gained by the animals known to ingest these plants.

Results

We identified 260 plant species that were used by the Kani tribals for treatment of various ailments (Table 1). Of these 260 medicinal plant species recorded, 114 were consumed by wild animals (Table 1) and of the 45 ailments we accounted for, animals consumed plants pertaining to 29 ailments (Table 2). Among the recorded species, 83 were trees, 77 herbs, 56 shrubs, 42 climbers and two were grasses. We found that the dry forests had 94 species of medicinal plants, which was the highest, followed by 82 species in wet evergreen forests, and 72 species in the moist deciduous, while savannah and woodlands had only 13 species of known medicinal value. With an exception for the dry forests, where the numbers of climbers were greater, tree species were found to be comparatively higher (Table 1). Among the plant species we recorded, 57 are commonly distributed (Table 1), 121 are frequently distributed, 55 are sparsely distributed and 25 are rare species, 10 among which are rare and endemic (Table 1, Figure 1). Approximately 7.7% of medicinal plants were endemic, of which 4 are found throughout Western Ghats, 4 occurs in central to southern Western Ghats, and 12 species remains restricted to southern Western Ghats (Nayar 1996) (Table 1). Some of these species includes, *Amorphophalus smithsonianus*, *Anaphyllum wightii*, *Arenga wightii*, *Aristolochia indica*, *A. tagala*, *Hopea utilis*, *Piper brachystachyum*, *Calamus thwaitesii*, *C.travancoricus*, *Corallocarpus epigaeus*, *Garcinia gummu-gutta*, *Poeciloneuron pauciflorum*, *Tabernaemontana hyneana*, *Trichopus zeylanicus* and *Vateria* indica, 10 of them falling under rare and endemic category (IUCN Red Data List, 2007) (Figure 1).

Among the Kani tribals interviewed, most knew the therapeutic uses of many plant species, however, there were only four specialised healers who also could cure a variety of ailments. More than 50 different ailments are treated using herbal medicines. Fever (various kinds), skin disease, rheumatism and jaundice were found to be the most prevalent ailments among the local people. Kani tribals used 29 species of wild plants for fever, 28 species for skin diseases, 18 for rheumatism and 7 for jaundice (Table 2).

Table 1. Habit, distribution, abundance, medicinal plant parts used by Kani tribe, medicinal plant parts used by wild animals (as food), and endemism of 260 plant species in the Mundanthurai range of Kalakad-Mundanthurai Tiger Reserve

Name of species	H	Ha	A	M	P	E*
Acacia caesia Willd.	C	DD	F	L- Fever	L- CL	-
A. sundra DC.	S	MD	F	Pith- Stomach-ache	L- NL	-
Acalypha fruiticosa Forsk.	H	DD	C	L-Skin dis.	L- C, S	-
Acronichia laurifolia Bl.	T	WE	C	L- Body pain	-	-
Adenia palmata Engl.	C	MD	C	Rt- Skin dis.	-	-
Adina cordifolia Hk.f.	T	MD	F	B-Fever	-	-
Aerva lanata Juss.	H	DD	F	WP-Urinary inf.	-	-
Aganosoma cymosa G.Don.	C	DD	F	Fl-Eye dis.	L-C, S	-
Ageratum conyzoides L.	H	DD	C	L- Wounds	-	-
Aglaia eleagnoidea Hiern.	T	WE	F*	Fr- Skin dis.	L- NL, LTM, BM	SWG
Aglaia roxburghiana Bedd.	T	DD	F	Fr- Skin dis.	L- C, S, NL; Fr- Ci, Ba, BM	-
Ailanthus excelsa Roxb.	T	DD	F	B- Asthma	L- NL	-
Alangium salvifolium Wang.	T	D	S	L-Rheumatism	-	-
Albizzia odoratissima Benth.	T	MD	F	B- Ulcer	L- NL	-
Allophyllus serratus Radlk.	T	WE	F	Rt- Diarrhoea	-	-
Alphonsea sclerocarpa Thw	T	MD	C	L-Skin dis.	Fr - C	-
Alstonia scholaris R.Br.	T	MD	F	B- Fever	-	-
Alysicarpus monilifer DC	H	DD	C	WP- Bleeding -	-	-
Amorphophallus smithsonianus Sivadasan	H	DD	R*	WP- Piles	L - S	SWG
Anaphyllum wightii Schott.	C	WE	R*	WP- Piles	-	SWG
Andrographis alata Nees.	H	DD	S	WP- Skin dis.	L - S	-
Anisochilus carnosus Wall.	H	DD	F	L- Cold	-	-
Anogiessus latifolia Wall.	T	DD	C	B- Bowel mvmt	L- NL	-
Ancistrocladus hyneanus Wall.	C	WE	F	L- Bronchitis	-	-
Antiaris toxicaria Lesch.	T	MD	S	B- Heart dis.	-	-
Antidesma diandra Roth.	S	WE	S	Fr- Stomach-ache	Fr - LTM	-
Apama siliquosa Lam.	S	WE	F	Rt-Antivenom	-	-
Arenga wightii Griff.	T	WE	R*	YL- Jaundice	-	WG
Argyreia speciosa Sweet.	C	MD	F	L- Boils	-	-
Arisaema leschenaultii BL.	H	WE	R	Tu-Piles	-	-
Aristida setacea Retz.	H	DD	C	WP-Skin dis.	L- C, S	-
Aristolochia indica L.	C	DD	R	Rt-Snake bite	-	-
Aristolochia tagala Cham.	C	WE	R	Rt-Snake bite	S- LTM	-
Asclepias currasavica L.	H	WE	F	Rt-Avomin	-	-
Aspargus racemosus Willd.	S	DD	F	Rt-Tonic	L- S	-
Asystasia gangetica T.And.	H	DD	F	L-Wounds	-	-
Atlantia monophylla Corr.	S	DD	F	L-Snake bite	L- NL, S, Fr- Ci, Ba	-
Baccaurea courtrallensis M.Arg.	T	WE	C*	Fr- Digestive	-	CSWG
Balanophora indica Wall.	S	WE	C	WP-Cold	-	-
Bambusa arundinacea Willd.	H	MD	C	L-Bowel mvmt	L- C, S	-
Barleria prionitis L.	H	MD	C	Rt-Toothache	-	-

Table 1. (Continued)

Name of species	H	Ha	A	M	P	E[¥]
Basella rubra L.	H	MD	F	L-Urinary dis.	-	-
Bauhinia racemosa Lam.	T	SW	F	B- Diarrhoea	L - C, S, NL, BM, Ba	-
Begonia floccifera Bedd.	H	MD, WE	S	L-Tonic	-	-
B. malabarica Lam.	H	WE	S	L-Tonic	-	-
Biophytum sensitivum DC.	H	DD	C	WP-Urinary dis	L - C	-
Bischofia javanica BL.	T	WE	S	L-Wounds	L- NL	-
Blachia calycina Benth.	S	DD	C*	L-Wounds	-	SWG
Blepheris boehaaviaefolia Pers.	H	DD	C	WP-Bone fract.	L - C, S	-
Boerhaavia diffusa L.	H	DD	C	Rt-Asthma	L- C	-
Bombax malabarica DC.	T	DD	F	Juice-Bleeding -	L- C, NL, BM; Fr- NL, BM	-
Borreria hispida K.Sch.	H	DD	C	L-Jaundice	L- C, S	-
Breynia patens Rolfe.	S	MD	F	L-Soar throat	-	-
Bridelia retusa Spr.	T	SW	F	B-Antihelm.	-	-
Bryonopsis laciniosa Naud.	C	MD	S	L-Fever	-	-
Buchanania lanzan Spr.	T	SW	F	Sd-Skin dis.	-	-
Cadaba trifoliata W. and A.	T	DD	F	L-Skin dis.	L- C, S	-
Calamus rotang L.	C	WE	F	Rt-Fever	S- El	-
C. thwaitesii Becc.	C	WE	R*	Rt-Fever	S- El	SWG
C. travancoricus Bedd.	C	WE	R*	Rt-Fever	S- El	SWG
Callicarpa lanata L.	S	SW	F	B-Fever	-	-
Calycopteris floribunda Lam.	C	WE	F	Fr- Jaundice	-	-
Calophyllum austroindicum Kosterm.	T	WE	F*	Sd- Rheumatism	-	SWG
C. decipiens W.	T	DD	R*	Sd- Rheumatism	L- NL	SWG
Calotropis gigantea R.Br.	S	DD	F	Fl- Asthma	-	-
Canarium strictum Roxb.	T	WE	F	Gum-Rheumatism	L- LTM	-
Capparis diversifolia W. and A.	S	DD	C*	Fr-Digestive	L- C, S	SWG
C. monii W.	S	DD	F	L- Eear dis.	-	-
Caralluma adscendens R Br.	S	DD	R	WP-Tonic	-	-
Carissa carandas L.	S	DD	C	Fr-Cooling	L- C, S, NL	-
Careya arborea Roxb.	T	SW	S	B-Ulcer	L- C	-
Caryota urens L.	T	WE	S	Sd-Headache	Fr- BM, El- Ba	-
Cassia auriculata L.	S	DD	C	Fl- Diabetese	-	-
C. fistula L.	T	DD	C	Fl- Skin dis	L- NL, Ba; Fr- Ci, GS	-
C. tomentosa Willd.	S	MD	C	L-Skin dis.	-	-
C. tora L.	H	DD	C	Sd- Ringworm	-	-
Cayratia pedata Juss.	C	MD	F	Tu- Piles	-	-
Celastrus paniculata Willd.	S	MD	S	Sd-Brain tonic	-	-
Celtis cinnamomea Lindl.	T	WE	F	Wd- Body pain	-	-
Centella asiatica Urb.	H	WE	F	L-Tonic	L- C, S	-
Ceropegia juncea Roxb.	H	WE	S	WP-Thirst	-	-

Name of species				M	P	E
Chlorophytum tuberosum Bak.	H	MD	S	Tu-Int. wounds	-	-
Chomelia asiatica O. Ktz.	S	DD	C	L-Urinary dis.	-	-
Cinnamomum zeylanicum Bl.	T	WE	F	L-Digestive	-	-
Cipadessa baccifera Miq.	S	MD	F	L-Ulcer	-	-
Cissampelos pareira L.	H	MD	C	Rt-Fever	L- C, S	-
Cissus quadrangularis L.	C	DD	F	WP-Digestive	L- C, S	-
Clerodendron infortunatum L.	S	MD	C	Rt-Fever	-	-
C. serratum Spr.	H	SW	F	Rt-Fever	-	-
Coccinia indica W. and A.	H	DD	F	L-Diabetese	-	-
Name of species	H	Ha	A	M	P	E[¥]
Cocculus hirsutus Diels.	S	DD	F	L-Cooling	L- C, S	-
Combertum ovalifolium Roxb.	C	MD	F	L-Wounds	Fr- BM, L- NL	-
Corallocarpus epigaeus Hk.f.	C	DD	R	Tu-Skin dis.	-	-
Cordia obliqua W.	T	MD	F	B-Bowel mvmt	L- C	-
Coscinium fenestratum Colebr.	C	WE	S	Sd-Fever	-	-
Costus speciosus Sm.	H	WE	R	Rt-Fever	-	-
Crinum latifolium L.	H	SW	S	Bulb-Corns	-	-
Crossandra undulifolia Salisb.	H	MD	S	Rt-Jaundice	-	-
Crotalaria striata DC.	H	DD	F	Sd-Skin dis.	-	-
C. verrucosa L.	H	MD	F	L-Scabies	-	-
Cryptolepis buchanani R.and S.	C	MD	F	Rt-Antivenom	-	-
Curculigo orchioides Gaertn.	H	DD	C	Rt-Tonic	L- C, S	-
Cycas circinalis L.	S	MD	F	Pith-Tonic	Fr- Ci, P	-
Cyclea peltata Cooke.	C	MD	F	Rt-Body pain	-	-
Cymbopogon flexuosus Wats.	G	SW	C	Oil-Body pain	-	-
Cynodon dactylon Pers.	G	DD	C	WP-Urinary dis.	L- C, S	-
Cyperus rotundus L.	H	DD	C	Nut-Fever	-	-
Desmodium gangeticum DC.	H	MD	F	Rt-Fever	L- C, S	-
Dichrostachys cineria W. and A.	S	DD	F	L-Skin dis.	L- C, S	-
Didymocarpus tomentosa W.	H	WE	F	WP-Urinary dis.	-	-
Drymaria cordata Willd.	H	WE	F	WP-Laxative	-	-
Dioscorea oppositifolia L.	C	MD	F	Tu-Tonic	-	-
D. pentaphylla L.	C	DD	F	Tu- Tonic	-	-
Diospyros melanoxylon Roxb.	T	DD	C	Fr- Bone fract.	-	-
D. peregrina Gurke.	T	DD	S	Fr- Bone fract.	-	-
Diploclisia glaucescens Diels.	C	WE	F	Rt-Body pain	-	-
Dodonaea viscosa L.	S	DD	C	L-Ext. Swelling	-	-
Dracaena terniflora W.	S	MD	F	Rt-Diuretic	-	-
Drosera burmanni Vahl.	H	DD	R	WP-Asthma	-	-
D. indica L.	H	DD	R	WP-Asthma	-	-
Ehretia microphylla Lam.	S	MD	F	Rt-Skin dis.	L- C, S	-
Elaeocarpus serratus L.	T	WE	F	L-Rheumatism	-	E[¥]

Table 1. (Continued)

Name of species	H	Ha	A	M	P	E¥
Elephantopus scaber L.	H	MD	C	WP-Stomach-ache	-	-
Emblica officinalis Gaertn.	T	SW	F	Fr-Tonic	Fr- NL	-
Entada scandens Benth.	C	MD	F	Sd-Fever	-	-
Eriocaulon lanceolatum Miq.	H	WE	F	WP-Fever	-	-
Erythropalum populifolium Mast.	C	WE	F	L-Rheumatism	-	-
Erythroxylon lanceolatum Hk.f.	S	WE	S	Wd-Skin dis.	-	-
E. monogynum Roxb.	S	DD	C	Wd-Skin dis.	L- C, S; Fr- Ci	-
Euphorbia antiquorum L.	S	DD	F	Sd-Purgative	L- S	-
Evolvulus alsinoides L.	H	DD	C	WP-Fever	L- C, S	-
Excoecaria crenulata W.	S	WE	S	L-Rheumatism	-	-
Fagraea obovata Wall.	S	WE	S	L-Fever	-	-
Ficus racemosa L.	T	MD	F	B-Diabetese	L- NL, BM	-
F. retusa L.	T	DD	F	B-Diabetes	L- C, NL, BM	-
Fluggea virosa Baill.	S	MD	C	L-Ulcer	-	-
Garcinia gummi-gutta (L.) Roxb.	T	WE	R*	Fr-Stomach ache	Fr- NL, GS	-
G. echinocarpa Thw.	T	WE	R*	Fr-Stomach ache	-	-
Gardenia gummifera L.f.	S	MD	S	Gum-Sinus	-	-
Gelonium multiflorum A. juss.	S	DD	F	B-Toothache	-	-
Name of species	H	Ha	A	M	P	E¥
Gloriosa superba L.	H	DD	F	Tu-Skin dis.	-	-
Glycosmis pentaphylla Corr.	S	DD	C	Rt-Fever	L - S; Fr- Ci	-
Gmelina arborea Roxb.	T	MD	S	B-Nerves pain	-	-
Gnetum ula Brogn.	C	WE	S	Sap-Jaundice	Fr- Ci	-
Gymnema sylvestre R. Br.	C	DD	F	L- Diabetese	-	-
Heckeria subpeltata Kunth.	S	WE	S	L-Digestive	-	-
Heracleum rigens Wall.	H	WE	R	Fr-Digestive	-	-
Heynea trijuga Roxb.	T	WE	S	B-Skin dis.	-	-
Hiptage madablota Gaertn.	C	MD	F	L-Asthma	-	-
Holoptelia integrifolia Pl.	T	MD	S	B-Body pain	-	-
Homonoia riparia Lour.	S	WE	S	Rt-Urinary dis.	-	-
Hopea parviflora Bedd.	T	WE	F*	Resin-Bleeding	L- S, NL	CSWG
H. utilis Bedd.	T	WE	S*	Resin-Bleeding	L- C	SWG
Hydnocarpus wightiana Bl.	T	WE	F	Oil-Skin dis.	-	-
Hydrocotyle javanica Thunb.	H	WE	F	WP-Tonic	-	-
Ichnocarpus frutescens R. Br.	C	DD	C	Rt-Tonic	L- C, S	-
Indigofera longeracemosa Boiv.	S	DD	F	L-Snake Bite	-	-
Justicia betonica L.	H	MD	F	L-Rheumatism	-	-
Justicia simplex D.Don.	H	DD	C	L-Rheumatism	L- C	-
Kingiodendron pinnatum Harms.	T	MD	F*	Oil-Joint Pain	L- NL	CSWG
Klugia notoniana A. DC.	H	WE	R	Rt-Dog Bite	-	-
Knema attenuata Warb.	T	WE	S*	B-Wounds	Fr- GS	WG
Leea sambucina Willd.	C	WE	F	Rt-Stomach-ache	-	-

Leportea crenulata Gaud.	S	WE	S	L-Rheumatism	-	-
Leptadenia reticulata W. and A	S	DD	S	L-Milk secretion	L- S	-
Leucas aspera Spr.	H	DD	C	L-Cough	L- S	-
Litsea floribunda Gamb.	T	WE	S	B-Bowel mvmt.	L- LTM	-
Lobelia nicotianaefolia Heyne.	H	WE	R	L-Asthma	-	-
Loranthus longiflorus Desv.	S	DD	F	B-Wounds	L- C, S	-
Maba buxifolia Cl.	S	DD	R	Rt-Body pain	-	-
Macaranga peltata M. Arg.	T	WE	S	Gum-Skin dis.	-	-
Madhuca latifolia Macbride.	T	SW	F	Oil-Rheumatism	-	-
Mallotus philippinensis M. Arg.	T	MD	C	Fr-Antihelmen.	B- El	-
Mangifera indica L.	T	WE	S	B-Venereal soars	L- NL,LTM; Fr- GS, Ba	-
Mappia foetida Miers.	T	WE	R	B-Anti-cancer.	-	-
Melia composita Willd.	T	MD	C	B-Skin dis.	Fr- GS	-
Memecylon edule Roxb.	T	DD	F	Rt-Mens. Dis.	L- C, S	-
Mesua ferrea L.	T	WE	F	B-Fever	Fr- GS, LTM	-
Mimosa pudica L.	H	MD	C	L-Diarrhoea	L- C, S	-
Mimusops elengi L.	T	MD	S	B-Fever	-	-
M. hexandra Roxb.	T	MD	F	B-Wounds	L- S	-
Mucuna artopurpurea DC.	C	MD	S	Sd-Tonic	-	-
Mundulea suberosa Benth.	S	DD	C	B-Fish poison	L- S, B- GS	-
Murraya exotica L.	S	MD	F	L-Antivenom	L- S	-
Musa paradisiaca L.	H	WE	R	Juice-Snake Bite	Fr and Fl- Ba	-
Mussaenda laxa Hutch.	S	MD	S	Fl-Jaundice	-	-
Myristica malabarica Lam.	T	WE	F*	Sd-Rheumatism	Fr- NL, LTM	WG
Naravelia zeylanica DC.	C	MD	F	Rt- Sinus	-	-
Name of species	H	Ha	A	M	P	E¥
Ocimum sanctum L.	H	DD	C	L-Cold and Cough	L- S	-
Oldenlandia umbellata L.	H	DD	C	Rt- Bl. vomiting	L- C, S	-
Ophiorhiza mungos L.	H	MD	F	L-Dog bite	-	-
Oxalis corniculata L.	H	DD	F	L-Cooling	-	-
Pachygone ovata Miers.	C	MD	F	Fr- Fish Poison	L- C, S	-
Passiflora incarnata L.	C	WE	C	Fr- Digestive	L- LTM	-
Pavonia odorata Willd.	C	DD	F	Fr- Cooling	-	-
Peperomia reflexa A. Dietr.	S	WE	S	L-Stomachache	-	-
Peristrophe bicalyculata Nees.	H	DD	F	L-Snake bite	-	-
Phoenix humilis Royle.	T	SW	F	Fr- Tonic	Fr- Ci, SB, Ba	-
Phyllanthus niruri L. sensu Hk. f. .	H	DD	C	L-Jaundice	L- C, S	-
Piper attenuatum B. Ham.	C	WE	F	Fr-Digestive	-	-
P. brachystachyum Wall.	C	WE	R	Fr-Cough	-	-
Plantago asiatica L.	H	WE	F	Sd- Laxative	-	-
Plectranthus coleoides Benth.	S	WE	C	L-Aromatic	-	-
Plectronia didyma Kurz.	S	MD	S	B-Fever	-	-

Table 1. (Continued)

Name of species	H	Ha	A	M	P	E[¥]
Poeciloneuron pauciflorum Bedd.	T	WE	R*	B-Rheumatism	-	SWG
Polygala javana DC.	H	DD	F	L-Antivenom	-	-
Polygonum chinense L.	H	WE	F	WP-Tonic	-	-
Pongamia glabra Vent.	T	DD	F	Oil-Skin dis.	L- S, NL	-
Premna tomemtosa Willd.	T	MD	S	L-Rheumatism	-	-
Pseudarthria viscida W. and A.	H	MD	S	Rt-Nerve dis.	L- C, S	-
Pterocarpus marsupium Roxb.	T	SW	F	Wd- Diabetes	L- C; B- GS	-
Putranjiva roxburghii Roxb.	T	MD	S	L-Fever	-	-
Remusatia vivipera Schott.	H	WE	F	C-Piles	-	-
Randia dumetorum Lam.	S	DD	C	Fr- Avomin-	L and Fr- C, S	-
Rubus elipticus Sm.	S	WE	S	Fr-Digestive	-	-
Santalum album L.	T	MD	F	Wd-Cooling	L- C, BM; Fr- Ba	-
Sapindus emarginatus Vahl.	T	WE	F	Fr-Cough	L- C, S	-
Sarcostemma brevistigma W. and A.	C	DD	F	Sd-Sedative	-	-
Schefflera wallichiana Harms.	S	WE	S	B-Skin dis.	-	-
Sida acuta Burm.	H	DD	C	Rt-Tonic	L- C, S	-
Schleichera trijuga Willd.	T	MD	F	Oil-Rheumatism	L- C, S, NL	-
Sida cordifolia L.	H	DD	C	Rt-Tonic	L- S	-
S. rhombifolia L.	H	MD	C	Rt-Tonic	L- C, S	-
Smilax zeylanica L.	C	WE	F	Rt-Skin dis.	-	-
Solanum indicum L.	H	MD	F	Rt-Nerves dis.	-	-
S. melongena Pr. var insanum	H	DD	S	Rt-Nerves dis.	Fr- C, L- S	-
S. verbascifolium L.	S	MD	F	Fr- Antihelm.	-	-
Spilanthes acmella Murr.	H	WE	S	Buds- Toothache	-	-
Spondias mangifera Willd.	T	MD	S	Fr- Bowel mvmt	-	-
Stenosiphonium confertum Nees.	S	WE	C	Rt- Cl. uterus	-	-
S. wightii Bremek.	S	MD	C*	Rt- Cl. uterus	-	SWG
Stephania wightii Dunn.	C	WE	F	Tu-Skin dis.	-	-
Sterculia guttata Roxb.	T	MD	S	Gum-Toothache	-	-
Stereospermum tetragonum DC.	T	MD	S	Rt-Fever	-	-
Streblus asper Lour.	T	DD	F	B-Fever	L- C, S, NL	-
Strychnos potatorum L. f.	T	DD	S	Sd-Tonic	-	-
Symplocos cochinchinensis	T	WE	F	B- Uterus Bldg -	Fr- LTM	-
Name of species	H	Ha	A	M	P	E[¥]
Syzygium cumini L.	T	DD	C	Sd-Diabetese	L- NL; Fr- Ba, S, BM	-
Tamarindus indica L.	T	DD	C	Fr-Laxative	L -NL; Fr- GS, BM	-
Tabernaemontana heyneana Wall.	T	WE	S*	L- Fever, Headache	-	WG

Tectona grandis L.f.	T	DD	C	Sd-Hair growth	L- GS, NL ; Fr- GS, M,B- El	-
Tephrosia purpurea Pers.	H	DD	F	Rt-Spleen enl.	L- S	-
Terminalia bellerica Roxb.	T	MD	F	Fr-Tonic	L- NL; FR- Ci	-
T. chebula Retz.	T	SW	F	Fr- Tonic	L- NL; FR- Ci	-
Toddalia asiatica Lam.	C	MD	F	Rt-Fever	L- C, S	-
Trichopus zeylanicus Gaertn.	H	WE	S	WP-Tonic	-	-
Urena lobata L.	H	MD	F	Fr-Urin. inf.	L- C	-
Vallaris solanacea O.Kze.	C	MD	F	Latex-Ulcer	L- C	-
Vanda tessellata Hk.	H	MD	S	Rt-Rheumatism	-	-
Vateria indica L.	T	WE	R*	Resin-Rheumatism	-	CSWG
Ventilago madraspatana Gaertn.	C	DD	F	Rt-Fever	L- S	-
Vernonia cineria Less.	H	DD	F	L-Piles	L- C	-
Vicoa indica DC.	H	DD	F	L-Anitcancerous	L- C	-
Vitex altissima L.f.	T	MD	F	L-Swelling	L- S	-
Walsura piscidia Roxb	T	DD	S	B-Skin dis.	L and Fr- C	-
Waltheria indica, L.	H	DD	F	Rt-Bleeding -	L- S	-
Wrightia tinctoria R.Br.	T	DD	F	L-Toothache	L- C	-
Zanthoxylum flavescens Roxb.	S	WE	S	B-Toothache	-	-
Ziziphus xylopyrus Willd	S	DD	C	L-Scabies	L - C, SB, Fr- C,	-
Zornia diphylla Pers.	H	DD	C	L-Scabies	-	-

* = endemism assigned according to Nayar 1996.

H = Habit: H= Herb, S= Shrub, C= Climber, T= Tree; G= Grass; Ha = Habitat type: DD = dry deciduous, MD = moist deciduous, SW = savannah woodland, WE = wet evergreen; A = Abundance: C= Common, F= Frequent, S= Sparse, R= rare; *Endemic species; M = Medicinal use: dis = disease / disorder, ext = external, inf = infection, fract.= fracture); P = Part used: L= Leaves, Fr = fruits, B= Bark, Fl = Flowers, Rt = Root, Sd= Seed, Tu = Tuber, WP = Whole plant, WD = Wood; YL = Young Leaves; Animals: C = Chital, S = Sambar, SB= Sloth bear, NL = Nilgiri langur, LTM = Lion tailed macque, BM = Bonnet macque, CL = Common langur, Ba = Bat, El= Elephant, Ci= Civet, GS= Giant squirrel; E = endemism, WG = Western Ghats, CSWG = central and southern Western Ghats, and SWG = southern Western Ghats

About 12 species were used as anti venom agents against snake, scorpion and dog bites. Only a single species was found to be used for diseases related to eyes, ears, throat, heart, menopause, corn, venereal sores and vomiting of blood.

Among the mammalian wildlife within Mundanthurai range, *Axis axis* (chital deer) is restricted to the Mundanthurai plateau, and is known to feed on 162 species of plants (Johnsingh and Shankar, 1994) of which 55 (34%) are of medicinal value. From our observations, *Cervus unicolour* (sambar deer) fed on 56 and *Elephas maximus* (Asian elephant) on 6. The primates in our study are two endemic primates, *Trachypithecus johnii* (Nilgiri langur) and *Macaca silenus* (lion-tailed macaque), which fed on 30 and 9 species of medicinal plants respectively, while *Macaca radiata* (bonnet macaque) diet consisted of 11 species of plants (Table 1). Fruit bats (a few species, which was not identified) fed on 10 species of medicinal plants, *Ratufa indica* (giant squirrel) on 10, *Paradoxurus hermaphroditus* (palm civet) on 9 and *Melurus ursinus* (sloth bear) were observed to feed on two species of medicinal plants (Table 1), besides various other food plants.

Some of the major ailments and the herbal drugs used, by both the Kani tribals and wild mammals for their cures are as follows:

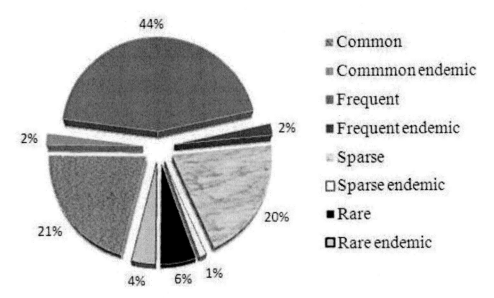

44%

2%

2%

20%

21%

4%   6%   1%

- Common
- Commmon endemic
- Frequent
- Frequent endemic
- Sparse
- Sparse endemic
- Rare
- Rare endemic

Figure 1. Conservation status of medicinal plant species within Mundanthurai range.

Fever – Around 29 species are used by the Kani tribals against fever. Among these, bark of species like *Alstonia scholaris, Adina cordifolia, Mesua ferrea* and *Streblus asper*; leaves (5 species) of species like *Acacia caesia, Putranjiva roxburghii*; roots (12 species) of species like *Toddalia asiatica, Desmodium gangeticum, Evolvulus alsinoides, Glycosmis pentaphylla*; seeds of *Coscinium fenestratum* and *Entada scandens* are consumed as a cure for fever. The green leaves of *Tabernaemontana hyneana*, besides action against fever, are also effective for severe headaches.

Among these plants, *G. pentaphylla, D. gangeticum, E alsinoides* are used by wild herbivores like the sambar and chital. Elephants were seen to feed on the roots of *Calamus spp* and bark of *Streblus asper*. The Nilgiri langur was seen to feed on the leaves of *S. asper*, while lion tailed macaques fed on the leaves of *Mesua ferrea*.

Skin disease and snakebites – Other than normal skin eruptions, bites of ticks, leeches, insects and snakes cause allergic reactions and infections are treated by the Kani tribe. For such ailments, 36 species of plants were found to be used by the Kani's for treatment (Table 1). Leaves of *Acalypha fruiticosa, Alphonsea sclerocarpa, Cadaba trifoliata*; fruits of *Aglaia roxburghiana, A. eleaeagnoidea*; flowers of *Cassia fistula*, oil of *Pongmia glabra;* tubers of *Stephania wightii* are used for skin eruptions and infections. The leaves of species like *Crotalaria verrucosa, Zizyphus xylopyrus* and *Zornia diphylla* are known to be very effective for scabies. Six plant species were found to be used as treatment for snakebites. Most important among them were the roots of *Aristolochia indica* and *A. tagala* and juice of *Musa paradisiaca*. The roots *of Cryptolepis buchanani, Apama siliquosa*, and leaves of *Murraya exotica* and *Polygala javana* also have anti-venom properties. The decoction of the bark of an endemic species, *Hopea utilis,* is also known to give relief from leech bites.

Table 2. List of different ailments that are treated by Kani tribal people, number of medicinal plant species used by the Kani tribals for these ailments, number of medicinal plants species consumed by wild animals, number of medicinal plant species used by humans and wild animals, and common names of the species of wild animals observed to feed on these overlapping Medicinal Plant Species.

Ailments	Humans	Animals	Humans and animals	Animal species
Anticancerous	27	1	1	Ch
Antihelminthic	3	1	0	---
Antivenom	4	1	1	S
Asthma	7	2	0	---
Avomin	2	1	1	Ch
Blood vomitting	1	1	0	---
Bleeding	5	4	1	Ch, Nl, Bm
Bone fracture	3	1	1	Ch, S
Bowel movement	5	4	1	Ch, S
Cough and cold	6	3	2	S
Cooling	5	3	1	Ch, S
Diabetes	7	4	0	---
Diarrhoea	3	2	1	Ch, S
Digestive	9	3	1	Ch, S
Eye disorder	1	1	0	---
Fever	29	12	2	Ch, S
Fish Poison	2	2	1	Gs
Hair growth	1	1	1	Gs
Headache	1	1	1	Bm
Jaundice	7	3	3	Ch, S, Ci
Joint pain	1	1	0	---
Laxative	3	1	1	Gs, Bm
Menstural disorder	1	1	0	---
Mild secretion	1	1	1	S
Nerve disorder	3	2	0	---
Piles	6	2	1	S
Purgative	1	1	0	---
Rheumatism	17	5	2	Ch, Nl, LTM
Ringworm	1	0	0	---
Scabies	3	1	1	Ch, Sb
Sedative	1	0	0	---
Sinus	1	0	0	---
Skin disease	27	13	5	Ch, S, Ci, B, Bm
Snake bite	6	3	1	S, Nl
Spleen enlargement	1	1	0	---
Stomach ache	7	3	2	Nl, Gs, LTM
Swelling	1	1	1	S
Tonic	22	12	5	Ch, S, Ci, B, Nl, Sb
Toothache	6	1	1	Ch
Ulcer	5	3	1	Ch
Urinary disorder	6	2	2	Ch, S
Urinary infection	2	1	0	---
Uterine bleeding	1	1	0	---
Venereal soars	1	1	0	---
Wounds	8	5	2	Nl, Gs

Animal species: 'Ch' for chital, 'S' for sambar, 'Nl' for Nilgiri langur, 'Bm' for bonnet macaque, 'Gs' for giant squirrel, 'Ci' for civet species, 'LTM' for Lion-tailed macaque, 'Sb' for sloth bear and 'B' for different species of bats

Bonnet macaques and fruits bats were found to feed voraciously on the fruits of *A. roxburghiana*, while the endemic primates were seen to prefer *A. monophylla* and *A. tagala*. The ripe fruits and leaves of *Zizyphus xylopyrus* were highly fed on by both chital and sambar deer in the Mundanthurai plateau.

Rheumatism and joint pains – The Kani tribals use 17 species of wild plants as a cure for rheumatism (Table 2), among which species like *Callophyllum austroindicum, C. decipiens* and *Myristica malabarica* deserve special mention. The seeds of these species that are also preferred food plants of Nilgiri langurs and lion-tailed macaques (Table 1, 2). Bark of *Poeciloneuron pauciflorum*, leaves of *Elaeocarpus serratus, Alangium salviflorum, Erythropaulum populifolium*, and resin and gum of *Canarium strictum* and *Vateria indica* are used for rheumatic diseases by the local people.

Jaundice – Jaundice is one of the major ailments occurring among the Kani tribals, and we found 7 plant species to be effective against it and used by the Kani tribe (Table 1). Chital and sambar were found to feed on the mature leaves of *Borreria hispida* and *Phyllanthus niruri* which is well known for the treatment of jaundice among the local people. The sap of a gymnosperm climber *Gnetum ula*, which was found to be fed on by civets was also utilised for the same purpose by humans.

Toothache – Among the 6 species used for toothache the leaves of *Wrightia tinctoria* is believed to be effective (Table 1). Other than this, the bark of *Zanthoxylum flavescens* and *Gelonium multiflorum*, gum of *Sterculia guttata,* and roots of *Berleria prionitis* are also used for the same purpose by the tribals. Wild ungulates were found to be feeding preferably on *W. tinctoria* and *B. prionitis*.

Tonic – Twenty one species of herbal drugs are consumed as tonics (Table 1, 2). Among these the most notable one is *Trichopus zeylanicus* which is also know as the wonder drug "Arogya Patchcha". Consumption of the unripe fruits of this herb brings energy and vigour to the Kani tribals. The roots of species like *Asparagus racemosus, Curculigo orchioides, Ichnocarpus fruitescens, Sida cordifolia, S. acuta* are also used to maintain normal health. Intake of the fruits of *Emblica officinalis, Terminalia bellerica, T. chebula* also help to increase immunity against coughs and colds. In addition to the above mentioned ailments, one shrub (*Mundulea suberosa*) and one climber species (*Pachygone ovata*) is used very frequently by the local people as a fish poison (not medicinal) to catch fish from the local reservoirs, and were also consumed by giant squirrels as a part of their diet (Table 2).

Our observations showed that wild animals consumed the highest number of plant species, which were also used by the local people against skin disorders and infections (Table 2), followed by those used for fever, as tonics, rheumatism and wounds. We also found that the plant parts used by humans and animals were not similar in most of the cases (Table 2), yet the overlap that occurs (44%), is of great interest. This overlap is mainly for ailments such as skin disorders, as tonics, jaundice, stomach ache, wounds and urinary disorder (Table 2).

Discussion

Wild animals get infected with parasites and pathogens, and while they may not always show external signs or symptoms, they can treat themselves by modifying their diets to a certain extent and benefit from their anti-parasitic qualities (Huffman, 2003; Huffman, 2006).

Janzen (1978) had noted that Indian tigers, wild dogs, civets, bears, and jackals feed on species (*Carea arborea, Dalbergia latifolia*), which helps in the elimination of their intestinal parasites. In the present study, plant parts used by both humans and animals, it may be quite likely that by ingesting similar plant parts, animals may be benefiting from similar therapeutic value as the humans. Nevertheless, without any chemical constituent analysis it is difficult to draw any further conclusion about whether the overlap in plant parts used by humans and animals were for similar ailments or just as a diet. But, this information will provide a baseline for detail future study in such aspects.

Currently, no large-scale exploitation of the medicinal plants was noticed within the study area. Among 260 species, 57 (22%) were commonly distributed and small-scale extraction by the local Kani tribals was noted. Among the 20 endemic species, 55% are consumed by the wild animals. Albeit, at present no large-scale commercial exploitation is noticed within the area, occasional collection of valuable herbs like, *C. thwaitesii* (also for commercial purpose), *G. gummi-gutta*, *T. zeylanicus*, *V. indica*, from certain parts of Kalakad-Mundanthurai Tiger reserve was noted. Similar to other ecosystems of the world, this area face problems of habitat and biodiversity loss, and conservation measures for these threatened species should be the foremost priority for park management.

Kalakad-Mundanthurai Tiger reserve, which was established in 1987 (as a nature reserve) for conservation of regional biodiversity, is currently undergoing efforts to document the resource-use patterns of wild animals and the threats to flora and fauna (Johnsingh, 2001). Such attempts have helped to achieve widely documented information on medicinal plant species used by local people, though, till now, public awareness regarding over exploitation of medicinal plants for commercial purposes is not brought under notice. In today's world, where human attention has been drawn more towards organic food and herbal medicines, the commercialization of botanical drugs is feared to caused threats to some of these species (Ved and Goraya, 2008), especially rare and endemic ones. Hence, our study provides important baseline information on these botanical drugs, so that conservation and protection efforts can be directed towards these species. Both conventional and community-based participatory methods are necessary (Iqbal et al., 2005) to ensure the future of these threatened species. This study will also aid future studies looking at chemical properties of these plant species, correlating them to their animal use, for better understanding of plant-animal interactions and human-animal conflicts in these forests.

Conclusion

By exploring the folklore and experience of Kani tribals within the Mundanthurai range of Kalakad-Mundanthurai Tiger reserve, we found 260 plant species of medicinal importance that are commonly used by this tribe. Interestingly, we found 44% of these plant species were consumed by wild animals. We also found that Kani tribals used 20 species of endemic plants for medicinal purposes, 12 among these are exclusively found in the southern Western Ghats, seven among which are more restricted endemics are also consumed by the wild mammals. Our study suggests that monitoring the status of these widely used, rare and threatened medicinal species will be crucial for their future conservation.

Acknowledgments

We are thankful to Manoharan and Manikanthan, our local Kani tribal field assistants and Boodhathan, another Kani tribal (Forest Department employee), for their immense help in field survey and collection of plant materials and information. We acknowledge the valuable suggestions by V. Gopalan of the Botanical Survey of India, Southern Circle, Coimbatore. We wish to thank S.K. Mukherjee (ex-Director, WII), and V. K. Melkani (Field Director, Kalakad-Mundanthurai Tiger reserve) for providing various facilities to carry out the research. We thank Sarbari Ray and Shomen Mukherjee for their valuable suggestions in the manuscript.

References

Anonymous (1976). *Wealth of India: A dictionary of Indian raw materials and industrial products*. Vol 1. 569 p.

Ali, R. and Pai, A. (2001). Human use areas in Kalakad-Mundanthurai Tiger reserve. *Current Science* 80: 448-452.

Carrai, V., Borgognini-Tarli, S.M., Huffman, M. A. and Bardi M. (2003). Increase in tannin consumption by sifaka (*Propithecus verreauxi verreauxi*) females during the birth season: a case for self-medication in prosimians? *Primates*, 44: 61-66.

Champion, H.G. and Seth, S.K. (1968). *A Revised Survey of Forest Types of India*. Govt. of India, Delhi.

Cousins, D. and Huffman, M.A. (2002). Medicinal properties in the diet of gorillas- an ethno pharmacological evaluation. *African Study Monographs*, 23: 65-89.

Huffman M. A. (1997). Current evidence for self-medication in primates: a multidisciplinary perspective. *Year Book of Physical Anthropology*, 40: 171-200.

Huffman, M.A. (2003). Animal self-medication and ethno-medicine: exploration and exploitation of the medicinal properties of plants. *Proceedings of the Nutrition Society*, 62: 371-381.

Huffman, M.A. and Seifu, M. (1989). Observations on the illness and consumption of a possibly medicinal plant *Vernonia amygdalina* (Del.), by a wild chimpanzee in the Mahale Mountains National Park, Tanzania. *Primates*, 30: 51-63.

Huffman, M.A. (2006). Primate Self-Medication. In: Primates in Perspective. C. Campbell, A. Fuentes, K. MacKinnon, M. Panger, S. Bearder (eds.) pp. 677-689. University of Oxford Press, Oxford.

Huffman, M.A. and Caton, J.M. (2001). Self-induced increase of gut motility and the control of parasitic infections in wild chimpanzees. International *Journal of Primatology*, 22: 329-346.

Huffman, M.A., Gotoh, S., Izutsu, D., Koshimiz, K. and Kalunde, M.S. (1993). Further observations on the use of *Vernonia amygdalina* by a wild chimpanzee, its possible effect on parasite load, and its phytochemistry. *African Study Monographs*, 14: 227-240.

Iqbal, Z.A., Jabbar, A., Akhtar, M.S., Muhammad, G. and Muhammad, L. (2005). Possible use of ethnoveterinary medicine in poverty reduction in Pakistan: use of botanical anthehelmintics as an example. *Journal of Agriculture and Social Sciences*, 1: 187-195.

Jain, S. K. and Mudgal, V. (1999). *A Handbook of Ethnobotany*. India, Bishen Singh Mahendra Pal Singh. Dehra Dun.

Janzen, D.H. (1978). Complications in interpreting the chemical defences of trees against tropical arboreal plant-eating vertebrates, In: *Ecology of Arboreal Folivores*. Montgomery, G. (eds.) pp. 73-84. The Smithsonian Institute Press, Washington DC.

Johnsingh, A.J.T. (2001). The Kalakad-Mundanthurai Tiger reserve: a global heritage of biological diversity. *Current Science*, 80: 378-388.

Johnsingh, A.J.T. and Sankar, K. (1994). *Food plants of chital, sambar and cattle on Mundanthurai plateau, Tamil Nadu, south India*. Mammalia, 55: 56-65.

Kent, M. and Coker, P. (1994). *Vegetation description and analysis: a practical approach*. John Wiley and Sons, England.

Krishnamani, R. and Kumar, A. (2000). Phytoecology of Lion-tailed macaque (*Macaca silenus*) habitats in Karnataka, India: floristic structure and density of food trees. *Primate Report*, 5: 27-56.

Mueller-Dombois, D. and Ellenberg, H. (1974). *Aims and methods of vegetation ecology*. John Wiley and Sons, New York.

Myers, N., Mittermeirer, R.A., Mittermeirer, C.G., de Fonseca G.A.B. and Kent, J. (2001). Biodiversity hotspots for conservation priorities. *Nature*, 403: 854-858.

Nayar, M.P. (1996). *Hotspots of endemic plants of India, Nepal, and Bhutan*. Tropical Botanical Garden Research Institute, Thiruvananthapuram, Kerala, India.

Pate, H.R. (1917). Madras District Gazetters, Tirunelveli. Vol. I. Madras Government Press, Madras.

Pope, H.G. (1969). *Tabernanthe iboga*, an African narcotic plant of social importance. *Economic Botany*, 23:174-184.

Ramesh, B.R. (1996). *Vegetation map of Kalakad Mundanthurai Tiger Reserve*. French Institute, Pondicherry.

Ray, J. and Rawat, G.S. (2002). Patterns of plant species diversity and endemism in Kalakad-Mundanthurai Tiger reserve, Tamilnadu. In: *Perspectives of Plant Biodiversity*. A.P. Das (ed.) pp. 559-557. Bishen Singh Mahendra Pal Singh, Dehra Dun.

Rodriguez, E. and Wrangham, R. (1993). Zoopharmacognosy: The Use of Medicinal Plants by Animals. In: *Recent Advances in Phytochemistry*. K.P. Downum, J.T. Romeo and H.A. Stafford (eds). pp. 89-105. Plenum Press, New York.

Sunderraj, W. and Johnsingh, A.J.T. (1996). Impact of Flash Flood on the Gallery Forest and arboreal mammals of river Servalar, Mundanthurai Plateau, South India. *Journal of Wildlife Research*, 1: 89-94.

Ved, D.K. and Goraya, G.S. (2008). *Demand and Supply of Medicinal Plants in India*. Bishen Singh, Mahendra Pal Singh, Dehra Dun.

Wrangham, R.W. (1995). Relationship of chimpanzee leaf-swallowing to a tapeworm infection. *American Journal of Primatology, 37: 297-303.*

In: Medicinal Plants and Sustainable Development
Editor: Chandra Prakash Kala

ISBN 978-1-61761-942-7
© 2011 Nova Science Publishers, Inc.

Chapter 13

Diversity of Endemic Medicinal Plants in Kalakad Mundanthurai Tiger Reserve, Southern India

*M. Ayyanar** and S. Ignacimuthu*
Entomology Research Institute, Loyola College,
Chennai – 600 034, Tamil Nadu, India

Abstract

Kalakad Mundanthurai Tiger Reserve (KMTR) is a valuable repository of biodiversity in southern Western Ghats of Tamil Nadu, India with rich floral and faunal diversity, both in terms of species richness and endemism. Field surveys were carried out in KMTR during September 2004 to June 2006. Endemism of each medicinal plant was determined by field study, published literature and herbaria. More than 350 species of ethnomedicinal plants were recorded in our study with the support of tribal practitioners, of which 46 species were endemic. Euphorbiaceae and Rubiaceae were the dominant families with respect to number of endemic medicinal plants, 6 and 4 species respectively. *Begonia*, *Blachia*, *Biophytum* and *Psychotria* are reported with 2 species of endemic plants with ethnomedicinal importance. The majority of the plants of KMTR are rapidly getting threatened, because of the anthropogenic activities inside the forest areas by means of several pilgrim and tourist places. The biodiversity of KMTR is vulnerable, hence needs immediate conservation attention by involving local communities and forest representatives.

Keywords: Endemism; Medicinal plants; Tribal people; Threat factors; Western Ghats.

* Current Address: Division of Biodiversity and Biotechnology, Department of Botany, Pachaiyappa's College, Chennai – 600 030, Tamil Nadu, India, Phone: + 91 44 2664 0793 (Res), +91 99403 76005 (Mob), Email: asmayyanar@yahoo.com

Introduction

Plant resources are depleting globally at an alarming rate and a number of economically and medicinally important plant species will soon be extinct (Laloo et al., 2006). For example nearly 25% of the estimated 250,000 species of vascular plants in the world may become extinct within the next 50 years (Kala, 2000). The degree of threat to natural populations of medicinal plants has increased because more than 90% of medicinal plant raw material for herbal industries in India and also for export is drawn from natural habitat (Dhar et al., 2002). Endemism is a term used to indicate that a plant or animal taxon is restricted, in its geographical range, to a particular region and is commonly regarded as an important criterion for assessing the conservation value of a given area (Tchouto et al., 2006). In other terms, endemism is one of the most important criteria used in the identification of high-priority areas for conservation (Riemann and Ezcurra, 2005). The concept of endemism of a family, a genus or a species with reference to a particular region is varied.

The endemism in Indian biodiversity is very high and more than 30% of the country's recorded flora are endemic and are concentrated mainly in the North-East region, Western Ghats, North-West Himalaya and the Andaman and Nicobar islands and a small segment of endemism occurs in Eastern Ghats. According to Nayar (1996), there are 5725 species of vascular plants endemic to India, of which 2244 species are endemic to biodiversity hot spots of India and among them 186 species are of medicinal importance. Out of the estimated 17 500 species of vascular plants in India, around 15% are feared to be under threat. India is a home to thousands of ethno-medicinally important plant species and is ranked sixth among 12 mega diversity countries of the world (Semwal et al., 2007) and has second largest tribal population in the world after Africa. According to 2001 census, tribal people of India constitute 8.2% of the country's total population with more than 500 tribal communities. With enormously diversified living ethnic groups and rich biological resources, India represents one of the great emporia of ethnobotanical wealth (Pal, 2000). During the last few decades there has been an increasing interest in the study of medicinal plants and their traditional uses in different parts of India (Pattanaik et al., 2008; Hedge et al., 2007; Jagtap et al., 2006; Ayyanar and Ignacimuthu, 2005; Katewa et al., 2004; Jain, 2001; Jamir, 1999; Jain, 1991). The objectives of this paper is to identify endemic plants which are of ethnomedicinal importance in Kalakad Mundanthurai Tiger Reserve with their distribution in Tirunelveli hills and peninsular India and to discuss on the conservation measures to be taken up in the endemic medicinal plants.

Methods

Area of Study

Agasthiyamalai hills of Tamil Nadu occupy the forests of Tirunelveli and Kanyakumari districts of south Tamil Nadu and known as 'Tirunelveli hills'. The present study was conducted within the periphery of Kalakad Mundanthurai Tiger Reserve (KMTR, part of Tirunelveli hills) situated in southern tip of Western Ghats of Tamil Nadu (Figure 1) which covers an area of 895 sq. km and lying between the longitudes $77^0 10^'$ - $77^0 35^'$ E and latitudes

8^0 25' - 8^0 53' N. The hills in KMTR are characterized by numerous folds and extension engulfing small, narrow valleys and the elevation varies from 50 to 1869m (Manickam et al., 2004). It is the 17th Tiger Reserve in the country and it is a priority area for conservation of its rich floral and faunal diversity, both in terms of species richness and endemism (Melkani, 2001).

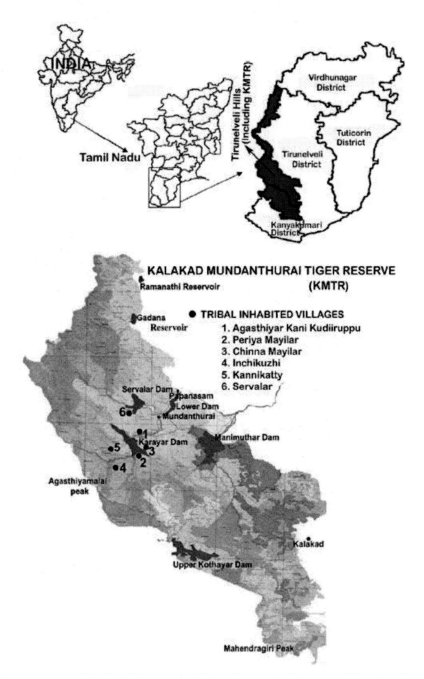

Figure 1. Location map of Kalakad Mundanthurai Tiger Reserve in Tirunelveli hills of southern Western Ghats, Tamil Nadu, India with tribal inhabited villages.

Table 1. Forest and Habitat types in Kalakad
Mundanthurai Tiger Reserve, Southern India

Forest types and altitude	Dominant species	Remarks
Southern Tropical Thorn Forests (200 m)	*Acacia* sps, *Albizia* sps, *Canthium* sps, *Capparis* sps, *Dodonaea viscosa* etc	It has three layered vegetation, such as the tree canopy, the undergrowth and the ground cover
Southern Tropical Dry Deciduous Forests (350 m)	*Anogeissus latifolia, Dillenia pentagyna, Pterocarpus marsupium, Terminalia chebula, Oryza granulata* etc	Most of the species found here are deciduous and the undergrowth is usually dense since enough light penetrates through the upper canopy
Southern Tropical Moist Deciduous Forests (500 m)	*Bambusa arundinacea, Acronychia pedunculata, Anamirta cocculus, Blachia calycina, Helicteres isora, Terminalia chebula* etc.	Evergreen elements dominating the lower storey giving the false impression of evergreen nature to these forests
Southern Tropical Semi Evergreen Forests (700 m)	*Antidesma menasu, Filicium decipiens, Mallotus philippensis, Entada pursaetha, Gnetum ula* etc.	Distributed in patches and belts wherever the moisture availability is adequate to support a semi-evergreen forest
Southern Tropical Wet Evergreen Forests (800 – 1500 m)	*Strobilanthes* and *Selaginella* sps.	The epiphytic orchids, aroids, ferns, mosses and lichens are common.
Subtropical Montane Forests (Above 1500 m)	*Aglaia elaegnoideaa, Euphorbia santapaui,* some of the *Impatiens spp., Lasianthus spp.* and an endemic palm *Bentinckia condapanna.*	The trees found here are evergreen, usually short-boled and of less than 12 m height with dense round crowns, coriaceous leaves and branches covered with epiphytes, mosses and lichens
Low level Grasslands (500 m)	*Buchanania lanzan, Mundelia sericea, Terminalia chebula* etc grow intermingled sporadically with grasses like *Cymbopogon coloratus* and *Themeda traindra* etc.	It occurs beyond scrub jungles and deciduous forests and these forests are very scattered and intermixed with the local forests and fire is common during the dry months
Grassy Swards at high altitudes (Above 1500 m)	*Arundinella purpurea, Chrysopogon orientalis, Themeda tremula, Zenkaria sebastinei* and etc.	It is composed of grasses, herbs and shrubs mixed in varying proportions and it covers large areas on mountain tops.

The vegetation is floristically rich when compared to other regions of Western Ghats (Henry et al., 1984) and represents several unique habitats, viz., Southern tropical thorn forests, Southern tropical dry deciduous forests, Southern tropical moist deciduous forests, Southern tropical semi evergreen forests, Southern tropical wet evergreen forests, Subtropical montane forests, Grassland at low altitudes and high altitudes (Table 1). Of the recorded 533 endemic plants of Tamil Nadu, 448 (84%) are found in KMTR and more then 50 species of plants are red listed (Annamalai, 2004) and many plants are assessed as strict endemic (Table 2). Many new plants have been described and several plants of geographical interest including threatened and endangered taxa were rediscovered from this area after a lapse of several decades (Henry and Gopalan, 1998).

Table 2. Strict Endemic Plants of KMTR*

Botanical name of the Plant	Family	Habit
Biophytum longibracteatum Tad. and Jacq.	Oxalidaceae	Herb
Corymborchis veratrifolia Bl.	Orchidaceae	herb
Dimorphocalyx beddomei (Benth.) Airy Shaw.	Euphorbiaceae	Tree
Elaeocarpus venustus Bedd.	Elaeocarpaceae	Tree
Eugenia rottleriana Wight and Arn.	Myrtaceae	Tree
Eugenia singampattiana Bedd.	Myrtaceae	Tree
Euphorbia santapaui A.N. Henry	Euphorbiaceae	Shrub
Evodia luna-akenda Gaertn.	Rutaceae	Tree
Glochidion ellipticum Wight	Euphorbiaceae	Tree
Hedyotis eualata (Gamble) A.N.Henry and Subram.	Rubiaceae	Shrub
Hedyotis gamblei A.N.Henry and Subram.	Rubiaceae	Shrub
Hedyotis ramarowii (Gam.) Rao and Hem.	Rubiaceae	Shrub
Hopea utilis Bedd.	Dipterocarpaceae	Tree
Hybanthus travancoricus (Bedd.) Melch.	Violaceae	Herb
Lasianthus blumeanus Wight	Rubiaceae	Shrub
Marsdenia tirunelvelica A.N.Henry and Subram.	Asclepiadaceae	shrub
Memecylon subcordatum Cogn.	Melastomataceae	Shrub
Memecylon subramanii Henry	Melastomataceae	Shrub
Micrococca wightii (Hk.f.) Prain	Euphorbiaceae	Shrub
Nothopegia aureo-fulva bedd.	Acanthaceae	Tree
Ophiorrhiza tirunelvelica A.N.Henry and Subram.	Rubiaceae	Herb
Phyllanthus singampattiana (Seb. and Henry) Kum. and Chandr.	Euphorbiaceae	Shrub
Piper barberi Gamb.	Piperaceae	Shrub
Psychotria nudiflora Wight and Arn.	Rubiaceae	Shrub
Sonerila kanniyakumariana Gopalan and A.N. Henry	Melastomataceae	Herb
Stenosiphonium wightii Bremek	Acanthaceae	Shrub
Syzygium beddomei (Duth.) Chitra	Myrtaceae	Tree
Teucrium plectranthoides Gamb.	Lamiaceae	Herb
Wendlandia angustifolia Wight ex Hook.f.	Rubiaceae	Tree

* Source – Annamalai, 2004.

Ethnology, Questionnaire Survey and Data Collection

The indigenous people inhabiting KMTR are called Kani or Kanikaran (Kanis), the oldest group of the branch of the ethnic group in South India (Southern states of Tamil Nadu and Kerala). They live in five villages of KMTR such as Agasthiyar Kani kudiiruppu, Chinna Mayilar, Periya Mayilar, Inchikuzhi and Servalar each consisting of 5–56 families disbursed in the deep forest areas. Frequent field surveys were carried out in KMTR in different seasons during September 2004 to June 2006. The Kani settlements were located through field surveys and tribal practitioners were consulted to gather medicinal information through questionnaire, interviews and discussions. Plants were collected by the method suggested by

Rao and Sharma (1990). The collected plants were identified by their vernacular names, photographed and sample specimens were collected for the preparation of herbarium and voucher specimens were deposited in the herbarium of Entomology Research Institute, Loyola College, Chennai. Endemism of the species was determined by field study, herbaria and the published literatures of Ahmedullah and Nayar (1986), Nayar (1996) and Annamalai (2004).

Table 3. Endemic plants[#] having ethnomedicinal value in KMTR

Botanical Name / Family	Availability in Tirunelveli hills	Distribution in peninsular India
Acrotrema arnottianum Wight. Dilleniaceae	Upper Kodayar	Western Ghats of Kerala, Travancore, Tirunelveli hills
Aglaia lawii (Wight) Saldanha Meliaceae	Papanasam and Sivagiri up to 800m	Konkan, Kanara, Malabar, Tirunelveli hills
Arenga wightii Griff. Arecaceae	Kalakad	Travancore, Attapadi valley to Tirunelveli hills upto 900m
Baccaurea courtallensis M. Arg. Euphorbiaceae	Courtallam, Papanasam, Upper Kodayar	South of Kanara, Travancore, Anamalais, Tirunelveli hills
Begonia fallox DC. Begoniaceae	Kalakad, Papanasam, Upper Kodayar, Mahendragiri	Southern Western Ghats
Begonia floccifera Bedd. Begoniaceae	Kalakad, Mahendragiri, Upper kodayar, Papanasam, Naraikadu, Thirukurangudi, Manjolai,	Travancore, Tirunelveli hills
Biophytum insignis Gamble Oxalidaceae	Papanasam	Tirunelveli hills
Biophytum longibracteatum Tad. and Jac. Oxalidaceae	Papanasam	Tirunelveli hills
Blachia calycina Benth. Euphorbiaceae	Throughout the hills	Western Ghats of Kerala, Karnataka and Tamil Nadu
Blachia umbellata Baill. Euphorbiaceae	Courtallam, Papanasam, Thirukurangudi	Southern Western Ghats
Calamus brandisii Baccari ex Hook.f.* Arecaceae	Naraikadu, Inchikuzhi, Kannikatty	North Canara to Tirunelveli hills
Capparis diversifolia Wight and Arn.* Capparaceae	Mundanthurai, Papanasam, Kalakad	Pondicherry, Anamalais, Travancore, Tirunelveli hills
Capparis rheedii DC.* Capparaceae	Papanasam	Western Ghats of Kerala and Tamil Nadu
Cayratia pedata (Lam.) Juss. ex Gagnep. var. pedata Vitaceae	Kalakad, Courtallam, Sivagiri, Upper Kodayar, Papanasam, Sivasailam, Thirukurangudi,	Southern Western Ghats
Coscinium fenestratum Gaertn. Menispermaceae	Kalakad and Petchiparai	Southern Western Ghats
Curcuma neilgherrensis Wigh. Zingiberaceae	Kalakad	Throughout Western Ghats at high altitudes
Dimorphocalyx lawianus Hook.f. Euphorbiaceae	Courtallam, Papanasam, Kalakad, Mahendragiri	All districts of western Ghats at an altitude of 1400m
Diotacanthus albiflorus Benth. Acanthaceae	Papanasam and Upper Kodayar	Travancore, Tirunelveli hills, South Western Ghats of Kerala
Eugenia singampattiana Bedd. Myrtaceae	Papanasam, Valayar, Singampatti	Endemic to Tirunelveli hills
Gordonia obtusa Wall. Ternstroemiaceae	Kalakad, Manjolai, Courtallam, Mahendragiri, Upper Kodayar	Throughout Konkan to Travancore
Grewia gamblei Drumm. Tiliaceae	Courtallam and Thirukurangudi	Southern Western Ghats, Wynaad, Nilgiris, Coimbatore
Hedyotis eualata (Gamb.) Henry and Subr. var. agasthyamalayana*	Inchikuzhi, Papanasam, Upper Kothayar	Agasthiyamalai hills of Kerala and Tamil Nadu

Rubiaceae		
Kingiodendron pinnatum Harms Caesalpiniaceae	Throughout the hills	South Kanara -Travancore, Nilgiris, Coimbatore, Deccan in Karnataka, Andhra Pradesh, Tirunelveli hills
Knoxia heyneana DC. Rubiaceae	Kalakad	Tirunelveli, Travancore hills, Dindigul hills of Tamil Nadu
Litsea ligustrina (Nees.) Hook.f. Lauraceae	Papanasam, Kalakad, Sivagiri, Upper kothayar	Deccan, Coimbatore hills, Nilgiris, Palnis, Tirunelveli hills
Botanical Name / Family	Availability in Tirunelveli hills	Distribution in peninsular India
Mallotus stenanthus Muell. Arg. Euphorbiaceae	Papanasam, Courtallam, Sivasailam, Upper Kodayar	Konkan, Kanara, Anamalais, Travancore, Tirunelveli hills
Meiogyne pannosa (Dalzell) Sinclair. Annonaceae	Mahendragiri, Courtallam, Kalakad	Throughout Western Ghats in the altitude of 600 – 1400 m
Memecylon malabaricum Cogn. Melastomataceae	Papanasam, Kalakad and Naraikadu up to 1500m	Coimbatore to Kanyakumari, Palni hills, Kanara, Nilgiris
Miliusa eriocarpa Dunn. Annonaceae	Papanasam, Mancholai, Sivagiri	Southern Western Ghats and in all districts of Tamil Nadu
Neanotis monosperma (Wall. ex. W and A.) W. H. Lewis var. *tirunelvelica* Rubiaceae	Kouthalai, Kothayar	Tirunelveli hills
Orophea thomsonii Bedd. Annonaceae	Kalakad, Sivagiri and Sivasailam	Travancore, Anamalais, Tirunelveli hills
Phyllanthus baillonianus M. Arg. Euphorbiaceae	Papanasam and Upper Kodayar up to 1000m	Southern Western Ghats
Piper hymenophyllum Miq. Piperaceae	Kalakad and upper Kodayar	Nilgiris, Travancore, Tirunelveli, Western Ghats of Karnataka
Polyalthia rufescens Hook.f. and Thomson* Annonaceae	Valayar	West Coasts, Cochin, Malabar to Travancore, Tirunelveli hills
Pouzolzia cymosa W. Urticaceae	Kalakad up to 600m	Nilgiris, Coimbatore, Kolli, Shevroy hills
Psychotria connata L. Rubiaceae	Kalakad, Papanasam, Courtallam, Upper Kodayar up to 1100m	Travancore, Tirunelveli hills
Psychotria flavida Blume. Rubiaceae	Kalakad and Papanasam	Konkan, Kanara to Travancore, Tirunelveli
Botanical Name / Family	Availability in Tirunelveli hills	Distribution in peninsular India
Pterospermum obtusifolium Wight. Sterculiaceae	Kannikatty and Inchikuzhi	Travancore, Tirunelveli hills, forests of central Tamil Nadu
Rauvolfia beddomei Hk. F. Apocynaceae	Kothayar	Southern Western Ghats of Kerala, Tamil Nadu
Scleria lithosperma (L.) Sw. Cyperaceae	Throughout the foot hills	Tirunelveli hills
Scolopia crenata Wight and Arn. Flacourtiaceae	Manjolai, Sivasailam, Papa-nasam, Courtallam, Sivagiri up to 500m	Tirunelveli hills, Tiruchirappalli surroundings of Tamil Nadu
Solanum vagum Heyne. Solanaceae	Courtallam and Papanasam up to 600m	Tirunelveli hills
Syzygium zeylanicum (L.) DC. var. *lineare* (Duthie) Alston Myrtaceae	Papanasam and Kalakad up to 1500m	Southern western Ghats
Trichopus zeylanicus Gaertn. Trichopodaceae	Kalakad and Papanasam up to 900m	Endemic to Agasthiyamalai hills
Trichosanthes cuspidata Lam. Cucurbitaceae	Kannikatty and Inchikuzhi	Travancore and Tirunelveli hills
Zehneria maysorensis (Wight and Arn.) Arn. Cucurbitaceae	Kouthalai	Southern Western Ghats of Tamil Nadu, Madurai

- Annamalai, 2004; * previously reported by Viswanathan et al. (2001).

Results and Discussion

Of the recorded vascular plants (approximately 2000) in KMTR, 601 species of plants are reported as medicinal plants (Annamalai, 2004). Among the collected 383 species of ethnomedicinal plants in KMTR in the present study (Ayyanar, 2008), 46 species are endemic (Table 3). For each species botanical name, family, distribution in Tirunelveli hills and Peninsular India are provided. Euphorbiaceae and Rubiaceae are the leading families with more number of endemic ethnomedicinal plants with 6 and 4 species respectively. The genus *Begonia*, *Blachia*, *Biophytum* and *Psychotri*a with 2 species of endemic plants have ethnomedicinal importance. *Begonia* is an endemic genus, since the genus is represented in India with 60 species, of which 23 species are found to be endemic. A large number of *Begonia* species have been sited from Northeastern India and Sikkim and seven endemic *Begonias* have been reported from peninsular India (Kumar and Bhattacharyya, 1992).

The plants such as *Eugenia singampattiana* and *Biophytum longibracteatum* are declared as strict endemic plants to KMTR.

Environmental or anthropogenic pressure on many rare plant species causes their distribution to so limited and wipe out the species (Karuppasamy et al., 2001). Sarcar et al. (2006) studied the total number of the species *Eugenia singampattiana* in two isolated fragmented populations such as Singampatti and Papanasam hills of Tirunelveli hills and they suggested that this species has narrow zones of endemism in the world and its status is required to be revised as a plant of Critically Endangered.

Most of the plants of KMTR are rapidly getting threatened, because of the disturbance of anthropogenic activities inside the forest areas. KMTR includes a number of religious places like Nambikoil in Thirukurangudi range, Karumandiamman and Pattarayan koils in Kalakad range, Amman koil in Ambasamudram range, Agasthiar and Sorimutthayyanar koil in Papanasam range, Lord Shiva temple in Mundanthurai range (foot hills), Golakanathan and Durga temple in Kadayam range. Among these Sorimutthayyanar koil and Nambikoil are the very famous pilgrimage places, which are visited by large number of persons in festival seasons (Annamalai, 2004).

A vast number of habitats in peninsular India are under threat due to mining, plantations, building of dams and other anthropogenic activities (Ahmedullah and Nayar, 1986). Likewise, during the last few decades the forests of KMTR was also subjected to various anthropogenic pressures such as agriculture, construction of hydro-electric project, raising of monoculture plantations, unscientific extraction of minor forest produce and other developmental activities (Swamy et al., 2000) and some major changes in habitat management have occurred in these forests. Shahabuddin and Raman (2007) suggested that, to ensure strict nature protection, there is an urgent need to develop alternatives to household and livelihood needs for plant products, of people living in and around protected areas.

While the demand for medicinal plants is increasing, their survival in their natural habitats is under threat and a number of medicinal plants have been assessed as endangered, vulnerable and threatened due to over harvesting in the wild (FRLHT). For example, *Aegle marmelos*, *Andrographis paniculata*, *Aristolochia tagala*, *Gloriosa superba*, *Madhuca longifolia*, *Piper nigrum*, *Rauvolfia serpentina* and *Terminalia arjuna* are known as common plants. Simultaneously, these plants are collected extensively by the traditional practitioners, plant collectors, traders and herbalists for their role in medicinal preparation and now they are in threat category. The different disturbance regime by the human population to environment has shrunken the biological diversity.

Conclusion

This study revealed that KMTR has rich diversity of plants with varied ethnomedicinal uses and a large amount of them are endemic. It is expected that some more species of medicinal plants are facing threat to their existence in the wild and some of them have become extinct (e.g. *Eugenia singampattiana*). Conservation of such medicinal plants is important for the protection of natural biodiversity. Hence, efforts must be taken to protect the biodiversity in this area by involving the local communities. Conservation measures targeted at the endemic and threatened plants as well as most important medicinal plants of the reserve will prevent destruction of natural vegetation. In addition, trainings should be given to the indigenous communities regarding the connection between the plants around their environment, the technique of identifying the endemic and red listed plants with medicinal importance. Destruction and reduction of habitats in the forest and surrounding areas diminish the loss in biodiversity; hence the conservation based forestry practices with the help of tribal people are essential to protect the forest and its environs.

Acknowledgments

The authors are thankful to ICMR, New Delhi for providing financial assistance; the Chief Wildlife Warden, Principle Chief Conservator of Forests, Chennai for giving permission to take up field trips in KMTR. We also grateful to the cooperation received from the local people who shared their knowledge on plants with us during field trips.

References

Ahmedullah, M and Nayar, M.P. (1986). *Endemic Plants of the Indian Region.* Vol. I Peninsular India, Botanical Survey of India, India.

Annamalai, R. (2004). *Flora of Kalakad Mundanthurai Tiger Reserve, Tamil Nadu Biodiversity Strategy and Action Plan - Forest Biodiversity.* Tamil Nadu Forest Department, Government of India, Chennai, India.

Ayyanar, M. (2008). *Ethnobotanical Wealth of Kani Tribe in Tirunelveli Hills.* Ph. D. Thesis, University of Madras, Chennai, India.

Ayyanar, M. and Ignacimuthu, S. (2005). Traditional knowledge of Kani tribals in Kouthalai of Tirunelvelli hills, Tamil Nadu, India. *Journal of Ethnopharmacology*, 102: 246 – 255.

Dhar, U., Manjkhola, S., Joshi, M., Bhatt, A., Bisht, A.K. and Joshi, M. (2002). Current status and future strategy for development of medicinal plants sector in Uttaranchal, India. *Current Science*, 83: 956–964.

FRLHT (Foundation for Revitalization of Local Health Traditions), Bangalore, India. http://envis.frlht.org.in.

Hegde, H.V., Hegde, G.R. and Kholkute, S.D. (2007). Herbal care for reproductive health: Ethno medicobotany from Uttara Kannada district in Karnataka, India. *Complementary Therapies in Clinical Practice,* 13: 38-45.

Henry, A.N. and Gopalan, R. (1998). Kalakad - Mundanthurai Tiger Reserve, Tamil Nadu - A floristic assessment. In: *Plant Diversity in Tiger Reserves of India.* Hajra, P.K., Gangopadhyay, M. and Chakrabarty, T. (Eds.). pp. 5-12. Botanical Survey of India, Kolkata.

Henry, A.N., Chandrabose, M., Swaminathan, M.S. and Nair, N.C. (1984). Agasthiyamalai and its environs: A potential area for a biosphere reserve. *Journal of Bombay Natural History Society*, 82: 282–290.

Jagtap, S.D., Deokule, S.S. and Bhosle, S.V. (2006). Some unique ethnomedicinal uses of plants used by the Korku tribe of Amravati district of Maharashtra, India. *Journal of Ethnopharmacology*, 107: 463-469.

Jain, S.K. (1991). *Dictionary of Indian Folk Medicine and Ethnobotany.* Deep publications, Paschim Vihar, New Delhi.

Jain, S.K. (2001). Ethnobotany in Modern India. *Phytomorphology,* Golden Jubilee Issue: 39-54.

Jamir, N.S. (1999). Ethnobiology of Naga tribe in Nagaland: I. Medicinal herbs (India). *Ethnobotany,* 9: 101-104.

Kala, C.P. (2000). Status and conservation of rare and endangered medicinal plant in the Indian trans-Himalaya. *Biological Conservation,* 93: 371-379.

Karuppasamy, S., Rajasekaran, K.M. and Karmegam, N. (2001). Endemic flora of Sirumalai hills, South India. *Journal of Economic and Taxonomic Botany*, 25: 367–373.

Katewa, S.S., Chaudhary, B.L. and Jain, A. (2004). Folk herbal medicines from tribal area of Rajasthan, India. *Journal of Ethnopharmacology*, 92: 41-46.

Kumar, K.D. and Bhattacharyya, U.C. (1992). Endemic species of the family Begoniaceae of India. *Journal of Economic and Taxonomic Botany,* 16: 565–568.

Laloo, R.C., Kharlukhi, L., Jeeva, S. and Mishra, B.P. (2006). Status of medicinal plants in disturbed and the undisturbed sacred forests of Meghalaya, northeast India: population structure and regeneration efficacy of some important species. *Current Science,* 90: 225–232.

Manickam, V.S., Jothi, G.J., Murugan, C. and Sundaresan, V. (2004). *Check-list of the Flora of Tirunelveli hills, Southern Western Ghats, India.* Centre for Biodiversity and Biotechnology, St. Xavier's College, Palayamkottai, India. p. i –ii.

Melkani, V.K. (2001). Involving local people in biodiversity conservation in the Kalakad–Mundanthurai Tiger Reserve - An overview. *Current Science,* 80: 437–441.

Nayar, M.P. and A.R.K. Sastry. (1987 – 1990, Vol. I to III). *Red Data Book of Indian Plants.* Botanical Survey of India, Calcutta.

Pal, D.C. (2000). Ethnobotany in India. In: *Flora of India. Introductory volume - part II.* Singh, N.P., Singh, D.K., Hajra, P.K. and Sharma B.D. (eds). pp. 303–320. Botanical Survey of India, Calcutta.

Pattanaik, C., Sudhakar, C.S. and Murthy, M.S.R. (2008). An ethnobotanical survey of medicinal plants used by the Didayi tribe of Malkangiri district of Orissa, India, *Fitoterapia,* 79: 67-71.

Rao, R.R. and Sharma, B.D. (1990). *A Manual of Herbarium Collections.* Botanical Survey of India, Calcutta.

Riemann, H. and Ezcurra, E. (2005). Plant endemism and natural protected areas in the peninsula of Baja California, Mexico. *Biological Conservation,* 122: 141-150.

Sarcar, M.K., Sarcar, A.B. and Chelladurai, V. (2006). Rehabilitation approach for *Eugenia singampattiana* Bedd. - an endemic and critically endangered tree species of southern tropical evergreen forests in India. *Current Science,* 91: 472–481.

Semwal, D.P., Pardhasaradhi, P., Nautiyal, B.P. and Bhatt, A.B. (2007). Current status, distribution and conservation of rare and endangered medicinal plants of Kedarnath Wildlife Sanctuary, Central Himalayas, India. *Current Science,* 92: 1733–1738.

Shahabuddin, G. and Kumar, R. (2007). Effects of extractive disturbance on bird assemblages, vegetation structure and floristics in tropical scrub forest, Sariska Tiger Reserve, India. *Forest Ecology and Management,* 246: 175–185.

Swamy, P.S., Sundarapandian, S.M., Chandrasekar, P. and Chandrasekaran, S. (2000). Plant species diversity and tree population structure of a humid tropical forest in Tamil Nadu, India. *Biodiversity and Conservation,* 9: 1643–1669.

Tchouto, N.G.P., Yemefack, M., De Boer, W.F., De Walde, L.J.G., Maeswn, V.D. and Cleef, A. M. (2006). Biodiversity hotspots and conservation priorities in the Campo-Ma'anrain forests, Cameroon. *Biodiversity and Conservation,* 15: 1219-1252.

In: Medicinal Plants and Sustainable Development   ISBN 978-1-61761-942-7
Editor: Chandra Prakash Kala   © 2011 Nova Science Publishers, Inc.

Chapter 14

Indigenous Knowledge of Medicinal Plants among Rural Communities of Dhutatoli Forest Range in Pauri District, Uttarakhand, India

P. C. Phondani[1]*, R. K. Maikhuri[1], C. S. Negi[1], C. P. Kala[2], M. S. Rawat[3] and N. S. Bisht[4]

[1]G.B. Pant Institute of Himalayan Environment and Development
Garhwal Unit, Srinagar Garhwal– 246 174, Uttarakhand, India
[2]Ecosystem and Environment Management, Indian Institute of Forest Management,
Nehru Nagar, Bhopal– 462 003, Madhya Pradesh, India
[3]National Medicinal Plants Board, Janpath-110001, New Delhi, India
[4]H.N.B. Garhwal Central University, B.G.R. Campus Pauri
Garhwal–246001, Uttarakhand, India

Abstract

The present study documents the indigenous knowledge of medicinal plants that are used in surrounding Dhutatoli forest range of Uttarakhand state in India. Ethnomedicinal uses of 54 medicinal plant species along with botanical name, vernacular name, family, habitat and occurrence, part used and folk medicinal uses are presented. All these plants belong to 39 families and used to cure more than 47 types of different ailments. Out of 54 plants, 28 plant species used to cure more than one disease. In majority of the cases it was found that underground parts such as root, tuber, bulb, rhizome etc. are used in preparation of medicines for curing ailments. Most of the diseases are cured from the plants belong to herbaceous community. Approximately 70% population from the villages was found dependent on herbal treatment and preferred to visit Vaidyas (local medical practitioners) for curing common ailments. It is noticed that every elder both man and woman in the villages posses sound knowledge of locally available medicinal plants. The study emphasizes the potentials of the ethnobotanical research and the need

---

* E-mail: prakashphondani@gmail.com, pc.phondani@rediffmail.com for the documentation of traditional knowledge pertaining to the medicinal plant utilization for the greater benefit of mankind.

Keywords: Medicinal plants, indigenous knowledge, Himalaya, traditional herbal healers.

Introduction

Uttarakhand is one of the hilly states in the Indian Himalayan region. Because of its unique geography and diverse climatic conditions it harbours the highest number of plant species known for medicinal properties among all the Indian Himalayan states (Kala et al., 2004). The majority of the human populations in Uttarakhand state (65%) live in rural areas. There are very few primary health centres in the states. Each primary health centre caters more than 31,000 people although the stipulated norm of 20,000 is expected for the hilly region of Uttarakhand (Samal et al., 2004). Therefore, the rural inhabitants of Uttarakhand are still dependent on the *Vaidyas* (traditional herbal practitioners) for treating disease due to isolation being inhabited in remote and far flung areas and relatively poor access to modern medical facilities (Maikhuri et.al., 1998; Kala, 2002a, 2005). The Medicinal and Aromatic Plants (MAPs) and their products have a very long history of being utilized and traded in the Himalayan region. There has been a recent dramatic surge of interest of appears to be the result of emerging new strategy for economic development, health improvement and conservation and management of valuable plant species. Of the 2500 wild plant species of known medicinal value found in the Indian sub-continent (Kempanna, 1974), 300 species are used by 8000 licensed drug manufacturing units in India (Ahamad, 1993). It is reported that western Himalaya contains 50% of plant drugs mentioned in the British Pharmacopoeia. It caters to 80%, 46% and 33% of the Ayurvedic, Unani and Allopathic system of medicines, respectively and contributes a major share in the economy of the rural and traditional communities. Traditional system of medicine is a wise practice of indigenous knowledge system, which has saved the lives of poor people around the globe. Traditional knowledge system is of particular relevance to the poor in the following sectors: agriculture, animal husbandry and ethnic veterinary medicine, management of natural resources, primary health care and preventive medicine, psycho-social care, saving and lending, community development, poverty alleviation, etc. (Maikhuri et al., 2000). According to an estimate of the world Health Organization about 80% of the populations of developing countries rely on traditional medicine, mostly plant drugs, for their primary health care. One important common element of complementary or traditional medicine is that they encourage and elect self-healing. Therefore, an urgent need for a comprehensive analysis and documentation of indigenous knowledge of medicinal plants based traditional health care system of rural communities inhabited in remote and an isolated valley of Himalayan region becomes increasingly important.

Study Area

The present study was carried out in 14 villages in and around of Dudhatoli forest range in Pauri district of Uttarakhand state in India. The study area covers an altitudinal range of 1550 - 2700 masl and is located at the latitudes 30^0 00.993' to 30^0 03.764' N and longitudes 79^0 09.724' to 79^0 12.040' E. The climate of the study area can be divided into three distinct seasons, namely rainy (Jul to Sept), winter (Nov to Feb) and summer (Apr to Jun). The mean annual rainfall in the study area was recorded as 1652 mm and temperature remains cool and pleasant all around the year. Mean minimum monthly temperature ranged between 6.4 °C - 15.0 °C whereas; mean maximum monthly temperature ranged between 13.20 °C - 27.0 °C. All the study villages are situated within 1-11 Km. away from the road head where the primary health care centres are rarely exit or are in very poor conditions. The major economic activities of the people inhabited in rural landscape are collection of non-timber forest products, agriculture and animal husbandry. The local people of these areas depends on traditional system of medicine for curing different ailments they suffer from, and the region is famous for its rich biodiversity, socio-cultural, tradition and mythology.

Methodology

An extensive literature survey (Kala, 2002; Maikhuri et al., 1998; Gaur, 1999) was carried out to gather information on locality, local names, altitude range, habitat, and plant parts used for curing different ailments by local communities of the study area. The information related to ethnobotany was collected using questionnaires, interviews and group discussion in the fields. Extensive field visits was made with traditional herbal practitioners to gather information on the identity and occurrence of medicinal plants and mode of their utilization. Randomly selected households in the study site were surveyed to gather information on medicinal plants used in other purposes. The perception of local people about knowledge of medicinal plants used in traditional health care system and prefer to visit *Vaidyas* for curing ailments were analysed within the different groups of people belonging to different age class i e. young, elder and old (Kala, 2004, 2010). The information related to quantity/dosage of medicine prepared from different medicinal plants and prescribed to the patient for particular period of time was obtained from the traditional herbal practitioners. The data obtained was analyzed carefully in MS Excel spread sheet were utilized to make simple calculations, determine proportions and other related information. The plant species collected was maintained in to herbarium specimens, and were identified with the help of literature, regional floras (Gaur, 1999; Naithani, 1985) and taxonomical experts of the HNB Garhwal Central University and other RandD Institutions. Specimens of each species identified were brought to the G.B. Pant Institute (Garhwal Unit) herbarium for scientific identification where they were subsequently deposited.

Table 1. Medicinal plants used by local people for curing different Ailments

S.No.	Name of plants	Vernacular name	Family	Habit	Part used	Folk medicinal uses
1.	*Achyranthes aspera*	Latjira	Amaranthaceae	Climber	Whole	Ring worm, Asthma
2.	*Aconitum hetrophyllum*	Atis	Ranunculaceae	Herb	Root	Fever, Stomach ache
3.	*Acorus calamus*	Buch	Araceae	Herb	Whole	Cough, Dyspepsia
4.	*Adhatoda vasica*	Vashika	Acanthaceae	Shrub	Leaves	Fever, Bronchitis
5.	*Allium sativum*	Lashun	Liliaceae	Herb	Bulb	Stomach disease
6.	*Aloe vera*	Ghirt kumari	Liliaceae	Herb	Leaves	Diabetes, Skin disease
7.	*Angelica glauca*	Choru	Apiaceae	Herb	Root	Fever, Gastric
8.	*Arnebia benthami*	Balchari	Boraginaceae	Herb	Root	Hair disease
9.	*Asculus indica*	Pangar	Hippocastanaceae	Tree	Root, Bark	Rheumatic pain
10.	*Asparagus racemosus*	Jhirna	Liliaceae	Shrub	Root	Epilepsy
11.	*Berberis aristata*	Chatru	Berberidaceae	Shrub	Root	Eye disease
12.	*Bergenia ciliata*	Silphori	Saxifragaceae	Herb	Root	Kidney stone, Piles, Paralysis
13.	*Brassica compestris*	Sarsoo	Brassicaceae	Herb	Leaves, Seed	Anemia, Skin disease
14.	*Cannabis sativa*	Bhang	Cannabaceae	Herb	Leaves	Piles
15.	*Capsicum annuum*	Mirch	Solanaceae	Herb	Fruit	Rabies, Snake bite
16.	*Cedrus deodara*	Devdar	Pinaceae	Tree	Bark	Rheumatism, Back pain
17.	*Centella asiatica*	Brahmi	Apiaceae	Herb	Leaves	Leucorrhea, Epilepsy, Mental
18.	*Citrus aurantifolia*	Kaghzi Nimbu	Rutaceae	Tree	Fruit	Common cold
19.	*Coriandrum sativum*	Dhaniya	Apiaceae	Herb	Leaves	Stomach disorder
20.	*Cucumis sativus*	Kakree	Cucurbitaceae	Climber	Seed	Urinary disorder
21.	*Curcuma domestica*	Haldi	Zingiberaceae	Herb	Rhizome	Blood purifier, Eye disease
22.	*Cynodon dectylon*	Dub ghass	Poaceae	Creeper	Whole	Vomiting, Dysentery, Powerful
S.No.	Name of plants	Vernacular name	Family	Habit	Part used	Folk medicinal uses
23.	*Daucus carota*	Gajar	Apiaceae	Herb	Root, Seed	Anemia, Abortifacient
24.	*Eupatorium perfoliatum*	Bashya	Asteraceae	Shrub	Leaves	Cuts
25.	*Ficus semicardata*	Khina	Moraceae	Tree	Fruit, Milk	Provide strength, Baldness
26.	*Hedychium spicatum*	Van-Haldi	Zingiberaceae	Herb	Rhizome	Asthma, Energetic
27.	*Juglans regia*	Akhrot	Juglandaceae	Tree	Embryo	Pregnancy
28.	*Lyonia ovalifolia*	Anyar	Ericaceae	Tree	Buds	Itching
29.	*Macrotyloma uniflorum*	Gaheth	Fabaceae	Herb	Seed	Kidney stone

#	Scientific name	Local name	Family	Habit	Part used	Uses
30.	*Mentha arvensis*	Podina	Lamiaceae	Herb	Leaves	Stomach disorder
31.	*Momordica charantia*	Karela	Cucurbitaceae	Climber	Fruit, Seed	Rheumatic, Stomachache
32.	*Musa paradisca*	Kela	Musaceae	Tree	Spadix	Cough, Cold
33.	*Myrica esculenta*	Kafal	Myricaceae	Tree	Fruit	Cardiac disorder
34.	*Ocimum sanactum*	Tulsi	Lamiaceae	Herb	Leaves	Bronchitis, Constipation
35.	*Phyllanthus emblica*	Anowla	Euphorbiaceae	Tree	Fruit, Bark	Blood purifier, Throatache
36.	*Picrorhiza kurrooa*	Kutak	Scrophulaceae	Herb	Root	Typhoid fever, Jaundice
37.	*Pinus wallichiana*	Kail	Pinaceae	Tree	Resin	Arthritis
38.	*Piper nigrum*	Kali mirch	Piperaceae	Herb	Fruit	Common cold
39.	*Prunus persica*	Aaru	Rosaceae	Tree	Leaves	Wormosis
40.	*Quercus leucotrichophora*	Banj	Fagaceae	Tree	Seed	Snake bite
41.	*Raphanus sativa*	Muli	Brassicaceae	Herb	Root	Jaundice
42.	*Reinwardtia indica*	Phiunli	Linaceae	Herb	Petal	Tounghwash
43.	*Rhododendron anthopogon*	Awon	Ericaceae	Tree	Leaves	Ring worm
44.	*Rosa sinensis*	Gulab	Rosaceae	Shrub	Flower	Eye disease
45.	*Rumex hastatus*	Almoru	Polygonaceae	Herb	Leaves	Wounds, Bleeding
46.	*Sesamum orientale*	Til	Pedaliaceae	Herb	Seed, eaves	Aphrodisiac, Body pain
47.	*Swertia chirata*	Cheraita	Gentianaceae	Herb	Whole	Fever, Diabetes
48.	*Taxus baccata*	Thuner	Taxaceae	Tree	Bark	Anti- cancer, Bone fracture
49.	*Thalictrum javanicum*	Peeli jari	Ranunculaceae	Herb	Root	Diabetes, Jaundice
50.	*Tinospora sinensis*	Gilai	Menispermaceae	Climber	Whole	Fever, Leprosy, Urinary
51.	*Valeriana hardwick*	Tagar	Valerianaceae	Herb	Root	Urinary disorder, Joint pain
52.	*Verbascum Thapsus*	Akulbeer	Scrophulaceae	Herb	Whole	Bronchitis, Asthma
53.	*Vigna mungo*	Kali dal	Fabaceae	Climber	Seed	Bone fracture
54.	*Zanthxylum armatum*	Timru	Rutaceae	Shrub	Bark	Toothache

Results and Discussion

The results showed that the rural communities of this region possess immense knowledge and make use of 54 medicinal plant species belonging 39 families used for medicinal purposes for curing 47 different ailments. About 28 plant species is used to cure more than one disease. Among the plants used remedies they are categorized as per their use parts and used underground parts (27.7%), leaves (24.1%), fruits (12.9%), seeds (9.2%), bark (9.3%), flower (5.6%) and whole (11.2%) of medicinal plant species contributes in curing a verity of diseases. In addition to this, out of the total medicinal plants used majority of them belonged to herbaceous community (51.8%) followed by trees (25.9%), shrubs (11.2%), climber (9.2%) and creeper (1.8%), collected from forest and alpine meadows (Table 1). However, many of these medicinal plant species are also used for other purposes such as cereals (3.2%), legumes (2.7%), vegetables (7.0%), fruits (10.7%), fibres (2.0%), timbers (5.7%), spices (7.7%), oils (5.0%), and other/none (55.7%) by the local people and only 1-2% medicinal plant species used more than two purposes (Figure 1).Approximately 70% population was found dependent on herbal treatment and maximum people preferred to visit *Vaidyas* for curing common ailments. It was found that besides *Vaidyas*, the old aged people both men and women in the villages had sound knowledge about medicinal values of some specific plants, especially those species which are very oftenly used for common diseases like cough, cold, fever, viral fever, headache, stomach ache, diarrhoea, dysentery, minor wounds and cuts. This could be said as wisdom of age because the younger were poor in knowledge of medicinal plants but still they had faith in the efficacy of these medicines. As per the survey conducted in the villages regarding percentage of people preferred to visit *Vaidyas* for curing ailments reveals that about 68% veteran category of Kimwadi village prefers to visit *Vaidyas* for curing ailments. The percentage of young and elder category of local people visiting *Vaidyas* is very less in all the villages as compared to old (Table 2). Among the people surveyed regarding knowledge of medicinal plants in different age groups showed that about 53% of the age old people have good knowledge of traditional health care system followed by elders (31%), where as younger have very less (16%) knowledge (Figure 2).

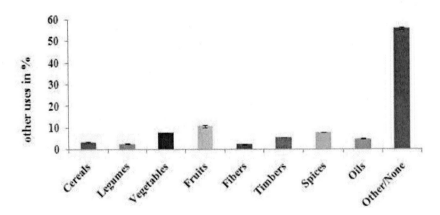

Figure. 1. Other uses of medicinal plant species (%) by the local people in traditional health care system.

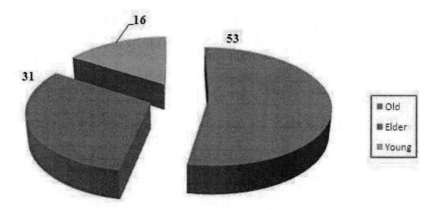

Figure. 2. Age wise percentage of traditional knowledge of medicinal plants used in traditional health care system.

Table 2. Perception of local people (more than 40%) in different age groups preferred herbal treatment for curing Ailments

S. No.	Villages	Young (15-30) (%)	Elder (31-50) (%)	Old (≥51) (%)
1.	Daida	44±4.4	58±2.9	66±6.0
2.	Tolnlyon	43±5.8	61±0.9	61±5.4
3.	Kimwadi	45±6.0	63±1.7	68±6.6
4.	Than	39±6.0	58±1.1	61±3.7
5.	Chaunda	42±6.0	61±1.4	64±6.0
6.	Sunder gaon	45±4.4	59±1.7	64±4.7
7.	Pokhri	42±1.9	47±2.5	54±1.6
8.	Kandie	46±3.7	58±2.2	61±2.4
9.	Massou	38±6.5	59±2.3	66±7.5
10.	Riksal	36±4.6	50±1.6	54±4.9
11.	Jaiti	41±1.6	46±1.5	50±2.2
12.	Syousal	42±2.7	50±2.5	56±3.8
13.	Mansari	45±5.0	58±3.1	62±5.3
14.	Magrown	36±4.6	51±2.1	57±5.6

People preferred to go *Vaidyas* to diagnose their problem although they know some medicinal plants themselves. They said the effectiveness of the herb was connected to the knowledge of the exact nature of diseases. They also added that dose response differs from person to person and also for the same person from time to time because the cause and effect varies. It was found difficult to extract indigenous knowledge base particularly related to medicinal plants from these communities. The younger generations show no interest in learning about this indigenous knowledge preferring modern medicine instead.

Thus, most of the young people are ignorant regarding the use of medicinal plants in curing ailments, however, they do know about the importance of these plants with respect to market.

The use method of the plants varies according to the nature of the disease. In some cases most of the plant species are not used alone but are mixed with other herbs in specific amounts. The medicines are mostly consumed in a powdered form, as the local people believe this form is considered to be more effective than any other form i.e. as pills, tablets etc. In majority of the cases, a decoction of leaves, stem, fruits and root/tuber is drunk or rubbed on the body to cure a disease or diseases. Most of the decoctions were made just by crushing the plant parts with the help of the mortar and pestle, but some were made by boiling plant parts with water, decanting of the liquid and drinking after cooling.

Some plant decoctions were used directly on the wound or the infected part of the body. In some cases the patient is bathed in the decoction made by boiling with water. Generally bathing with the decoction was found common to cure skin diseases.

Paste of some plants was plastered to set dislocated or fractured bones or muscular pain. Some of the diseases like headache, cuts, wounds, burns, boils and skin disease were treated through external application. It was also found that garland made of either the root or the stem was also worn to cure diseases like fever.

In these garlands the numbers of species of the plant part remain fixed. Some herbs are taken empty stomach for its best results and in others there are some restrictions of food for the period of medication.

Conclusion

The documentation of indigenous knowledge and evaluation of the use of plants for a variety of purposes assumes greater significance not just to store it, but also to keep it alive and make it available for future use because of rapid socio-economic and cultural changes that are taking place across the rural st-up of the region. This implies maintaining the ecosystems or natural habitat as well as the socio-cultural organizations of the local people. However, this would conflict with the autonomy of the people introduced. It seems that the only alternative is to carefully record the knowledge and insights of the people living within these traditional societies. Knowledge of herbs, traditional practices and wisdom is in the hands of the older generation particularly the local medical practitioners known as *Vaidyas*. However, this wisdom, and certain medicinal plants, their distribution, important attributes, harvesting and management practices and the extraction of useful properties from them are fast disappearing due to various reasons. Some of them are due to lack of interest of the younger generation, abandonment of apprenticeship with *Vaidyas* which has broken the continuation of knowledge flow to the younger generations, deforestation and illegal collection, which has significantly reduced the availability of herbs in their natural habitat. The so-called scientific outlook has demoralized local practitioners and the drastic change in lifestyles and food habits have necessitated the need to look for alternative methods of relief.

Acknowledgments

The authors are thankful to all local people for their kind co-operation and active participation in this study. We are also thankful to the National Medicinal Plants Board (NMPB), Govt. of India for financial support.

References

Ahmad, R.U. (1993). Medicinal plants used in ISM – their procurement, cultivation, regeneration and import/export aspects – a report. In: *Glimpes in Plant Research Vol.X. Medicinal Plants: New Vistas of Research*. Part 1. (Eds.) Govil, J.N., Singh, V.K. and Shamima Hashmi. pp. 221-258. Today and Tomorrow Publishers and Printers, Delhi.

Gaur, R.D. (1999). *Flora of the District Garhwal North West Himalaya with Ethnobotanical Note*. Trans media, Srinagar Garhwal.

Kala, C.P. (2002). Indigenous knowledge of Bhotia tribal community on wool dying and its present status in the Garhwal Himalaya, India. *Current Science,* 83: 814-817.

Kala, C.P. (2004). Revitalization traditional herbal therapy by exploring medicinal plants: A case study of Uttaranchal state in India. In: *Indigenous Knowledge: Transforming the Academy*. pp. 15-21. Proceedings of an International Conference, Pennsylvania State University, Pennsylvania, USA.

Kala, C.P. (2005). Indigenous uses, population density and conservation of threatened medicinal plants in protected areas of the Indian Himalayas. *Conservation Biology,* 19: 368-378.

Kala, C.P. (2010). *Medicinal Plants of Uttarakhand: Diversity, Livelihood and Conservation*. Biotech Books, Delhi.

Kala, C.P., Farooquee, N.A. and Dhar, U. (2004). Prioritization of medicinal plants on the basis of available knowledge, existing practices and uses value status in Uttarakhand, India. *Biodiversity and Conservation,* 13: 453-469.

Kempanna, C. (1974). Prospects for Medicinal Plants in Indian Agriculture. *World Crops,* 26: 166-168.

Maikhuri, R.K., Nautiyal, S., Rao, K.S. and Saxena, K.G. (1998). Role of medicinal plants in the traditional health care system: A case study from Nanda Devi Biosphere Reserve, Himalaya. *Current Science,* 75 (2): 152-157.

Maikhuri, R.K., Nautiyal, S., Rao, K.S. and Semwal, R.L. (2000). Indigenous Knowledge of medicinal plants and wild edible among three tribal sub-communities of the Central Himalayas, India. *Indigenous Knowledge and Development Monitor,* 8: 7-13.

Naithani, B.D. (1985). *Flora of Chamoli*. Botanical Survey of India. Dehradun. Vol. 2: 595.

Samal, P.K., Shah, A., Tiwari, S.C..and Agrawal, D.K. (2004). Indigenous health care practices and their linkage with bio-resources conservation and socio-economic development in central Himalayan region of India, *Indian J. Traditional Knowledge,* 3 (1), 12-26.

In: Medicinal Plants and Sustainable Development   ISBN 978-1-61761-942-7
Editor: Chandra Prakash Kala   © 2011 Nova Science Publishers, Inc.

Chapter 15

Use of Medicinal Plants for Curing Urogenital Disorders

Chandra Prakash Kala

Ecosystem and Environment management,
Indian Institute of Forest management, Nehru Nagar, Bhopal,
Madhya Pradesh, India

Abstract

Some traditional *Vaidyas,* the practitioners of Ayurveda, claims to cure the number of chronic diseases. In view of understanding such claims, two major uro-genital diseases – leucorrhea and spermatorrhea were selected, and herbal formulations as used by traditional *Vaidyas* for curing these disorders were studied in the remote rural areas of Uttarakhand state in India. The study indicates that despite the availability of effective herbal medicine with some rural traditional *Vaidyas* for curing the selected disorders, people were less aware of this fact and thus hardly approach to these knowledgeable *Vaidyas* for successful treatments. Providing proper incentives to such *Vaidyas* and developing suitable infrastructure may help to revitalize the traditional herbal therapy and also to mitigate the severity of such chronic diseases.

Keywords*:* Herbal therapy, leukorrhea, spermatorrhea, herbal formulations.

Introduction

The use of plants for therapy is evolved with the social and cultural groupings of human beings and this valuable knowledge is perfected over the period of time through innumerable trials and errors (Kala, 2005a). The evolution and recognition of Ayurveda across the world witnesses such facts related to medicinal properties and efficacies of plant species. The practitioners of Ayurveda are known as *Vaidyas*. A sizeable part of this medical system has been documented, yet there is still unrecorded knowledge in oral form on herbal therapy, which has not been documented. The transfer of occupied knowledge to only some specified persons through generations has restricted this valuable knowledge to the limited number of people (Kala, 2006a, 2006b). Simultaneously with the spread of Allopathy, its popularity and process of urbanization, the frequency of use of herbal formulations began to decline and thus not only stopped the further growth of several traditional herbal therapies but also poses threats to their existence (Kala, 1998, 2010a). In rural areas the dependency of local people for therapy on the traditional *Vaidyas* keeps alive the tradition in almost its original form (Kala, 2006c, 2009, 2010b; Phondani et al., 2010; Semwal et al., 2010). This knowledge needs to be documented and standardized through experiments in laboratory for its wide acceptability.

There are number of examples in traditional system of herbal therapies that claim to cure some chronic diseases. It has been observed that many traditional *Vaidyas* claim to cure successfully some chronic uro-genital disorders including leukorrhea and spermatorrhea. In order to understand such claims, this chapter deals with the analysis and documentation of such specialized indigenous knowledge prevalent in remote rural societies of Uttarakhand state in India.

Methods

Semi-structured questionnaire survey was conducted among knowledgeable traditional *Vaidyas* with a view to document the knowledge on the preparation of traditional medical formulations, especially associated with curing of urogenital disorders. After gathering such information from 56 traditional *Vaidyas* resided across various parts of Uttarakhand, five knowledgeable *Vaidyas* were selected randomly for validation of 2 major traditional home made herbal formulations used for curing 2 major disorders – leukorrhea and spermatorrhea. People undergone treatments for these two uro-genital disorders were also interviewed on monthly basis for understanding their views on the effects of the treatments.

Results

Of the total 56 *Vaidyas* interviewed, 6 were young (16-25 years), 14 were adult (26-45 years) and 26 were old (>46 years). The less number of *Vaidyas* in lower age group indicates that there is a decline in this traditional knowledge through generations. At present, the herbal medical knowledge is scattered in the society and many females are quite familiar with some specific treatments, however the profession is basically male dominated. Among the two selected urogenital disorders, the highest number of unhealthy people visited to *Vaidyas* for the treatment of leukorrhea, followed by spermatorrhea (Table 1). Apart from the common formulations used by *Vaidyas*, there was a special herbal drug used by a few *Vaidyas* for the treatment of leucorrhea. About 24 species of medicinal plants are mixed up in a definite proportion to prepare this herbal formulation. *Mucuna pruriens, Plantago depressa, Chlorophytum tuberosum, Tinospora cordifolia, Aegle marmelos, Holarrhena antidysenterica* and *Curculigo orchioides* were the major species used in high proportion for preparing this herbal drug. Besides, some endangered medicinal plant species, such as, *Nardostachys jatamansi, Dactylorhiza hatagirea* and *Crocus sativus* were also used for enhancing the efficacy of this herbal drug.

Table 1. Urogenital disorders and herbal formulations as prescribed by traditional *Vaidyas* for treatment

Name of Disease	Herbal Medicinal Formulation	No. of Patient Treated (monthly)
Leukorrhoea	Half spoon juice of Satawari (*Asparagus racemosus* Willd.) root, half spoon juice of Giloi (*Tinospora cordifolia* L.) and 10 gm refined sugar is mixed up with 250 gm cow milk. This dose is given 2 times in a day morning and evening.	30-35
Spermatorrhea	About 25 gm juice of Semal (*Bombax ceiba*) bark and 25 gm of mishri is given with 250 gm milk two times in a day (morning and evening) before having meals.	25-30

Discussion

In the study area, the traditional healers cure the human diseases by two different methods - chanting 'mantras' during treatment and prescribing only some herbal medicine. Some ailments such as Jaundice, malarial fever, snake bite, stomachache, psychological and some sort of dermatological problems are being cured basically by 'mantras' as well as by the use of some herbs (Kala, 2005a, 2006a). For curing such diseases the patients generally consult the specific healer who has the expertise in mostly curing some particular disorder. Rests of diseases are cured with the help of home-made herbal formula by *Vaidyas*. Snake bite, jaundice and some other similar diseases are cured free of cost.

There is a belief that the potency of healing reduces if fees is taken in its return. In past, there was a similar notion in Tibetan Medical System of therapy (Kala, 2002, 2005b). The other type of *Vaidyas*, who cured almost all the ailments do not visualize any harm in charging the fees for treatment. Earlier, patients used to procure some ration to *Vaidyas* in return of treatment that is now changed to receive cash in return of the treatment. Apart from this, there have been several other changes in the doctrine of this system and also in the processing of formulations.

Now most of the certified *Vaidyas* (*Vaidyas* having formal training and education), mostly purchase the medicine from market that is prepared in pharmaceutical company. The collection of plants from the wild is mainly done by traditional healers living in remote areas. Some *Vaidyas*, who collect the raw material from the wild or purchase it from the market for preparation of home-made formulations, are approached by patients from both urban and rural areas due to the potential positive effects of the prescribed medicine.

Conclusion

Among several ailments and disorders prevalent in the society the urogenital disorders are common. There are high number of patients of leukorrhea and spermatorrhea, and mostly *Vaidyas* are consulted to cure these ailments in the present study area – the Uttarakhand state of India. According to *Vaidyas* there are more than 65% of women suffering from leucorrhea in the rural areas of the study area. Besides many herbal formulations, there is an effective traditional herbal formulation that is used by some specific herbal healers for curing the leucorrhea even if it has become chronic. This chapter also depicts that even the availability of herbal medicine with some rural *Vaidyas* people are less aware of this fact and thus hardly approach to these *Vaidyas* for successful treatment. If the proper incentives are given and infrastructure is made to such traditional healers, this indigenous knowledge can be made useful for the large number of patients suffering from various chronic diseases.

Acknowledgments

I acknowledge the *Vaidyas* of Uttarakhand for their support and cooperation during the fieldwork in various hill districts of Uttarakhand.

References

Kala, C.P. (1998). Ethnobotanical Survey and Propagation of Rare Medicinal Herbs for Small Farmers in the Buffer Zone of the Valley of Flowers National Park, Garhwal Himalaya. Technical Report. International Centre for Integrated Mountain Development, Kathmandu, Nepal.

Kala, C.P. (2002). *Medicinal Plants of Indian Trans-Himalaya*. Bishen Singh Mahendra Pal Singh, Dehradun, India.

Kala, C.P. (2005a). Current status of medicinal plants used by traditional Vaidyas in Uttaranchal state of India. *Ethnobotany Research and Applications*, 3: 267-278.

Kala, C.P. (2005b). Health traditions of Buddhist community and role of amchis in trans-Himalayan region of India. *Current Science*, 89 (8): 1331-1338.

Kala, C.P. (2006a). Preserving Ayurvedic herbal formulations by Vaidyas: The traditional healers of Uttaranchal Himalaya region in India. *HerbalGram*, 70: 42-50.

Kala, C.P. (2006b). Medicinal plants: Potential for economic development in the state of Uttaranchal, India. *International Journal of Sustainable Development and World Ecology*, 13 (6): 492-498.

Kala, C.P. (2006c). Problems and prospects in the conservation and development of the Himalayan medicinal plants sector. *International Journal of Sustainable Development*, 9 (4): 370-389.

Kala, C.P. (2009). Medicinal plants conservation and enterprise development. *Medicinal Plants*, 1 (2): 79-95.

Kala, C.P. (2010a). *Medicinal Plants of Uttarakhand: Diversity, Livelihood and Conservation*. Biotech Books, Delhi.

Kala, C.P. (2010b). Assessment of availability and patterns in collection of Timroo (*Zanthoxylum armatum* DC.): A case study of Uttarakhand Himalaya. *Medicinal Plants*, 2 (2): 79-84.

Phondani, P.C., Maikhuri, R.K. and Kala, C.P. (2010). Ethnoveterinary uses of medicinal plants among traditional herbal healers in Alaknanda catchment of Uttarakhand, India. *African Journal of Traditional, Complementary and Alternative Medicine*, 7 (3): 195-206.

Semwal, D.P., Kala, C.P. and Bhatt, A.B. (2010). Medicinal plants and traditional health care knowledge of vaidyas, palsi and others: A case study from Kedarnath valley of Uttarakhand. *Medicinal Plants*, 2 (1): 51-57.

D. Medicial Plants
and Sustainable Development

In: Medicinal Plants and Sustainable Development   ISBN 978-1-61761-942-7
Editor: Chandra Prakash Kala   © 2011 Nova Science Publishers, Inc.

Chapter 16

Community-Based Entreprises, Local Health Care Promotion and Women Empowerment: An Innovative Case Study from Southern India

Maria Costanza Torri [*1], *Thora Martina Herrmann* [2]
and Maria Luiza Schwarz [3]

[1]University of Toronto Scarborough, Department of
Social Sciences, Canada
[2]Canada Research Chair in Etynoecology and Biodiversity
Conservation, Université de Montréal, Canada
[3]Department of Geography, Université de Montréal, Canada

Abstract

Gender, the socially constructed roles and characteristics assigned to women and men in a specific culture, plays a key role in people's access to, use of and control over biodiversity. This is especially relevant in the case of medicinal plants, as in numerous societies, it is mainly women who are wild plant gatherers and managers, home gardeners and plant domesticators, herbalists and healers, as well as seed custodians.

Yet, in many countries women's knowledge and practices are neglected as insignificant and gendered realities are not acknowledged in many development and plant conservation initiatives. This results in serious inequities in the distribution of the benefits of biodiversity and affects its sustainable management. We will show, through the analysis of an innovative study case, represented by the women-lead cooperative GMCL in India the link between gender and medicinal plants biodiversity uses, sustainable management and access.

We will explore in detail the link between women-based businesses in herbal products and sustainable rural development in a challenging environment counting on limited resources. Finally, our paper shall give an understanding of the key role that

---

[*] E-mail: mctorri@yahoo.it

women entrepreneurship centred upon the herbal sector can play in reinforcing local health care and promoting empowerment poor rural indigenous and tribal women.

Keywords: development, empowerment, gender, commercialization, biological resources, traditional knowledge, local communities, India.

Introduction

World demand for *natural health products* (NHP)- including herbal products of medicine value, food supplements, neutraceuticals, natural and organic food- and *functional food*[1] (FF) has been growing steadily (WHO, 2002). This global market is estimated at around US$16 billion (Planning Commission, 2002). In Canada, the NHP and FF industry is very dynamic and is growing rapidly and is currently making a transition from its niche market status to the main stream.

Despite the growing performance of this sector, the local communities, including the indigenous communities worldwide, who have traditionally been related to natural resources and are too often marginalized. For that reason, there is a concern that an important opportunity for rural communities to increase their livelihoods is lost at the very moment when renewed effort is needed to reduce their marginalization.

Although medicinal plants have been used extensively in many countries, including Canada but also Mexico, especially in the context of traditional medicine as well as more recently by the natural products and phytotherapeutic industry, there are few studies that have focused on the commercial aspects of this phenomenon and its potential as productive engine of rural development and enhancement of livelihoods for the local communities living in semi-arid and arid zones. There is also a vacuum of information from a development perspective, where commercial factors, from small business creation and income generation are addressed.

Gender, the socially constructed roles and characteristics assigned to women and men in a specific culture, plays a key role in people's access to, use of and control over biodiversity (Howard, 2003). This is especially relevant in the case of medicinal plants, as in numerous societies, women have primary responsibility for health care at the household level. Literature shows that, worldwide, it is mainly women who are wild plant gatherers and managers, home gardeners and plant domesticators, herbalists and healers, as well as seed custodians (Howard-Borjas, 2002, Howard, 2003).

Yet, in many countries women's knowledge and practices are neglected as insignificant and gendered realities are not acknowledged in many development and plant conservation initiatives (Agarwal 2000). This results in serious inequities in the distribution of the benefits of biodiversity and affects its sustainable management (Deda and Rubian, 2004).

Previous work on this issue (Herrmann, 2003) has led to conclude that women's local knowledge in plant use, management and conservation is fundamental to guarantee livelihoods enhancement, as well as household and community health care, hence women's

---

[1] Functional foods as defined by Health Canada (1998) are similar in appearance to conventional food but are demonstrated to have physiological benefits and/or reduce the risk of chronic disease beyond basic nutritional functions.

involvement and empowerment are needed to secure sustainable management of biological resources, and to foster women's status and human welfare. This chapter aims to investigate, through the analysis of an innovative study case, represented by the women-lead cooperative GMCL (Gram Mooligai Limited), India, the possible link between gender and medicinal plants biodiversity uses, sustainable management and access. This chapter further explores in detail the link between women-based businesses in herbal products and sustainable rural development in a challenging environment counting on limited resources.

Finally, this chapter aims to obtain a throughout understanding of the key role that women entrepreneurship centred upon the herbal sector can play in reinforcing local health care and promoting empowerment poor rural women while integrating the sustainable use of local medicinal plants.

Role of Gender in Herbal Sector

Poverty alleviation together with gender equality has been placed high on the international development agenda following the adoption of the United Nations Millennium Development Goals (MDGs) in 2000. The first and foremost of these goals is to halve the proportion of people living on less than US$1 per day, and those suffering from hunger, by 2015 (UN Millennium Declaration, 2000). The third goal refers explicitly to gender highlighting the urgent need to "promote gender and empower women".

Yet, despite these global commitments, and the recognition of women's concerns by the international community, the equitable divisions of power, work, access to and control of resources between women and men are hardly ever addressed. The obligation to address the MDGs, together with the high levels of spatial concurrence between regions rich in biodiversity and the majority of the world's rural poor (WRI, 2000), has compelled scholars and practitioners operating at the environment–development interface to seek solutions to poverty that include natural resource-based activities while enhancing gender equality in the same time (Deda et al., 2004, Brewster et al., 2006, Adams et al., 2004, Bird and Dickson, 2005; FAO, 2003, Oksanen and Mersmann, 2003, Roe, 2004, World Bank, 2002, WRI, 2005) The commercialization of natural products is seen as an important potential vehicle for achieving this (Scherr, White and Kaimowitz, 2004). Priority has thus been placed on understanding more fully the contribution biodiversity and the natural product trade can make to achieving the goals of poverty alleviation, gender equality with examination of the links between the use and trade in natural products, livelihood security, and environmental sustainability (MDG 7) forming a focal area for research attention (Roe, 2004).

Numerous studies have left little doubt that natural products derived from biodiversity contribute to the well-being and, sometimes, the very survival of millions of poor rural households (Arnold, 2002, Belcher et al., 2005, Fischer, 2004, Godoy et al., 2000, Narendran et al., 2001, Scherr et al., 2004). The processing and sale of natural products certainly offers a low barrier to entry and widely available option to generate cash income that is progressively being taken up by rural dwellers in many countries, including South Africa, as a means to cope with economic hardship. Indeed, in some situations, such as in the dry woodlands of southern Africa, the trade in natural products may be one of the few accessible local income generating options available to the rural poor, and women in particular (Campbell et al., 2002 and Shackleton, 2004). These products may be harvested for subsistence purposes and/or as commodities that can be offered for sale in the market in raw or processed form. The use and sale of products may take place on a regular basis, seasonally as a gap filler, or only in times of emergency providing an important fallback option or safety net (McSweeny, 2004, Takasaki et al., 2004). Natural product markets have been shown to be significant in assisting rural households to realize some, if not all, of their cash requirements (Marshall and Newton, 2003, Marshall et al., 2006, Narendran et al., 2001, Ndoye et al., 2001), and are particularly crucial for the most marginalized and vulnerable segments of society (Beck and Nesmith, 2001, Cavendish, 2000), women included.

While this "picture" of the significance of the natural product trade for livelihoods exists, the situation in reality is complex and variable, and limited empirical data from across a range of regions, vegetation types, and socio-economic contexts are available to assess the ability of these products to create lasting opportunities for local livelihood enhancement (FAO, 2003). Indeed, the refocusing of the development agenda on poverty has led to recent reassessment of the role that biodiversity plays in livelihoods and poverty alleviation. A profusion of new commentary has emerged. Many authors note that the most disadvantaged populations are less likely to succeed in the herbal market (Arnold and Ruiz-Perez 2001). Generally the members of these communities selling plants species including medicinal ones and derived products receive a minimum percentage of the price paid by consumers.

This poses many fresh questions, and, to some extent, tempers previous optimism regarding the ability of this sector to make a difference by providing a more subtle and complex picture of livelihood–biodiversity linkages (e.g., Arnold, 2002, Belcher, 2005, Koziell, 2001, Lawrence, 2003, Ros-Tonen and Wiersum, 2005, Scherr et al., 2004, Wunder, 2001). Central to these new enquiries is a more perceptive and nuanced appreciation of (a) the links between natural resource dependence and the potential of the natural product trade to provide pathways out of poverty;" and (b) the extent to which opportunities associated with natural product production and sale can be made more pro-poor and thus contribute to the efforts to combat poverty and vulnerability (FAO, 2003) and Koziell, 2001). A key area of debate is whether the trade in natural products can assist in improving livelihoods and income, or alternatively, whether it offers limited options serving only as a last resort, possibly contributing to persistent poverty (Belcher, 2005, Ros-Tonen and Wiersum, 2005 and Wunder, 2001).

This chapter aims to demonstrate, through the analysis of the GMCL that the creation of women- lead enterprises active in the herbal sector can play important and stimulating roles in mobilizing resources for sustainable, lasting and more equitable income generating. Besides, it can reveal a better and deeper understanding of the contribution of commercial activities led by rural poor women to strengthen local health care, to encourage women empowerment, and to maintain biodiversity and ecosystem conservation while taking into account the sociocultural perceptions related to them.

In the last two decades there has been an increase in funds from Governments and international development agencies to create micro- enterprises formed by women. This is in large part because there is an increasing recognition of women's contribution to family income and because according to a current trend, the women who are the single heads of the households and breadwinners amount to ¼ of the households in the world (Mayoux 1995, UNFPA 2004).

The sector of herbal products could represent an interesting area for establishing rural women's entrepreneurship. The increase in the natural products industry is helping to spread the use of plants to other sectors of society, so that the use of medicinal plants has been transformed from being an activity confined to local gatherers and traditional healers to a prosperous business (Hersch-Martinez 2006:47). The estimated amount of aromatic and medicinal species in the international market is around 25,000 species (Schippmann, Leaman et al. 2003). New trends in health care and the search for natural products, meaning those who have no additional chemicals and are made with artisanal methods, has become a growing niche market with great potential for rural development.

Although, the herbal market is becoming more and more receptive, in some cases the plant population is too small or vulnerable to respond to this demand. This is particularly the case in fragile ecosystems such as semi-arid areas that count on limited vegetation cover. In India, between 80 and 90% consumed in medicinal plants the country are harvested from the wild. Concern about the conservation of medicinal plants can be seen at two levels: at the level of species and at the level of ecosystems. On the one hand the problems related to the over-exploitation of certain species with high commercial value have been identified, and on the other hand there are those who identify the changes in the uses of land, the deforestation and degradation of ecosystems as the biggest threat. In short, the major problem is that several species of economic value on the market are being overexploited, while a larger number of species with no-commercial value utilized by local communities for health care, are threatened due to rapid increase in the degradation and loss of natural ecosystems (Bodeker, 1999). The study looks carefully at the issue of conciliation and commercial uses and conservation o medicinal plants and their ecosystems from gender perspective.

The Case Study

Active since 2000, GMCL supplies medicinal herbs to Indian pharmaceutical enterprises (such as Himalaya Drug Company, Natural Remedies, Ompharma etc.) playing an intermediary role between these companies and the local farmers. It also commercialises ayurvedic medicines produced by local communities under the brand of *"Village Herbs"*. Although GMCL has only been operational for a short time, its turnover jumped from $140,000 in 2005-2006 up to $180,000 in 2008, contributing an average of $90 annually to the livelihoods of some 1300 families in Karnataka and Tamil Nadu. GMCL was established by a network of Indian NGOs, particularly FRLHT (Foundation for the Revitalization of Local Health Traditions) and CCD (Covenant Centre for Development), as an attempt at developing participatory management for poor women. The shareholding of the company is represented by female cultivators and gatherers of medicinal plants organised into 72 local groups called *Sanghas[2]*, distributed in 80 villages in Karnataka and Tamil Nadu. GMCL presents a formally established and agreed decision-making structure where all problems connected with the running of the enterprise (for example raw material supplies and prices, technical and managerial problems, wage levels) are discussed at regular meetings of an elected board of directors composed of both managers and representatives of *Sanghas*. These

---

[2] "Sangha" is a Sanskrit word that can be translated roughly as "association" or "assembly" "company" or "community" with common goal, vision or purpose.

latter are elected among the members of the *Sanghas*. GMCL plays the role of a marketing/commercial entity. Its main functions are liaising, selling the raw material and negotiating the commercial conditions with pharmaceutical sector and expanding the market share for the final product. CCD ensures the liaison between GMCL and the local communities, thus acting as a facilitator and action catalyst. Its role involves an *organizational* dimension (facilitating the constitution of *Sanghas* and their coordination), a *communication* dimension (facilitating the flux of information between the different levels of the organization) and a *capacity building* dimension (facilitating the acquisition of knowledge and know-how and the spread of information inside the *Sanghas*).

The Foundation for Revitalization of Local Health Traditions (FRLHT) is a non-governmental organisation established in 1993 in Bangalore (Karnataka). FRLHT seeks to revitalize Indian local health traditions through a range of field activities and research and extension programs.

The main areas of action are:

- conservation of the natural resources used by traditional medicine system.
- demonstration the contemporary relevance of the theory and practice of traditional medicine system
- revitalization the social processes (institutional, oral and commercial) for the transmission of traditional knowledge of healthcare and promotion of its wider use and application.

FRLHT has carried out several botanical and ecological surveys with the aim of cataloguing the medicinal plant species in India. These studies have been alternated by conservation projects, following an action research approach typical of this organization.

One of FRLHT's major projects has been to conserve species of medicinal plants in Indian forests in conjunction with of State governments and the participation of local communities[3].

Another NGO which has played an important role has been CCD (Covenant Centre for Development). CCD is based in Madurai (Tamilnadu) and was promoted in 1988 by a team of professionally trained social work students and teachers.

This NGO has gained considerable experience in mobilizing rural communities in the past 15 years, notably in the context of micro-credit with the creation of Self Help Groups (SHGs) and other village organizations. Working with women-led groups has given CCD insights into the priorities and needs of local communities and has helped the establishment of linkages of trust between the fieldworkers and these rural communities.

---

[3] This initiative has resulted in the setting up of a network of 55 Medicinal Plant Conservation Areas (MPCA) across different forest types and altitude zones in these five states of peninsular India. The most important purpose of this network of MPCAs is that it serves as the gene bank of medicinal plant resources of the region. The network of MPCAs captures the inter and intra specific medicinal plant diversity of peninsular India. The MPCAs capture around 2000 medicinal plant species, which represent 50% of the medicinal plant diversity of the five states, and significantly includes over 75% of the RED Listed Species of these states. For all the MPCA sites, detailed floristic studies on medicinal plant diversity including the threatened, traded and endemic plants have been undertaken.

Methodology

The field study took place in India, in the State of Tamil Nadu, in the districts of Dindugal and Virudhanagar Ramanad over a period of four months in 2007 and 2008. The data was collected through formal individual and group interviews. To complement the data collected in the interview process, I have also used participatory observations, such as attending village organizations' meetings, observing how their members cultivated, gathered and used local medicinal plants. My ethnographic approach is thus based on systematic observations, partly through participation and partly through various types of conventional interviews.

The first set of interviews was carried out with a sample of 15 FRLHT and CCD members, including the directors, programs officers and field officers. These in-depth interviews focused on the main characteristics and the perceived outcomes of this partnership initiative in terms of creation and dissemination of innovation stemming from TM, the contribution of the different network partners and the present and future challenges in the implementation and development of this initiative. The interviews, which consisted of open questions, lasted approximately 60 to 90 minutes.

The second set of interviews consisted of individual and group interviews with the villagers of three village organizations (*Sangha*, *Kalasam* and *MahaKalasam*) who were taking part in the FRLHT and CCD initiative. A sample of 20 members of each village organization was interviewed. In order to ensure a representative sample of the village society, parameters such as age, caste belonging and economic conditions were taken into account. The individual interviews consisted of structured and semi-structured components. The villagers were selected using a snow-ball technique in some of the CCD workers who worked in the area were asked to point us to some members of the village institutions whom I could interview. Their suggestions were based on the active involvement of these persons right from the outset of the initiatives organized by FRLHT and CCD and who, for this reason, were considered knowledgeable resources. Since the villagers to interview were pointed out by the main NGOs involved in the study, I have extended the sample in order to reduce the risk of bias. Half of the total sample was matched with a sample of randomly selected villagers who were taking part in the village organizations. While selecting interviewees, I tried to keep a balance between the socio-economic variables deemed relevant (e.g. age, caste, economic background).

Two focus groups with members of two different village organizations randomly selected were also carried out in order to complement and cross-check the data previously collected through individual interviews. In order to facilitate interaction between members, each focus group consisted of 12 members from the organizations that were not been previously interviewed.

The topics for the above-mentioned focus groups were centred on the role of local institutions in the FRLHT-CCD initiative, on the interrelations between village organisations and the other network partners. In these interviews, I also discussed the future challenges at the community level and put a particular focus on the maintenance of knowledge on traditional medicine.

I also conducted ten interviews in the villages with local folkhealers that are taking part in the initiative. This has enabled us to take into consideration local expert (or guided) knowledge on healing and hence gain some general insights into the local health system and the role played by the folkhealers in the initiative and in the conservation of traditional medicine. The folkhealers were asked to give their opinion on the importance attributed to their practices and knowledge by the villagers.

To analyze the interview transcripts, I have used content analysis. The themes that emerged from the data were grouped in categories such as capacity building, participation in the process of knowledge creation and diffusion, interrelationships with external organisations (in particular with FRLHT and CCD), degree of interest and acceptance of younger generations towards ethnomedicine and related future challenges (ecological constraints, folk healer acceptance, integration of local and scientific knowledge).

Economic Empowerment

The status of women is intimately connected with their economic position, which in turn depends on opportunities for women for participating in economic activities (Liedholm, 2002; Servet, 2006). Women's ability to save and access to bigger income would give them an economic role not only within the household but, may be, outside it as well.

The villagers have emphasized an increase of revenue as the major outcome of the GMCL activity.

A woman, who became a sales representative of GMCL affirms: "Before I used to struggle to make two ends meet. I collected a few rupees earnings to get through the day and I depended on my family for anything that I needed. Now I can give my contribution to support my family with my earnings".

In reference to the raw herbs, the gatherers interviewed stressed how the association with GMCL has allowed them to get better prices from those offered previously by local traders. In the past the villagers pointed out that they had to bear costs of transporting the raw material to the local market. Price fluctuation was a major problem, so that the gathering activity was not profitable for them.

A 40 years old woman from the village of Palavanatham recalls the past:

" Before becoming a member of GMCL, I had to trudge to the towns of Madurai to sell the herbs that I had collected. It was quite a long journey, around 50 Km from my village and I had to go by bus. This was quite expensive. The traders were never satisfied with the quality of my product and used to pay me very little…".

The members of some *Sanghas* still supply few species of plants to the local traders. Nevertheless, their negotiation capacity is increased since when they have become associated with GMCL. A villager from Kurayur explains:

"We supply 5 herbs species to GMCL. After we have decided to be associated with GMCL, some traders still come to my village and ask us to sell them some herb species. We say that we are not interested, that we have already a commitment with GMCL. They usually insist, some of them are ready to offer even a higher price then the one we currently get".

As the finished products are being sold through sales representatives who get a trade commission of 35% on their sales, GMCL has been able to provide the women with an additional form of income. The sales representatives interviewed affirm that the profit on their sales amounts to 20-25%. In tourist places such as B. R. Hills or in rural towns such as Sante Marally, the sales amount to an average of 2000-3000 Rs per month.

A sale representative from the village of Sante Marally affirms:

"Earlier I used to earn around 200-300 Rs everyday. But now I earn up to 1000 Rs and sometimes, even 5000 Rs to 10,000 Rs everyday. Further I can also save more now. I am also able to take care of my parents who stay with me. I also give some money to my son".

In order to examine the economic impact of GMCL, the income generated from taking part in GMCL activity was collated with the total monthly family income. The contribution of GMCL income to total family income is found to be significant indicating the positive impact of the strategy. In spite of the tendency among beneficiaries to underreport income, most of them stated to have generated a monthly income ranging from Rs 1500 to Rs 2000.

After the intervention of GMCL, the villagers are able to increase their savings as a consequence of the reduction of expenditures for medicines. A sales representative affirms:

"if someone has cough I gave her the sugam syrup. If she approaches an allopathic doctor for the same problem, she would have to shell out much money for her consultation. But if she comes to us, they can directly get treated for their problem without wasting much money, especially for older women because the Government hospital is 3 km away".

The advantage of reducing the expenditures in the household for the purchase of medicine is also emphasized by another sale representative from Maddur. She affirms:

"the problem is that we need to pay 20 Rs to the doctor to get a drug worth 2 Rs. By coming to us, people get free advice and they have to spend money only for the medicine. Further, this venture is not illegal because the medicines are all over-the-counter ones".

It is remarkable to note that GMCL has been able to enhance local entrepreneurship and employment. A leader from Umlalli explains:

"Our venture helps create job opportunities for women. We do not involve doctors because then our venture will become centralized and money will get distributed. We want to ensure that the local profit is used locally".

This company, in synergy with other local organizations (such as a micro credit organization called the *Kalasam*) can be the starting point to promote other forms of entrepreneurship at village level.

The increase of the revenue at household level made possible by GMCL activity has enhanced the saving habit among villagers. This can encourage them to use their financial resources in starting up small business activities on which they can fall back during difficult times. This could be also done through the support of village micro credit institutions.

Some sales representatives such as Rajeswari, who have been able to start up their own business activity, represent an example of the reinforcement of local entrepreneurship.

Rajeswari is a young woman in her thirties from a small hamlet close to Sante Marally (Karnataka). Since the past 4 years she has been working full time as a sale representative for GMCL products and she has opened a petty shop in Sante Marally. As her income is on the increase, she is planning to open a bigger medical shop in the next future.

One third of the women interviewed, especially the young ones, have expressed their interest in opening their own medical shop in the future. However, in the Utchanendal village a member of the local *Sangha* pointed out that the sales of GMCL medicines by the sales representatives find the resistance of other members in the village community, especially those belonging to higher castes. The sale of medicines is hindered by the lower social status of sales representatives: the villagers belonging to higher castes are in some cases unwilling to purchase medicines or interact with them due to their inferior status.

This can vary from a village to another, based on the differences in social structure that characterize the village communities.

The sales representatives, especially the young ones, see this activity as a way to increase their revenue on the basis of the provisions they can get from the sales. Nevertheless, in the majority of the cases, this consideration is not separated from a conviction that their activity is socially useful to enhance the community health system.

As a sale representative from Elanduri village explains:

"I have associated with GMCL because I want to popularize Ayurveda. Ayurvedic medicines do not have many side effects. What is happening nowadays is that because we use allopathic medicines, we are inviting hundreds of other diseases while treating one disease. Now, by marketing our products, we are able to give a new lease of life to our ancient medical system and are able to popularize it. Since, this system is a part of our national heritage, we need to respect it and popularize it. Our effects are geared in this direction. As we know, this system developed in our villages. Hence, we should teach our villagers that by adopting this system, they can make use of natural resources available in their own environment and get rid of their diseases without side effects"

It is important to point out that this increase is household income does not mean automatically an increased capacity for women to decide its allocation between the different expenses. Women generally only control income with male permission, which may be withdrawn. Women's own cash earnings are often incorporated into these existing patterns of resource allocation rather than radically transforming them. Although women may control some of their own earned income, this is widely variable between cultures, within cultures between different social groups, and even between households within the same family (Taub, 1998, UNHCR, 2007).

Given the unequal patterns of intra-household income decisions, increases in women's income from taking part in GMCL activity may merely substitute for male expenditure on family needs, freeing more male income for their own personal luxury expenditure.

Another issue is represented by the delicate link between economic income, participation and sustainability of GMCL activity in the long term. Women's participation in GMCL activities tends to involve work done outside the home in a collective workshed. As noted above, poorer women are generally less restricted in their mobility outside the home because of the necessity to work, and they have generally built up considerable support networks. However, working outside the home in collective sheds often involves further expenditure in time and/or transport and may prevent them from engaging in other forms of simultaneous production (e.g. looking after livestock in the compound) as well as activities like child-care. Regular work outside the home may therefore be possible only where the income gains are sufficient to cover these losses.

Social Empowerment

The GMCL model has been successful in producing inside the villagers wider socio-economic outcomes than only economic benefits. This includes an enhanced a *social empowerment process* for women, notably through the improvement of social status of herbs gatherers who are generally landless or marginal farmers and of sales representatives in the villages. The process of empowerment has had as a result a better access to power and resources at community and household level and the creation of women' institutions (*Sanghas* and other informal meeting groups).

For the women, participation in and the decision to be active in the *Sanghas* has often been the first gateway to be crossed and their first empowered step. The fact of taking part in harvesting and commercial activities has undoubtedly enhanced the skills and position of those women who are most active. These women are often able to use the need to travel to meetings and for marketing as a means of breaking previous restrictions on their movements outside the home and to develop a range contacts outside their immediate family and community. Nevertheless, for most women this process has not been easy. In many rural societies, attempts to control women's movements outside the home further constrain their autonomy.

A *Sangha* woman in the village of Perunguri recalls

> "my husband told me to stay at home and look after the housework, in stead of going and gossiping. If I was late in cooking his dinner after a meeting, I was beaten."

As the women that participate in GMCL initiative are poor and belong to the lower castes, the pressures at home were further exacerbated by the fact that they were mobile in spaces traditionally reserved for men and in many cases for upper caste men only. In the initial days, *Sanghas* meetings were hesitantly organized inside members' homes with the fear of reprimand. From inside homes, the women slowly moved out to gather in the *thinnai* (porch), or even in the local temple. Then it became a common sight to see the women conduct their meetings and other proceedings in the community's public place, the '*Chavady*' of the village.

Becoming a member of the *Sanghas* or a sale representative has increased woman's social standing in the village in a visible manner: the women own and manage their own small business, meet number of people in and outside her village who value their ideas and contribution. Social recognition has gradually given way to respect in most villages and the changes most visible in the public domain. This issue of respect and recognition by the village community is a very critical marker of change for the women.

A sale representative called Rajeshvari affirms:

" I was earlier working in a dairy, then in a shop and finally have joined this enterprise. I have become so much self-reliant that I can go to the city alone and sell my wares. Further, earlier I was just some person. But now, people recognize me as Rajeshvari who can treat diseases. I have also improved my knowledge regarding diseases because I have to educate the public".

For a Sangha woman in Sante Marally, her knowledge of herbal medicine has changed her relationship with the landlord. "I could not enter the landlords house by the front door, but now that I have learnt to use herbs, he calls me 'doctor', and begs me to come to his house". The extent of empowerment varied with each aspect examined. For example, one third of them felt that their self-confidence had increased considerably. The groups' dynamics enhanced their pride particularly since they were able to generate income from the economic activities taken up by them after joining the groups. About half of the selected members agreed that their communication skills have improved significantly after joining the groups; but most of them happen to be group leaders. They strongly agree that they can now participate in non-family meetings, interact effectively in the public sphere, and enjoyed better mobility. The example of the small contribution made by members of *Sanghas* out of their limited incomes for the construction of a house for an old destitute widow shows the change that had come about in their social outlook. It is thus evident that empowerment in terms of social outlook has been fairly remarkable. The informal discussions we had with them also lend support to this conclusion. An important issue that we would like to raise is the difficult to overcome caste barriers. The interviews have emphasized how low caste and social status may inhibit entry into entrepreneurial occupations, reducing the range of activities open to poor women and limiting their economic activities. This social and cultural constraint prevents an increase in the participation of the women in GMCL activity and limits their empowerment. As among these village communities the herb gathering activity is associated with a low caste and tribal background, it represents a social stigma. In the village of Thimmapuran (Tamilnadu) only four villagers are engaged in collecting herbs activity. Although CCD informed the villagers on the possible economic returns of this activity, the villagers have not shown any interest in taking part in the collection of herbs.

Capacity Building in the Sanghas

A range of training programs for women have been organized by CCD and another NGO, the FRLHT. These act ivies, carried out in conjunction with local healers and village botanists, involved training on issues such as processing and marketing of herbal drugs, value addition activities and sustainable harvesting and collecting techniques for medicinal plants. Savings/credit provision and improvements in marketing skills and networks as also been an area of strategic importance in training as has increased women's capacity of selling and therefore their income.

In the purpose of educating villagers and increasing their knowledge of medicinal plants and traditional health practices, a Medicinal Plants Conservation Park (MPCP) has been developed by CCD in Madurai district in a campus named Sevayoor . The park consists of an

Ethno-Medicine Forest (EMF) spread over 33 acres with a collection of over 500 plants species. This park has been conceived as an open space where humans, in this case local villagers, other communities, students etc. can come to see all the medicinal plants available in the zone and to learn about their different therapeutical uses. Similar regional resource centres are also being set up at Natham and Nagapattinam, which function as Community Conservation Centres (CCC) as well, owned and managed by the local communities, facilitated by CCD. These environmental grassroots initiatives serve as supportive means in the process of sound medicinal plant conservation.

This helped women in recognizing and giving value to their local knowledge of medicinal plants and has enhanced a process of capacity-building centred on ethnomedicine knowledge. This has resulted in an increased capacity to study, document and monitor traditional knowledge on medicinal plants and their use, make an inventory of plants and local biodiversity through biodiversity registers etc. An increased capacity for gatherers and collectors to harvest in a sustainable way the plants, to master the different agro-techniques and to keep the accounts and records has also been observed.

The enhancement of the villagers' know-how in this respect has represented a prerequisite for the implementation of GMCL activity. The increase of capacity building in terms of medicinal plants (how to use, to recognize and protect them) that constitutes the result of the previous project, has allowed the future involvement of local communities in GMCL activity. This is the case especially for the activities related to the final products. The villagers, who were already familiar with the use and the importance of medicinal plants to enhance their local health system, have shown a greater interest in purchasing and selling GMCL products. This is particularly evident in the villages around Sevayor (Tamilnadu), where the creation of nurseries and herbal kitchen gardens in the past few years had already sensitized the villagers on the importance of using medicinal plants.

Through these training activities especially targeted to women, there has been a gradual passage from a form of *individual* knowledge (mainly possessed by the folk healers) towards a form of *more diffused* knowledge, which involved the women in *Sanghas*. The villages' organizations such as *Sanghas* can become key players in promoting a community-based health system and in sensitizing the villagers on the importance of traditional medicine.

Conclusion

As we have been illustrated in this chapter, in more recent debates on environmental and development issues, women have gradually become visible. The emerging importance of participatory approaches in the context of applied development and conservation initiatives has led to a growing interest in "indigenous" or "local knowledge" in resource management. However, in development work and nature conservation at the practical level, gender issues, are still quite often considered as "special issues" or "further aspects." At the beginning of this book we highlighted the Convention on Biological Diversity (which was signed at the Rio Earth Summit in June 1992), as an important impulse that stimulated interest in the linkages between gender and biodiversity conservation as it explicitly recognizes in its preamble "the vital role that women play in the conservation and sustainable use of biological diversity" and affirms "the need for the full participation of women at all levels of policy-making and implementation for biological diversity conservation" (Weinstein, 1999).

Nowadays, the integration of conservation with economic development for local communities, such as microcredit or community enterprises, is increasingly seen as a way to alleviate poverty, and promote community participation in conservation efforts (Virdi, 2004, Tenenbaum, 1996). Indigenous entrepreneurship has become an option to couple community development with environmental protection while strengthening the grassroots level women in sustainable natural resource management (Zhao and Aram, 1995). The major question is whether a market-oriented intervention such as a community enterprise like GMCL, can promote activities related to sustainable natural resource use. In the above sections we explored the impact of GMCL in the field of conservation, and management of genetic resources by adopting an actor-oriented approach, which conceptualizes women as social actors who attempt to solve problems, use their own strategies within an arena of limited environmental conservation opportunities, and participate in the societal process as decision makers and negotiators in resource management. We have found evidence that supports both positive and negative appraisal of community enterprises and biodiversity conservation.

The training programmes organized by FRLHT and CCD helped the women in recognizing and giving value to their local knowledge of medicinal plants. This has resulted in an increased capacity to study and document medicinal plants and their use, make an inventory of medicinal plants and local biodiversity through biodiversity registers etc.. Thus, an increased awareness of the importance of the medicinal plant resources and therefore its conservation has been observed among the GMCL member. Most women said that the understanding and consciousness of this natural resource have improved because of the community development programmes.

On the occasion of programs such as local healers' conventions and village botanists' workshops, local communities in village learned new skills of identification, herbarium preparation and new uses of medicinal plants. This has helped them in recognition of the importance of medicinal plant conservation and protection. Thus, GMCL contributed to a shift from a form of individual knowledge and awareness of resources conservation, mainly possessed by the folk healers, towards a form of collective knowledge and awareness of medicinal plant maintenance, more diffused at the wider community level.

Although GMCL in partnership with outside organisations succeeded in promoting solidarity among grassroots women in order to enhance their knowledge, and use of and access to over natural resources, their participation in the decision -making process as well as the equitable distribution of resources and benefits accruing from these resources, one has not to forget that GMCL could only develop thanks to the a availability of medicinal plant resources in the local area. Without this local availability, the constitution of this community-based enterprise would have been unlikely.

An important issue therefore to be monitored in the future concerns the sustainability of this resource. A diminution of this key resource can put this community-based initiative centred on ethnomedicine at risk. Thus, a particular emphasis must be given by GMCL to sustainable harvesting techniques in order to assure the long-term occurrence of local biodiversity resources which lies at the heart of community-based enterprises active in the sector of traditional medicine (Laird and Pierce, 2002). One option might be the cultivation of medicinal plants that are becoming or might become rare do to overharvesting in order to maintain their availability in the long run. However, this possible solution requires specific propagation techniques which are not always and easily available on the ground. There is also the problem of land tenure and availability, as most of the local farmers possess a limited surface of land. Moreover such conservation techniques must be harmonised with the sociocultural context in order to avoid imposing a western conservation approach which is far from local realities.

References

Adams, W. M., Aveling, R., Brockington, D., Dickson, B., Elliott, J., Hutton, J., et al. (2004). Biodiversity conservation and the eradication of poverty. *Science*, 306: 1146–1149.

Agarwal B. (2000). Conceptualising environmental collective action: Why gender matters. *Cambridge Journal of Economics*, 24 (3): 283-310.

Arnold, J. E. M. (2002). Clarifying the links between forests and poverty reduction. *International Forestry Review*, 4 (3): 231–234.

Arnold, J. E. M. and Ruiz-Perez, M. (2001). Can non-timber forest products match tropical forest conservation and development objectives?, *Ecological Economics,* 39: 437- 447.

Bandura, A. (1988). Organizational Application of Social Cognitive Theory. *Australian Journal of Management,* 13 (2), 275-302.

Belcher, B. (2005). Forest product markets, forests and poverty reduction. *International Forestry Review*, 7 (2), 82–89.

Beck, T., and Nesmith, C. (2001). Building on poor people's capacities: The case of common property resources in India and West Africa. *World Development*, 29 (1), 119–133.

Belcher, B., Ruiz-Pe´rez, M., and Achdiawan, R. (2005). Global patterns and trends in the use and management of commercial NTFPs: Implications for livelihoods and conservation. *World Development*, 33 (9), 1435–1452.

Bird, N., and Dickson, C. (2005). *Poverty reduction strategy papers: Making the case for forestry.* ODI Forestry Briefing (No. 7). London: Overseas Development Institute (ODI).

Bodeker, G. (1999). Valuing biodiversity for Human Health and Well-being: Traditional Health Systems. In: *Cultural and Spiritual Values of Biodiversity.* Posey, D.A. (Ed). London and Nairobi: Intermediate Tecnology Publications, United Nations Environment Programme.

Campbell, B., Jeffrey, S., Kozanayi, W., Luckert, M., Mutamba, M., and Zindi, C. (2002). *Household livelihoods in semi-arid regions.* Options and constraints. Bogor, Indonesia: Centre for International Forestry Research (CIFOR)

Cavendish, W. (2000). Empirical regularities in the poverty–environment relationship in rural households: Evidence from Zimbabwe. *World Development*, 28 (11): 1979–2003.

Deda P. and Rubian R. (2004). Women and biodiversity: The long journey from users to policy makers. *Natural Resources Forum,* 28 (3): 201-205.

FAO (2003). State of the world's forests 2003. Part II. Selected current issues in the forest sector. Rome: Food and Agricultural Organization (FAO).

Fisher, M. (2004). Household welfare and forest dependence in Southern Malawi. *Environment and Development Economics*, 9, 135–154.

Godoy, R., Wilkie, D., Overman, H., Cubas, A., Cubus, G., Demmer, J., et al. (2000). Valuation of the consumption and sale of forest goods from a Central American rainforest. Nature, 406, 62–63.

Gutierrez, M. and Betancourt, Y. (1999). El mercado de plantas medicinales en Mexico. Situacion actual y perspectivas de desarrollo. México D.F., Fondo de América del Norte para la Cooperación Ambiental (FANCA), Ecología y Desarrollo de Tlaxcala y Puebla A.C.

Hersch-Martinez, P. (2000). Plantas Medicinales: Relato de una Posibilidad Confiscada. El estatuto de la flora en la biomedicina mexicana. México, D.F., Instituto Nacional de Antropología e Historia.

Hersch-Martinez, P. (1997). Medicinal plants and regional traders in Mexico: physiographic differences and conservation challenge. *Economic Botany* 51(1): 107-120.

Howard P. (Ed) (2003). *Women and Plants: Gender Relations in Biodiversity Management and Conservation*, Zed Books, London and New York.

Howard-Borjas, P. and Cuijpers, W. (2002). Gender and the management and conservation of plant biodiversity, in H. W., Doelle and E. Da Silva (eds). Biotechnology, in *Encyclopedia of Life Support Systems* (EOLSS), Oxford, UK.

Hull, J. (2001). Les mères célibataires authochtones au Canada. Un profil statistique. Winnipeg: Affaires indiennes et du Nord Canada.

Institut canadien de recherches sur les femmes (ICREF). 2006. Elucider la problématique de la pauvreté et de l'excusion des femmes. Ottawa: ICREF.

Kellert, S.R. (1996). *The values of life. Biological diversity and human society.* Washington, D.C: Island Press/Sheanvater Books.

Koziell, I. (2001). Diversity not adversity. Sustaining livelihoods with biodiversity. London: International Institute for Environment and Development (IIED).

Laird, S. (2002). *Biodiversity and Traditional Knowledge: equitable partnerships in practice*, Earthscan Publications, London, UK.

Laird, S.A. and Pierce, A.R. (2002). Promoting sustainable and ethical botanicals: strategies to improve commercial raw material sourcing: results from the sustainable botanicals pilot project industry surveys, case studies and standards collection, Rainforest Alliance, New York.

Lawrence, A. (2003). No forest without timber? *International Forestry Review*, 5(2), 87–96.

Liedholm, C. (2002). Small firm dynamics : evidence from Africa and Latin America, *Small Business Economics*, 18(1-3) : 227-242.

Lozoya, X. (1996). Medicinal Plants of Mexico: A Program for Their Scientific Validation. *Medicinal Resources of the Tropical Forest. Biodiversity and Its Importance to Human Health.* M. Balick, A. Anderson and K. Redford. New York, Columbia University Press.

Mafra, M.S.H. and Stadler, H.H.C. (2007). Etnoconhecimento e conservaçao da biodiversidade em áreas naturais e agricolas no Planalto Sul Catarinense, International Society for the Sistems Sciences *ISSSBrasi-Usp, 13p*

Mayoux, L. (1995). *From vicious to virtuous circles? Gender and micro-enterprise development.* Occasional Papers. U. N. R. I. f. S. Development. Geneva., UNDP.

McSweeny, K. (2004). Tropical forests product sale as natural insurance: The effects of household characteristics and the nature of shock in Eastern Honduras. *Society and Natural Resources*, 17, 39–46

Marshall, E., and Newton, A. C. (2003). Non-timber forest products in the community of El Terrero, Sierra de Manantlan Biosphere Reserve, Mexico: Is their use sustainable? *Economic Botany*, 5(2), 262–278.

Marshall, E., Schreckenberg, K., and Newton, A. C. (Eds.) (2006). Commercialization of non-timber forest product: Factors influencing success. Lessons learned from Mexico and Bolivia and policy implications for decision-makers. Cambridge: UNEP World Conservation Monitoring Centre.

Narendran, K., Murthy, I. K., Suresh, H. S., Dattaraja, H. S., Ravindranath, N. H., and Sukumar, R. (2001). Nontimber forest product extraction, utilization and valuation: A case study from the Nilgiri Biosphere Reserve, Southern India. *Economic Botany*, 55(4), 528–538.

Oksanen, T., and Mersmann, C. (2003). Forestry in poverty reduction strategies—An assessment of PRSP processes in sub-Saharan Africa. In T. Oksanen, B. Pajari, and T. Tuomasjukka (Eds.), Forestry in poverty reduction strategies: Capturing the potential. EFI Proceedings (No. 47, pp. 121–158). Joensuu: European Forest Institute.

Posey A. D. and Dutfield G. (1996). *Beyond intellectual property rights: towards traditional resource rights for indigenous and local communities*. IDRCandWWF, OttawaandGland

Roe, D. (2004). *The millennium development goals and conservation. Managing nature's wealth for society's health*. London: International Institute for Environment and Development (IIED).

Ros-Tonen, M.A.F. and Wiersum, K.F. (2005). The scope for improving rural livelihoods through nontimber forest products: An evolving research agenda. *Forests, Trees and Livelihoods*, 15, 129–148.

Rothwell, N. (2002). Variation saisonnière de l'emploi en milieu rural. Bulletins d'analyse - régions rurales et petites villes du Canada. *Statistique Canada*. 3 (8).

SAGAR, (2008). La asociaciòn de municipios y relaciones de complementaridad ; una alternativa para generar desarrollo regional sustentable en el altiplano semiarido de Tamaulipas, Mexico, Gobierno del Estado de Tamaulipas, México.

Schippmann, U., D. Leaman, et al. (2003). *Impact of cultivation and collection on the conservation of medicinal plants: global trends and issues*. The Third World Congress o Medicinal and Aromatic Plants, Chiang Mai, Thailand, Acta Horticulturae. International Society for Horticultural Science.

Scherr, S. J., White, A., and Kaimowitz, D. (2004). *A new agenda for forest conservation and poverty reduction. Making markets work for low income producers*. Washington, DC: Forest Trends and Centre for International Forestry Research (CIFOR).

Shackleton, C. M., and Shackleton, S. E. (2004). The importance of non-timber forest products in rural livelihood security and as safety nets: A review of evidence from South Africa. *South African Journal of Science*, 100, 658–664.

Servet, J. (2006). Banquiers aux pieds nus, La microfinance, Paris, Ed.Odile Jacob, p. 511.

Stromquist, N. (1995). The theoretical and practical bases for empowerment, in Carolyn Medel- Anonuevo (ed.) Women, Education, and Empowerment: Paths towards Autonomy, Hamburg, UNESCO,

Takasaki, Y., Barham, B. L., and Coomes, O. T. (2004). Risk coping strategies in tropical forests: Floods, illnesses, and resource extraction. *Environment and Development Economics*, 9, 203–224.

Taub, R.P. (1998). Making the adaptation across cultures and societies: A report on an attempt to clone the Grameen Bank in southern Arkansas, *Journal of Developmental Entrepreneurship*, 3(1): 53-70.

Tenenbaum, D. (1996). Entrepreneurship with a social conscience. *Technology Review*, 99(4): 18- 30.

United Nations Millennium Declaration (2000). Millenium Development Goals. <http://www.developmentgoals. org/>

UNFPA (2004). Women and micro enterprise developments: report. OP-UN/2004Women. New York.

UNHCR (2007). Good Governance practices for the protection of human rights, UNHCR, Geneva.

Vera-Toscano, E., Phimister, E., and Weersink, A. (2004). Panel Estimates of the Canadian Rural/Urban Women's Wage Gap. *American Journal of Agricultural Economics,* 86 (4): 1138-1152.

Virdi, M. (2004). Wild plants as resource: new opportunities or last resort? Some dimensions of the collection, cultivation and trade of medicinal plants in the Gori basin. In: Alam, G., Belt, J. (Eds.), *Searching synergy: stakeholder views on developing a sustainable medicinal plant chain in Uttaranchal,* India, KIT Bulletin n° 359, KIT Publishers, Amsterdam, p. 41-54.

Weinstein, M. (1999). Railbirds, scouts, and independent booksellers: Towards a constructivist interpretation of new business formation, *Irish Marketing Review*, 12(1): 3-17.

Winthrop, R.H. (1991). *Dictionary of Concepts in Cultural Anthropology*. New York: Greenwood Press

World Bank (2002). *A revised forest strategy for the World Bank Group*. Washington, DC: World Bank Group.

WRI (2005). World Resources 2005. The wealth of the poor. Managing ecosystems to fight poverty. World Resources Institute, UNDP, UNEP and World Bank. Washington, DC: World Resources Institute (WRI).

WRI (2000). World resources report 2000–2001. People and ecosystems: The fraying web of life. World Resources Institute, UNDP, UNEP and World Bank. Washington, DC: World Resources Institute (WRI).

Wunder, S. (2001). Poverty alleviation and tropical forests—What scope for synergies? World Development, 29(11), 1817–1833.

Zhao, L. and Aram, J.D., 1995, Networking and growth of young technology-intensive ventures in China, *Journal of Business Venturing*, 10(5): 349-371.

In: Medicinal Plants and Sustainable Development   ISBN 978-1-61761-942-7
Editor: Chandra Prakash Kala   © 2011 Nova Science Publishers, Inc.

Chapter 17

Sustainable Development of Medicinal Plants and Livelihood Opportunities

Chandra Prakash Kala[*]

Ecosystem and Environment Management,
Indian Institute of Forest Management, P.B. No. 357, Nehru Nagar,
Bhopal - 462 003, Madhya Pradesh, India

Abstract

The indigenous sustainable management practices of medicinal plants, developed by local communities, have been overlooked normally with the passage of time and changing socio-economic conditions. Realizing the importance of medicinal plants in recent years countries across the world have shown interest in the medicinal plant sector, which they wish to strengthen in order to create additional income, livelihood opportunities and employment prospects.

At the same time, meeting sustained availability of medicinal plants for various purposes is one of the challenging tasks. The present chapter deals with various traditional and ongoing management and conservation practices with respect to the medicinal plants and their long-term sustainability.

Keywords: Medicinal plants, sustainable development, cultivation, management practices.

Introduction

Over the centuries of experiments, the rich wealth of medicinal plants has been discovered and, at present, about 52,885 species of plants are known for curing diseases (Schippmann et al., 2002). Today, medicinal plants have become a commodity with high added value. The World Health Organization (WHO) has estimated that the present demand for medicinal plants is about US $ 14 billion a year. The demand for medicinal plant-based

---

[*] E-mails: cpkala@iifm.ac.in; cpkala@yahoo.co.uk

raw materials is growing at the rate of 15 to 25% annually, and according to the WHO estimates, the demand for medicinal plants is likely to increase to US $ 5 trillion in 2050 (Sharma, 2004). This increasing demand for plant-based drugs is, however, causing the heavy pressure on some selected high value medicinal plant populations in the wild (Kala, 2004, 2005a; Kala et al., 2006). Moreover, many medicinal plant species have slow growth rates, low population densities and narrow geographic ranges (Kala, 2005b). On the other hand, the indigenous knowledge on the use of lesser-known medicinal plants is declining sharply. Realizing the importance of medicinal plants in recent years countries across the world have shown interest in the medicinal plant sector, which they wish to strengthen in order to create additional income, and livelihood and employment opportunities. In view of the growing interest in plant-based drugs, it is imperative to study and understand the sustainability of medicinal plants resources along with opportunities for development. Historically, the strategies of conserving medicinal plants have evolved with the accumulation of knowledge on the useful properties of various plant species. With the globalization, the indigenous knowledge on the use of medicinal plants is rapidly transforming into commercial gains. However, the indigenous conservation and management practices, adopted by local communities, have been overlooked with the passage of time and changing socio-economic conditions. Since the medicinal plants are important for health care, international treaties and national policies have been enacted and implemented across the world. The Convention on Biological Diversity and the Convention on International Trade in Endangered Species of Wild Fauna and Flora are the major treaties, which enable to regulate the over-exploitation of valuable biodiversity including rare and endangered species of medicinal values. In the above context, it is a need of hour to study and implement the various parameters of medicinal plants sustainability. The present chapter deals with various traditional and ongoing management and conservation practices with respect to the medicinal plants and their sustainability.

In-Situ Conservation of Medicinal Plants

Apart from enacting Acts, the provision of notifying certain areas for conservation of biological diversity helps in sustainability of the medicinal plant species (Sajwan and Kala, 2007). Medicinal plants growing in such protected areas are conserved in their natural habitats. These are the areas, which function as the last resort of such valuable plant resources. The anthropogenic pressures, mainly in the form of human-induced landuse change and overexploitation of medicinal plants for commercial gains, have the largest effects on medicinal plants survival in the natural habitats including biodiversity (Kala and Shrivastava, 2004; Wallington et al., 2005). Therefore, to minimize the impacts of such disturbances, the philosophy of setting protected areas network has been brought in. Realizing the need of conservation as well as the utilization of bio-resources, the legal status of protected areas varies with national parks, sanctuaries, reserve forests and biosphere reserves. The legal provisions that do not allow harvesting medicinal plants from the national parks and also regulating their harvest from the sanctuaries mainly help in conservation of these important species including rare and endangered categories. Studies conducted in the Himalayan region have claimed that the population of rare and endangered medicinal plants was higher in the protected areas compared to the adjacent unprotected areas (Kala, 1998, 2005c).

Ex-Situ Conservation
and Cultivation of Medicinal Plants

Apart from meeting the national and international demand, cultivation of medicinal plants at large scale may conserve the wild genetic diversity. Farming also permits the production of uniform material, from which standardized products can be obtained. Cultivation also permits better species identification, improved quality control, and increased prospects for genetic improvements. Selection of planting material for large-scale farming is also an important task. Establishing botanical gardens is one the important tools for conservation of medicinal plants. The botanical gardens serve as information centers for the scientists, general public and those whoever are interested in the medicinal plants. Botanical gardens also help in disseminating awareness on economical, ecological and ethical significance of medicinal plants conservation. *Ex-situ* is especially desirable in case of species where wild populations have dwindled to critical levels and viable populations for some of these species are not available for initiating *in-situ* conservation action. Establishing plantations of medicinal plant species of conservation concerns for use in the herbal-based industry is required. These plantations may also function as field Gene banks and as seed orchards for sourcing quality seeds.

Applications of biotechnological tools for germplasm conservation are required, particularly to the recalcitrant seeds or species that do not set seeds through *in-vitro* banks and have poor seed germination. There are many rare and endangered medicinal plant species, which need special care and conservation through applications of science and technology. Developing suitable propagation packages for mass production of planting materials, analysis of phyto-chemicals for quality control and large scale cultivation of rare species are some of the areas where one can achieve the goal of conservation as well sustainable utilization of medicinal plant species. Micro-propagation and cell culture techniques provide opportunities for genetic improvement and large-scale production of plant species. *In-vitro* propagation could produce new cultivars that are rich in active ingredients.

To make cultivation of medicinal plants lucrative, it is necessary to support the effort - both technically and financially. In India, a programme to support cultivation through subsidy has been implemented by the National Medicinal Plants Board (NMPB), an apex body dealing matters related to the medicinal plants sector. Though the programme has generally resulted in encouraging cultivation of many species of conservation concerns and those in high demand by the industry, a number of other species used in herbal medicine continued to be sourced from the wild (Kala, 2010). NMPB has supported the farmers to cultivate medicinal plants in 40,000 hectares of land. About 120 species of medicinal plants have been brought under cultivation, which include many rare and endangered species such as *Aconitum heterophyllum, Saussurea costus, Commiphora wightii, Gloriosa superba, Saraca ashoka, Swertia chirayita, Nardostachys jatamansi* etc (Kala and Sajwan, 2007). Most of the *ex-situ* conservation approaches of medicinal plants need basic ecological understanding of concerned species related to edaphic, agro-climatic and geographical conditions. Even to preserve the seeds for desired period of time in the cryobanks, it is important to determine the optimum temperature required for the viability of seeds of concerned medicinal plant species.

Ecological Considerations for Sustainable Development of Medicinal Plants

Medicinal plants and their supporting natural systems may be sustained by dynamic ecological patterns and processes. Medicinal plants and their associates evolve together over thousands of years, which made them to adapt for a particular climatic condition. Some medicinal plants may affect communities disproportionately to their abundance and biomass, while some survive only in the presence of other symbiotic species. Besides, the loss of habitat can reduce the survival rate and viability of medicinal plants and too much disturbance can lead to ecosystem collapse. All these factors are interlinked and some way or others helps in survival of the species (Wallington et al., 2005; Farrington et al., 2008). The various ecological characteristics such as climate, soil, habitats, geography, phyto-sociology etc., are important and decisive factors for conservation of medicinal plants. The distribution of medicinal plants, generally, varies with biogeographic zones. Some of the medicinal plants have wide geographic range and adaptability hence they inhabit in more than one biogeographic areas while others have narrow range of distribution and even endemic to particular locality (Kala, 2005c). *Coptis teeta*, endemic to the eastern Himalaya and *Declapis hamiltonii* endemic to south India are the examples of some of the important medicinal plant species. Many medicinal plants, such as, *Saussurea obvallata, Taxus baccata, Dactylorhiza hatagirea, Picrorhiza kurrooa* etc. have habitat specificity. Further, if such species are domesticated out of their natural habitat, the natural efficacy in the forms of medicinal and aromatic properties got diminished (Kala et al., 2006). It is important to conserve such species in their natural habitats by means of *in-situ* conservation. Further, conserving representative areas of medicinal plants in a biogeographic zone facilitate conservation of the majority of species. The heavy livestock grazing is mainly considered an important factor for the loss of medicinal plants, especially of threatened categories across the globe. This may result in habitat alteration, habitat destruction, change in plants assemblages and composition, and providing space for invasive species (Kala, 1998, 2004; Kala and Shrivastava, 2005). It is also presumed that medicinal plants have different responses to harvesting by humans and browsing by livestock. Ungulate grazing negatively affects population growth of medicinal plants such as ginseng in the absence but not in the presence of harvesting (Farrington et al., 2008). Therefore, conservation tactics may deal accordingly. In order to mitigate the pressure of livestock grazing rotational grazing is recommended, apart from managing the herd size of grazers and browsers. In order to conserve species including medicinal plants by means of ecological approach, it is necessary to monitor the changes in ecosystem and abundance of the concerned species in such ecosystems (Gadgil et al., 1993; Folke et al., 1998). Some medicinal plants grow in specific habitats and microhabitats hence such habitats must be protected. If the species holds low abundance and density, the total protection may be granted to such species. Besides, the vulnerable stages of the life history of important medicinal plants may be given protection for their survival. The temporal restrictions may be imposed on the harvesting of medicinal plants. The different ecological processes at multiple scales are required to be assessed and managed for conservation of medicinal plants.

Medicinal Plants Conservation Areas

To conserve the medicinal plants for long period of time in its natural habitats Medicinal Plants Conservation Areas (MPCAs) may be identified and established. Since each agro-climatic zone is unique in terms of rich diversity of medicinal plant species, MPCA is required to establish in each agroclimatic zone so that the maximum diversity of medicinal plants may be brought under *in-situ* conservation programmes. The number of MPCAs may be increased as per the diversity of habitats and microhabitats of the respective agro-climatic zone, as such areas require focused and more attention due to rich botanical diversity. The initiatives taken by the Foundation for Revitalization of Local Health Traditions (FRLHT) of India in building the concept of MPCAs is praiseworthy. The major objectives of establishing MPCA is (1. to conserve the diversity and richness of medicinal plants in natural habitats across various agro-climatic zones, (2. to disseminate and strengthen the values of medicinal plants, its significance and conservation education, (3. to develop long-term institutionalized mechanism for conservation of medicinal plants, assessing their degree of threat, population status along with identifying threatened medicinal plant species and undertaking measures for their recovery, (4. to develop dialogues and sharing of experiences among different stakeholders of the medicinal plants sector who are actively involved in the conservation, cultivation and sustainable utilization of medicinal plants and (5. to facilitate linkages between the medicinal plant conservation organizations and medicinal plant user groups. One of the major tasks of MPCA is to involve local communities and assure them for sharing of benefits accrued from the medicinal plants sector and MPCAs. This community-oriented policy is required realizing that rural and tribal communities are among the key custodians of medicinal plants. Identification of proper areas for establishing MPCA is one of the important tasks. Areas traditionally known for their medicinal plants richness, occurrence of endemic species, representative of the forest types, high density of prioritized medicinal plant species and minimum level of legal protection may be some of the deciding factors for selection of MPCAs. Apart from conservation aspects, many more activities may be taken up in MPCAs which includes, developing a complete set of database on each MPCAs. On the basis of such database the strategies may be developed for future course of action in developing such MPCAs.

Establishing Medicinal Plants
Facilitation Centres (MPFCs)

Medicinal plants being new to the farming systems, a lot of support by way of technology dissemination, capacity building, production of quality planting material and its certification is required. To meet these requirements, Medicinal Plants Facilitation Centre is required to establish, which may act as a one-stop shop for the problems of farmers and other stakeholders of medicinal plants. Medicinal Plants Facilitation Centre may organize training programmes and stakeholders meet. Developing database on medicinal plants resources and herbal gardens along with certification of quality planting material, developing publication material, technical appraisal and monitoring of cultivation may be the other activities of Medicinal Plants Facilitation Centre. The following activities may be taken by such centers:

- Authentication of quality raw materials on the basis of taxonomic identification and chemical standardization.
- Act as a clearing-house and certification agency for source authentication of medicinal plants (cultivated, not from the wild).
- Technical know how pertaining to cultivation, post harvest and value addition.
- To oversee/monitor production of quality planting material by various agencies.
- Creation of linkages with marketing agencies/industry for assurance of buyback arrangements and certification of quality materials/products
- Promotion of global marketing system.
- To organize workshops and training programmes for farmers and other stakeholders as and when required.

Developing Guidelines for Good Agricultural Practices

Information on good agricultural practices of many important medicinal plant species is either not available or meager. This information is important in view of quality assurance and safety of the products derived from medicinal plant species. The WHO has developed guidelines for good agricultural and collection practices; however, there is a need to develop country specific guidelines for such practices.

Many organizations and institutions are involved in developing the good agriculture of medicinal plant species; however the information is not yet put together in consolidated forms. The available information on agronomy of medicinal plants developed by some institutions is also not percolated to the farm level. Reasons could be many but the growers are raising the crop in an unorganized manner. In certain cases, the publications of certain cultivation aspects, seems to have no research backup, resulting in skewed information to the growers. Therefore, there is a need to consolidate the existing information and develop country specific guidelines for good agricultural and collection practices.

Identifying Demand and Supply of Medicinal Plants

The major part of the traditional systems of herbal medicine, which includes folk health tradition, has transformed into trade over the period of time. At present, the herbal health care system may be broadly differentiated into the resource, trade and consumption.

Since trade is one of the important parts of this tradition, there is a need to update the existing information on the demand and supply of medicinal plants. Within India, a total of 960 medicinal plant species are being traded for raw drugs, in which 176 species are consumed in excess of 100 MT per year (Ved and Goraya, 2007). About 90% of the medicinal plants products are collected from the wild, hence sustainable harvesting of these species are important factor for their long term availability.

Sustainable Harvesting of Medicinal Plants

The indigenous communities have developed their own knowledge on the sustainable harvesting of medicinal plants, which still remains an important instrument for the conservation. In most of the communities, the traditional herbal healers mainly adopt the selective harvesting of medicinal plants, which depends on numerous factors (Kala, 2005b, 2005d). In India, the traditional herbal healers mostly used to collect mature plants. Underground plant parts (root and rhizomes) of perennials were generally gathered after 2 or 3 years of growth. Tubers and bulbs of the annual species were collected at the end of the flowering or fruiting.

Young leaves of medicinal plants were gathered throughout the growing period to maximize the quality of active compounds. Fruits and seeds of medicinal plants were collected when mature. The bark was collected when trees and shrubs began to bud in spring and after leaves shed in autumn (Kaul, 1997; Kala, 2002). In the Himalayan region of Nepal, young leaves, if required, are harvested in the spring, flowers and mature leaves in the summer, and fruits, seeds and rhizomes are collected in the autumn (Table 1). In Tibetan Medicine System, the harvesting of medicinal plants is determined by the cultural and religious calendar. In late September or early October, when most of the alpine plants complete their life cycle, Amchi (medical practitioners of Tibetan Medical System) collect plants for preparing medicine (Ghimire et al., 2004; Kala, 2005b). It was perceived that the mistaken identity of plant during collection, particularly of plants with phenotypic similarity, might lead to accidental poisoning; therefore only the experienced herbal healers used to collect the medicinal plants. After collection, proper care was taken to dry and process the material. The sustainability of medicinal plants in the wild depends on many factors including the quantum of their harvesting.

Table 1. Traditional harvesting practices of medicinal plants in India and Nepal

Sl. No.	Plant parts	Traditional harvesting period/ season	
		India (Kaul, 1997; Kala, 2005a)	Nepal (Ghimire et al., 2004)
1	Tuber and bulbs	End of flowering and fruiting	Autumn
2	Young leaves	Throughout growing period	Spring
3	Fruit and seeds	At maturity	Autumn
4	Bark	Beginning of bud in spring and shedding of leaves in autumn	-
5	Whole herb	Beginning of flowering stage	Beginning of senescence

Harvesting medicinal plants for commercial use coupled with the destructive harvest of underground parts of slow reproducing, slow growing and habitat-specific species, are the crucial factors in meeting the goal of sustainability (Ghimire et al., 2004; Kala et al., 2006).

Different modes of harvesting affect not only the ecosystem properties but also the individual species to survive (Hall and Bawa, 1993; Ticktin, 2004). Harvesting underground plant parts such as root, rhizome and tubers enhances the mortality of concerned medicinal plants. Similarly, harvesting aboveground plant parts, such as, shoots and leaves influence the photosynthetic rate and may decline the photosynthetic capacity of the concerned medicinal plants as well as the potential for survival and effective propagation.

Since the medicinal plants forms a large group of species with variety of growth forms, responses to environment and life forms along with mode of their harvesting are also diverse. Similarly, after harvesting the recovery of species depends on various environmental and ecological factors. Medicinal plants tolerance to harvest varies with climatic conditions as the temperate herbs become highly vulnerable to harvest of individuals (Ticktin, 2004). Furthermore, rising demand with shrinking habitats may lead to the local extinction of many medicinal plant species. For instance, the current practice of gum collection from some medicinal plants, such as, *Commiphora wightii* and *Canarium strictum* is no more sustainable because of changes in traditional gum collection strategies and weakening of customary laws. Earlier, the natural fissures once appear on the *C. strictum* tree, the local people in south India chip the resin protruding from large tree (Varghese and Ticktin, 2008). Only few individuals collect resin regularly and fulfill the demand of rest of the villagers. Collection of resin from naturally formed fissures has proven advantage over the artificially formed incision on the tree (Varghese and Ticktin, 2008).

Studies conducted across various eco-regions have culminated to the point that indigenous methods of resource utilization are often more sustainable than most global and commercially oriented practices, hence traditional ecological knowledge is a powerful tool for conservation and management of natural resources, including medicinal plants.

Conclusion

To ensure the long-term sustainability of medicinal plants as an essential commodity, it is important to conserve their genetic diversity through restoration. Simply putting ban on harvesting of medicinal plant and notifying areas as national parks may not serve the purpose as evident from the conflicts looming large between protected area managers and local people on the ownership issues of natural resources. An integrated management approach is strongly felt in order to address the local people's concerns and to mitigate the conflicts while conserving the natural resources. The adaptive indigenous knowledge, practices and perceptions associated with surrounding complex environmental and ecological systems may cope-up with the uncertainty of the ecosystems and diminish the intensity of ongoing impacts.

There are also opportunities to incorporate the conservation policies for medicinal plants within the framework of existing legal instruments, such as, the Convention on Biological Diversity and the Convention on International Trade of Endangered Species of Wild Flora and Fauna. Since the Convention on Biological Diversity under Article 8 (j) has strongly recognized the importance of indigenous knowledge for conservation of biodiversity, the policy makers and academician may need to synergize the values of ethnic conservation practices and ecological knowledge in view of medicinal plants conservation. The participation of local communities through dialogues and negotiations may ensure the conservation of natural resources, especially medicinal plants.

Acknowledgments

The author thanks the Director, Indian Institute of Forest Management, India for help and support.

References

Farrington, S.J., Muzika, R., Drees, D. and Knight, T.M. (2008). Interactive effects of harvest and deer herbivory on the population dynamics of American ginseng. *Conservation Biology,* http://www3.interscience. wiley.com/journal/121572130/abstract?CRETRY =1andSRETRY=0

Folke, C., Berkes, F. and Colding, J. (1998). Ecological practices and social mechanisms for building resilience and sustainability. In: *Linking Social and Ecological Systems.* Berkes, F., Folke, C. and Colding, J. (eds.). pp. 414-436. Cambridge University Press. Cambridge.

Gadgil, M., Berkes, F. and Folke, C. (1993). Indigenous knowledge for biodiversity conservation. *Ambio,* 22 (2/3): 151-156.

Ghimire, S.K., McKey, D. and Aumeeruddy-Thomas, Y. (2004). Heterogeneity in ethnoecological knowledge and management of medicinal plants in the Himalayas of Nepal: Implications for conservation. *Ecology and Society,* 9 (3): 6. [Online] http://www.ecologyandsociety. org/vol9/iss3/art6/

Hall, P. and Bawa, K.S. (1993). Methods to access the impact of extraction of non-timber tropical forest products on plant populations. *Economic Botany,* 47: 234-247.

Kala, C.P. (1998). *Ecology and conservation of alpine meadows in the Valley of Flowers National Park, Garhwal Himalaya,* Ph.D. Thesis, Forest Research Institute, Dehradun.

Kala, C.P. (2002). *Medicinal Plants of Indian Trans-Himalaya.* Bishen Singh Mahendra Pal Singh, Dehradun, India.

Kala, C.P. (2004). Pastoralism, plant conservation, and conflicts on proliferation of Himalayan Knotweed in high altitude protected areas of the Western Himalaya, India. *Biodiversity and Conservation,* 13 (5): 985-995.

Kala, C.P. (2005a). Ethnomedicinal botany of the Apatani in the Eastern Himalayan region of India. *Journal of Ethnobiology and Ethnomedicine,* 1 (11): 1-12. [Online] http://www.ethnobiomed.com/content/pdf/1746-4269-1-11.pdf

Kala, C.P. (2005b). Health traditions of Buddhist community and role of amchis in trans-Himalayan region of India. *Current Science,* 89: 1331-1338.

Kala, C.P. (2005c). Indigenous uses, population density, and conservation of threatened medicinal plants in protected areas of the Indian Himalayas. *Conservation Biology,* 19: 368-378.

Kala, C.P. (2005d). Current status of medicinal plants used by traditional *Vaidyas* in Uttaranchal state of India. Ethnobotany. *Research and Applications,* 3: 267-278.

Kala, C.P. (2010). *Medicinal Plants of Uttarakhand: Diversity, Livelihood and Conservation.* Biotech Books, Delhi. 188 p.

Kala, C.P., Dhyani, P.P. and Sajwan, B.S. (2006). Developing the medicinal plants sector in Northern India: challenges and opportunities. *Journal of Ethnobiology and Ethnomedicine,* 2, 1-15.

Kala, C.P. and Sajwan, B.S. (2007). Revitalizing Indian systems of herbal medicine by the National Medicinal Plants Board through institutional networking and capacity building. *Current Science*, 93, 797-806.

Kala, C.P. and Shrivastava, R.J. (2004). Successional changes in Himalayan alpine vegetation: two decades after removal of livestock grazing. *Weed Technology*, 18: 1210-1212.

Kaul, M.K. (1997). *Medicinal Plants of Kashmir and Ladakh.* Indus Publishing Company, New Delhi, India.

Sajwan, B.S. and Kala, C.P. (2007). Conservation of medicinal plants: Conventional and contemporary strategies, regulations and executions. *Indian Forester,* 133 (4), 484-495.

Schippmann, U., Leaman, D.J. and Cunningham, A.B. (2002). *Impact of Cultivation and Gathering of Medicinal Plants on Biodiversity: Global Trends and Issues.* Inter-Department Working Group on Biology Diversity for Food and Agriculture, FAO, Rome, Italy.

Sharma, A.B. (2004). Global Medicinal Plants Demand May Touch $5 Trillion By 2050. *Indian Express.* Monday March 29, 2004.

Ticktin, T. (2004). The ecological applications of harvesting non-timber forest products. *Journal of Applied Ecology*, 41: 11-21.

Varghese, A. and Ticktin, T. (2008). Regional variation in non-timber forest product harvest strategies, trade, and ecological impacts: the case of black dammar (*Canarium strictum* Roxb.) use and conservation in the Nilgiri Biosphere Reserve, India. *Ecology and Society,* 13 (2): 11. [Online] http://www.ecologyandsociety.org/vol13/iss2/art11/

Ved, D.K. and Goraya, G.S. (2008). *Demand and Supply of Medicinal Plants.* Foundation for Revitalization of Local Health Traditions, Bangalore, India. 216 p.

Wallington, T.J., Hobbs, R.J. and Moore, S.A. (2005). Implications of current ecological thinking for biodiversity conservation: A review of the salient issues. *Ecology and Society*, 10 (1): 15. [Online] http://www. ecologyandsociety.org/vol10/iss1/art15/

In: Medicinal Plants and Sustainable Development   ISBN 978-1-61761-942-7
Editor: Chandra Prakash Kala   © 2011 Nova Science Publishers, Inc.

Chapter 18

Conservation and Cultivation of Medicinal Plants for Sustainable Development in Nanda Devi Biosphere Reserve, Uttarakhand, India

L. S. Kandari[1], K. S. Rao[2], R. K. Maikhuri[3] and Abhishek Chandra[4]*

[1]Research Centre for Plant Growth and Development, School of Biological and Conservation Sciences, Private Bag X01, Scottsville 3209, University of KwaZulu-Natal, Pietermaritzburg, South Africa
[2]Department of Botany, University of Delhi, Delhi-110007, India
[3]G.B. Pant Institute of Himalayan Environment and Development, Srinagar Garhwal, 246174, Uttarakhand, India
[4]Department of Environmental Science and Engineering, Guru Jambheshwar University of Science and Technology, Hisar, India

Abstract

The wild collection and cultivation of a variety of medicinal and aromatic plants (MAPs) species provide a critical source of income and livelihood to many tribal and rural communities living in remote and far-flung area. In the Himalaya, collection of medicinal plants from the wild has been an age-old subsidiary occupation of Bhotiya communities, especially in the present study area, the Nanda Devi Biosphere Reserve (NDBR) of Uttarakhand state in India. In this study, attempts have been made to address collection, domestication and *ex-situ* conservation of four species (*Angelica glauca* Edgew., *Arnebia benthamii* Wall. ex G. Don., *Rheum emodi* Wall. ex Meissn. and *Pleurospermum angelicoides* (DC.) C.B. Clarke) by using simple and cost effective technology such as, polyhouse and shade netting. The study suggests that belowground biomass of all the selected rhizomatous species under polyhouse conditions using farm yard manure was 3 fold higher, as compared to control conditions.

* luxkandari@gmail.com

Keywords: Cultivation, Himalaya, Medicinal and Aromatic Plants, Polyhouse, Rural biotechnology.

Introduction

Sustainable management of medicinal plant resources is important, not only because of their value as a potential source of new drugs, but also due to the reliance on traditional medicinal plants for health. The vast majority (70-80%) of the population in developing countries still rely on traditional medicinal practitioners (TMPs) for healthcare (Farnsworth et al., 1985).

Due to rapidly increasing population and degradation of medicinal and aromatic plants (MAPs), sustainable use of such resources has become a challenging task (Kotwal et al., 2008). During the recent past, rising commercial demand for herbal drugs and dependence on produce harvested from the wild has led to the rapid depletion of a number of MAPs (Maikhuri et al., 1998a; 2002; Nautiyal et al., 2002). The bulk of the medicinal plant is still harvested from the wild and only a very small number of species are cultivated (FAO, 1993). About 30% of the drugs sold worldwide contain compounds derived from the plants. Thus, it is now essential to focus on the conservation of natural resources, especially the biodiversity hotspots of the world.

The Nanda Devi Biosphere Reserve (NDBR) in the western Himalaya is one such diverse ecosystem and harbors a wide range of MAPs (Hajra and Balodi, 1995; Samant et al., 1996). MAPs are an essential part of traditional health care systems of the Bhotiya transhumance community of the Garhwal Himalaya inhabiting the northern most mountainous border areas of Chamoli and Uttarkashi districts of Uttarakhand state.

Collection of medicinal plants from the wild has been an ageold subsidiary occupation of Bhotiya communities, usually done while livestock graze in forest and pastures (Rao et al., 2003). The wild collection and cultivation of a variety of MAPs provide a source of income and livelihood for rural communities.

These tribal are rich in ethnobiological and traditional knowledge owing to their close liasion with the local traditions and vegetation (Maikhuri et al., 1998a). However, this traditional knowledge is eroding due to change in social values and non-participation of younger generation in collection and processing (Shalini et al., 2008).

Due to an increase in the demand of herbal and natural products, there is a lot of unsustainable harvesting of MAPs and other forest products. The commercial production of MAPs is attributed reducing gaps between demand and supply in the market by providing green health alternatives and other natural products for both domestic and industrial uses (Boedeker, 2002; Temptesa and King, 1994). Therefore, domestication through cultivation of these valuable MAPs is one of the viable options to meet the growing demand of pharmaceutical industries so as to reduce the existing pressure on their natural habitats (Kala, 2009).

In this study, attempts have been made to address collection, domestication and *ex-situ* conservation of four species (*Angelica glauca, Arnebia benthamii, Rheum emodi* and *Pleurospermum angelicoides*) using different agrotechnology (polyhouse, shade net etc.) in order to reduce pressure on these species in their natural habitats.

Study Area

The study was conducted in Dhauli Ganga catchment of Nanda Devi Biosphere Reserve (NDBR), which is located in Chamoli district of Uttarakhand (30°17' to 30°41' N latitude and 79°40' to 80°05'E longitude) (Figure 1).

It is one of the most important biologically diverse areas of the Uttarakhand Himalaya with a repository of large species of MAPs (Figure 2). The area consists of a total of 14 villages with a total population of 2253 (419 households).

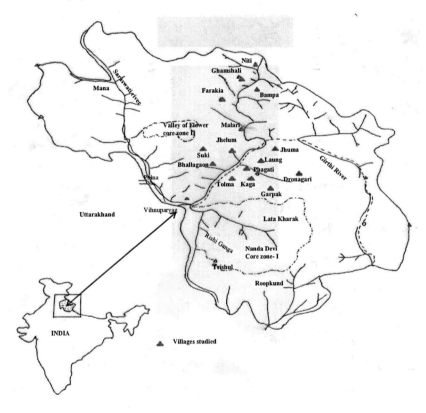

Figure1. Map of the study site in the Nanda Devi Biosphere reserve (Not to Scale).

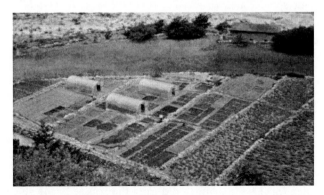

Figure 2. An overview of the study site (Photo by: L.S. Kandari).

Climatic Conditions

The daily temperatures were recorded using a thermometer for a period of January 2003 to December 2003. A monthly minimum and maximum temperatures were between 2 to 16 °C, and 15.3°C to 27.2 °C respectively. June and August are the hottest months of the year. The total annual rainfall is about 936.6 mm/year. About 43% of annual rainfall occurs over a short period of two months i.e., July and August with strong monsoonic currents (Figure 3).

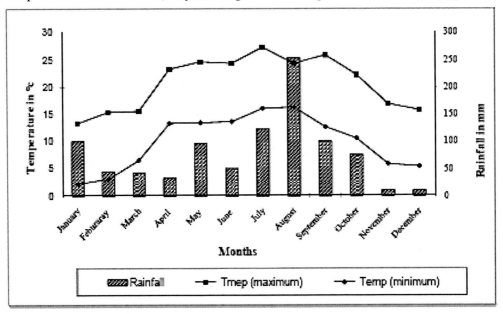

Figure 3. Climatic data of the study area.

Methodology

Ethnobotanical Study

An ethnobotanical survey was conducted in 14 villages of NDBR for the traditional and indigenous use of four species i.e., *A. glauca*, *A. benthamii*, *R. emodi* and *P. angelicoides*. Interviews with the local people, vaidyas, herbal practitioners, and older members of the community were conducted with the help of questionnaires. Information on local name of the plant, the local use and plant parts used for various purposes of each species was gathered.

Impact of Different Microclimatic Conditions and FYM on Belowground Biomass

Impact of polyhouse, shade net and farm yard manure (FYM) on below ground biomass of four selected species was also investigated during the course of the study. A polyhouse (10 X2 X3 m) was erected with the help of an iron frame and polythene sheet from all the sides.

A door was kept open in the front end of the polyhouse for access and ventilation. Shade net was made up with bamboo frame (10 X 2 X 3 m) and cover of a sheet of 50% Nelton agronets, which was obtainedfrom Parry and Co. Ltd Vadodara.

The top and sides were covered with 50% Shading net (green and black; Nelton agronets). Farm yard manure was prepared with a mixture of decomposed cow dung, sheep dung and decomposed leaves (leaf litter) in equal volume, *i.e.*, (1:1:1v/v). An open field space without any cover or modification was considered as control conditions. No manure was added in control beds.

Results

Sustainable Approach towards Maps Cultivation in NDBR

Even before and after the creation of Uttarakhand, medicinal plant cultivation and conservation was clearly identified as potential resources for uplifting the state's economy. Uttarakhand Government had already prioritized potential species for the state (Table 1) and signed a memorandum of understanding (MoU) with several companies/industries for the assured buy-back arrangements. With a change in the development paradigm, which is bringing people to the centre of all activates, the issues of medicinal plants cultivation has been prioritized. It was estimated that 60% of thecollected MAPs species were consumed by villagers in NDBR themselves for a variety of purposes. The local people knew a few medicinal plants, which they used to cure various diseases (Table 2).

**Table 1. Medicinal and aromatic plants species listed for promotion
of cultivation by the Uttarakhand Government.**

Local name	Botanical name
Kutki	*Picrorhiza kurroa* Benth.
Sarpagandha	*Rauvolfia serpentina* Benth.
Lavender	*Lavendula angustifolia* Mill.,
Atish	*Aconitum heterophyllum* Wall. ex Royle.
Tagar	*Pleurospermum densifolium* DC.
Jatamansi	*Nardostachys jatamansi* DC.
Chiraiyta	*Swertia chiraiyta* Karsten.
Kuth	*Saussurea costus* (Falc) Lipsch.

(Maikhuri et al., 2005

Due to imposition of conservation policies, many farmers of NDBR, using their indigenous knowledge, are now slowly shifting towards cultivation of high value and low volume MAPs in their kitchen garden *i.e.*, *Angelica glauca*, *Arnebia benthamii*, *Pleurospermum angelicoides* and *Allium* spp. Mostly some of the rhizomatous parts are usually sundried. After sun drying, it becomes easier to carry to the market and also it prevents rhizomes from decaying.

Table 2. Indigenous uses of few selected medicinal plants used by local people for their Daily Use

S. No	Species	Family	Local name	Part used	Indigenous uses
1	*Aconitum ferox* Stapf.	Ranunculaceae	Bish	Root	Tuberous roots used in cough, asthma and leprosy
2	*Aconitum heterophyllum* Wall. ex Royle,	Ranunculaceae	Atish	Root	Fever, cold and cough, diarrhea, piles
3	*Allium stracheyi* Baker	Alliaceae	Jimbu pharan	Leaves	Spice, jaundice and cough
4	*Allium humile* Kunth	Alliaceae	Ladum pharan	Leaves	Spice, jaundice and cough
5	*Angelica glauca* Edgew.	Apiaceae	Choru	Rhizome	Spice, stomachdisorder, diarrhea,
6	*Arnebia benthamii* (Wall. ex G. Don)	Boraginaceae	Baalchadi	Rhizome	Baldness
7	*Bergenia ciliata* (Haworth) Sternb.	Saxifragaceae	Pakhanbed	Roots	Kidney stones, cuts and wounds
8	*Betula utilis* D. Don.	Betulaceae	Bhojpatra	Bark	The bark is used in roofs for wood protection from soil and also used for packing.
9	*Carum carvi* Linn.	Umbeliferae	Kala zira	Seeds	Seeds used as spice, carminative, back pain, liver problem and stimulant
10	*Nardostachys jatamansi* DC.	Valeriananceae	Jatamansi	Roots	The root used for blood purification, stomach disorder, cardiac problems and jaundice. Local people use root as incense.
12	*Picrorhiza kurroa* Benth.	Scrophulariaceae	Kutki	Roots	Used as blood purification, stomach disorder, cardiac problems
13	*Pleurospermum angelicoides* (DC.) C.B.Clarke	Apiaceae	Chippi	Rhizome	Decoction of the root is used to cure stomach disorder, headache, typhoid, rheumatism. Also used as a spice and condiment.
14	*Podophyllum hexandrum* Royle.	Podophyllaceae	Bankakri	Fruit and Seed	Used in wounds/cuts, tuberculosis and constipation
15	*Potentilla fulgens* Wall.ex Hk.	Rosaceae	Bajradanti	Roots/leaves	The root powder is considered to cure toothache & pyorrhea.
16	*Rheum emodi* Wall. ex Meissn.	Polygonaceae	Dolu	Root/leaves	Used in internal injury, cold and cough. .
17	*Saussurea costus* (Falc) Lipsch.	Asteraceae	Kuth	Roots	Roots used as cuts and wounds, rheumatism.
18	*Taxus baccata* L.	Taxaceae	Thunear	Bark	Local people use the bark as a substitute for tea.

Collection from the Wild

All the selected four plant species i.e., *A. glauca*, *A. benthamii*, *R. emodi* and *P. angelicoides*, are used for medicines, aromatic, spicing and condiments purposes. *A. glauca* was collected at volume of between 210 kg/year to 150 kg/year by the villagers of Garpak and Tolma, respectively. *R. emodi* and *A. benthamii* were collected in less quantity due to their low economic return since their uses were limited among tribes. *R emodi* extracted maximum (20 kg/year) in Tolma village, followed by 15 kg/year in Rewing village. However, about 22.5 kg/year of *A. benthamii* was collected by the people of Malari village followed by 18.75 kg/year in Rewing village from forest (Figure 4).

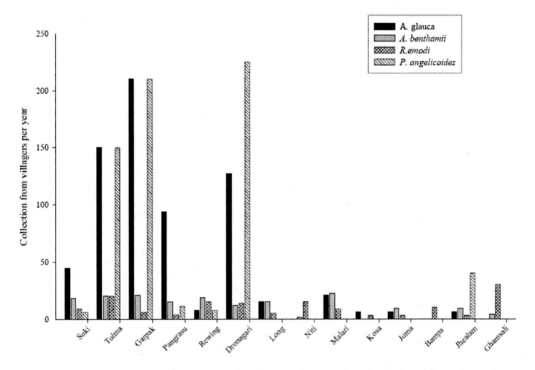

Figure 4. Collection of *R emodi*, *A glauca*, *A benthamii* and *P angelicoides* (kg/year) from the study site.

Cultivation in the Kitchen Garden

The area under the kitchen garden is very small in all buffer zone villages. Overall conditions from the kitchen garden by different species vary according to the priority of the species *i.e.,* economic potential and market value. Due to limited cultivated land area, 47% families in Dronagari and Garpak villages cultivate only *P. angelicoides*. Only 27-40% of families of Tolma and Garpak village cultivate *A. benthamii*, *A. glauca* and *R. emodi* (Figure 5).

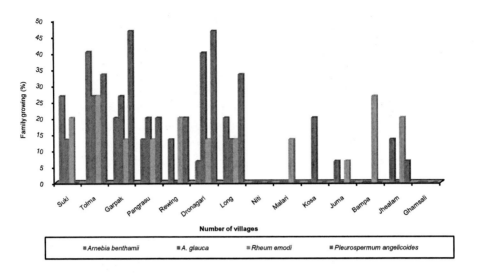

Figure 5. Cultivation of *A. glauca, A. benthamii, P. angelicoides* and *R. emodi* in the kitchen garden.

Estimation of Belowground Biomass

Polyhouse conditions have a remarkable effect on belowground biomass of these rhizomatous species. In *A. glauca* the maximum belowground biomass obtained is 71.7 ± 0.98 g/plant dry .wt. with FYM treatment, under polyhouse conditions. In *A. benthamii,* the maximum belowground biomass using FYM under polyhouse conditions was 225.1 ± 12.8 g/ dry.wt. followed by FYM treatment in open conditions. In the case of *R. emodi* belowground biomass using FYM treatment in polyhouse conditions was estimated 840 ± 4.02 g/ dry. wt. In *P. angelicoides*, the maximum belowground biomass using FYM treatment was 88.8 ± 12.5g/ dry. wt. under polyhouse (Figure 6).

Discussion

In the present study belowground biomass of all the rhizomatous species under polyhouse conditions using FYM was three-fold higher as compared to control conditions.

Chauhan and Nautiyal (2005) also found that economic yield of *Nardostachys jatamansi* increased with the addition of manure (FYM) in all the treatments and altitudes compared to control. Several workers have also supported addition of biofertilizer for the improvement of soil quality (Kostov et al., 1996; Kasera and Sharan, 2002). Therefore, *ex-situ* conservation of MAPs and management through various techniques along with establishment of the herbal gardens can be used to protect MAPs population from extinction.

Cultivation of medicinal herbs is an incentive to reduce human pressure on the high-altitude forest, providing enough time for these forest to regenerate after severe degradation due to anthropogenic impacts in the recent past (Babu et al., 1984; Moench, 1989; Zhou, 1993; Rao and Saxena, 1994; Farooque and Saxena, 1996; Kala et al., 1997; Maikhuri et al., 1998b; Kala, 2005).

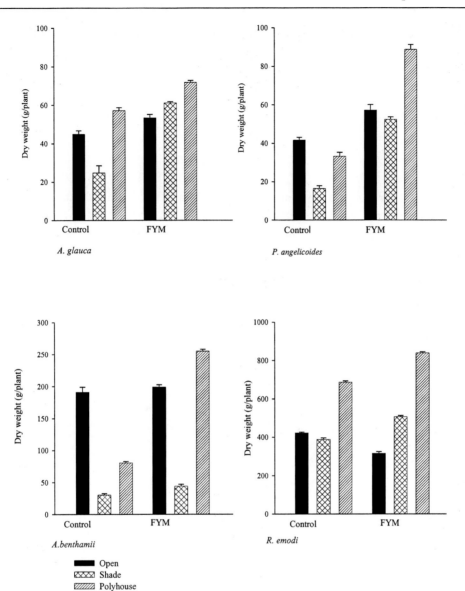

Figure 6. Belowground biomass under different microclimatic conditions.

MAPs also have a huge potential to generate employment opportunities in this hilly region, where lack of alternative employment opportunities make people migrate to the lower plains, (Silori and Badola, 1999, 2000; Farooque, 1994; Hoon, 1996). Farmers may be encouraged to cultivate these species, which have huge economic potential.

Conservation priority should also be given to multipurpose plants (plants with more diversified medicinal uses), as this could indicate high intensity of harvest, which could lead to overexploitation. Maikhuri et al., (1998b), projected that the productivity of medicinal herbs could be subsequently increased by more advanced techniques and proper management.

Therefore, a suitable cost effective agrotechnology for cultivation would be helpful for the sustainable conservation of these MAPs of the region. *In-situ* conservation measures are also required on those medicinal plants, which are found to be scarce in the study area, but are still harvested from the wild only.

Local people and farmers may be encouraged to undertake cultivation of MAPs in order to reduce the pressure on natural population and also reduce illegal extraction activity in the area.

Conclusion

The area under MAPs cultivation in the study area is still quite less, and people mostly cultivate those species in their marginal land, which has low volume and high cost. The present study shows that cultivating medicinal plants in polyhouses is beneficial to some extent. The productive yield of all four species (i.e., *A. glauca, A. benthamii, R. emodi* and *P. angelicoides*) increased 3 to 4 times in polyhouse condition, as compared to control conditions. This low cost agrotechnology is one of the viable methods for multiplication and conservation of MAPs. At present, due to increase in tourism, especially for trekking and mountaineering, the preferences of local youths have shifted from farming to tourism. There is also a decline in the numbers of practitioners who practice and possess knowledge of herbal care. Awareness programmes related to conservation of bioresources focusing MAPs should be initiated in this area. People should be made aware about collection, cleaning, drying and storage techniques about MAPs. Since about 70% of MAPs in the NDBR are harvested from the wild, there is a need to develop adequate strategy and action plan for the conservation and management for these bio-resources.

Acknowledgments

Authors are thankful to the Director, G.B. Pant Institute of Himalayan Environment and Development, Kosi-Katmal, Almora and Indian Council of Agriculture Research (ICAR), New Delhi for providing financial support.

References

Babu, C.R., Gaston, A.J., Chauduri, A. and Khandwa, R. (1984). Effect of human disturbance in the three areas of west Himalaya deciduous forest. *Environmental Conservation*, 11: 55-60.

Boedeker, G. (2002). *Medicinal Plants: Towards Sustainability and Security*. IDRC Medicinal Plants Global Network Sponsored Discussion Paper for WOCMAP III, Chiang Mai, Thailand.

Chauhan, R.S. and Nautiyal, M.C. (2005). Commercial viability of cultivation of an endangered medicinal herb *Nardostachys jatamansi* at three different agroclimatic zones. *Current Science*, 9: 1481-1488.

Farnsworth, N.R. Akerele, O. and Bingel, A.S. (1985). Medicinal plants in therapy. *Bulletin of World Health Organisation*, 63: 965–981.

Farooque, N.A. (1994). Transhumance in the Central Himalaya: A case study of its impacts on environment [Ph.D thesis]. HNB Garhwal University, Srinagar Garhwal, India.

Farooque, N.A. and Saxena, K.G. (1996). Conservation and utilization of medicinal plants in high hills of the central Himalayas. *Environmental Conservation*, 23: 75-80.

Food and Agriculture Organisatation (1993). *International trade on Non-Wood Forest Products. An overview*. FAO, Rome.

Hajra, P.K. and Balodi, B. (1995). *Plant wealth of Nanda Devi Biosphere Reserve*. Botanical Survey of India, Calcutta.

Hoon, V. (1996). *Living on the Move. Bhotiya tribe of Himalaya*. Sage Publications, New Delhi.

Kala, C.P. (2005). Indigenous uses, population density and conservation of threatened medicinal plants in protected areas of the Indian Himalayas. *Conservation Biology*, 19: 368-378.

Kala, C.P. (2009). Medicinal plants conservation and enterprise development. *Medicinal Plants*, 1 (2): 79-95.

Kala, C.P., Rawat, G.S. and Uniyal, V.K. (1997). *Ecology and Conservation of the Valley of Flower National Park, Garhwal Himalaya*. Wildlife Institute of India, Dehradun, India.

Kasera, P.K. and Sharan, P. (2002). Economics of Evolutions alsinoides (sankhpusphi) from Indian Thar Desert. *Annals of Forestry*, 10: 167-171.

Kostov, O. Tzvetkov, Y., Kalonianova, N. and Cleemput, V. (1996). Production of tomato seedlings on compost of vine branches, grape pruning, husk and seeds. *Compost Science and Utilization*, 4: 55-61.

Kotwal, P.C., Omprakash, M.D., Kandari, L.S., Mali, K.P., Badyal, M. and Mishra, A. (2008). Sustainable forest management through community participation. *Current Science*, 95: 1015-1017.

Maikhuri, R.K., Nautiyal, S., Rao, K.S. and Saxena, K.G. (1998a). Medicinal plants cultivation and Biosphere Reserve Management.: A case study from Nanda Devi Biosphere Reserve, Himalaya. *Current Science*, 74: 157-163.

Maikhuri, R.K., Nautiyal, S., Rao, K.S. and Saxena, K.G. (1998b). Role of medicinal plants in the traditional health care system: a case study from Nanda Devi Biosphere Reserve, Himalaya. *Current Science*, 75: 152-157.

Maikhuri, R.K., Rao, K.S., Chauhan, K., Kandari, L.S., Prasad, P., Negi, G.S. Nautiyal, S, Purohit, A., Rajasekaran,C and Saxena, K.G. (2002). *Cultivation and Conservation of higher Himalayan medicinal plants through participation and action research: A case study from the central Himalaya (Uttarakhand), India*. Proceeding of the Regional Workshop on wise Practices and Experiential learning in Conservation and Management of Himalayan Medicinal Plants. December, 15-20, Kathmandu, Nepal.

Maikhuri, R.K., Rao, K.S., Kandari, L.S., Joshi, R. and Dhyani, D. (2005). Does the outreach programme make an impact? A case study of medicinal and aromatic plants cultivation in Uttarakhand. *Current Science*, 88: 1480-1486.

Moench, M. (1989). Forest degradation and the structure of biomass in a Himalayan foothills village. *Environmental Conservation*, 16: 137-146.

Nautiyal, S., Rao, K.S., Maikhuri, R.K., Negi, K.S. and Kala, C.P. (2002). Status of medicinal plants on way to Vashuki Tal in Mandakini Valley, Garhwal, Uttaranchal. *Journal of Non-Timber Forest Products*, 9: 124-131.

Rao, K.S. and Saxena, K.G. (1994). *Sustainable Development and Rehabilitation of Degraded village Lands in Himalaya*. Bishen Singh Mahendra Pal Singh, Dehradun, India.

Rao, K.S., Semwal, R.L., Maikhuri, R.K., Nautiyal, S., Sen, K.K., Singh, K., Chandrasekhar, K. and Saxena, K.G. (2003). Indigenous ecological knowledge biodiversity and sustainable development in the central Himalayas. *Tropical Ecology*, 44: 93-111.

Samant, S.S., Dhar, U. and Rawal, R.S. (1996). Natural resources uses by some native within Nanda Devi Biosphere Reserve in west Himalaya. *Ethnobotany*, 8: 40-50.

Shalini, M., Maikhuri, R.K., Kala, C.P., Rao, K.S. and Saxena, K.G. (2008). Wild leafy vegetables: A study of their subsistence dietetic support to the inhabitants of Nanda Devi Biosphere Reserve, India. *Journal of Ethnobiology and Ethnomedicine*, 1-9.

Silori, C.S. and Badola, R. (1999). *Nanda Devi Biosphere Reserve: A case study on Socio-economic aspects for the sustainable development of dependent population*. Wildlife Institute of India, Dehradun, India.

Silori, C.S. and Badola, R. (2000). Medicinal Plant cultivation and Sustainable Development: A case study in the buffer zone of the Nanda Devi Biosphere Reserve, Western Himalaya, India. *Mountain Research and Development,* 20: 272-279.

Temptesa, M.S. and King, S. (1994). Tropical Plants as a Source of New Pharmaceuticals. In: *Pharmaceutical Manufacturing International: The International Review of Pharmaceutical Technology Research and Development.* Barnacal, P.S. (ed.). Sterling Publications Ltd., London.

Zhou, S. (1993). Cultivation of *Amomum villosum* in tropical forests. *Forest Ecology and Management*, 60: 157-162.

List of Contributors

Gabriela Růžičková
Department of Crop Science,
Breeding and Plant Medicine,
Faculty of Agronomy,
Mendel University, Zemědělská 1, 61300
Brno, The Czech Republic

Prokop Šmirous
AGRITEC, Research,
Breeding & Services, Ltd.,
Zemědělská 16, 78701
Šumperk, The Czech Republic

Blanka Kocourková
Department of Crop Science,
Breeding and Plant Medicine,
Faculty of Agronomy,
Mendel University, Zemědělská 1, 61300
Brno, The Czech Republic

Antonín Vaculík
AGRITEC, Research,
Breeding & Services, Ltd.,
Zemědělská 16, 78701 Šumperk,
The Czech Republic

Ricardo Gomez-Flores
Departamento de Microbiología e
Inmunología,
Laboratorio de Inmunología y Virología,
Facultad de Ciencias Biológicas,
Universidad Autónoma de Nuevo León,
San Nicolás de los Garza, N. L., México.

Patricia Tamez-Guerra
Departamento de Microbiología e
Inmunología,
Laboratorio de Inmunología y Virología,
Facultad de Ciencias Biológicas,
Universidad Autónoma de Nuevo León,
San Nicolás de los Garza, N. L.,
México.

Arun M Dixit
Centre for Environment and Social Concerns
(CESC),
Ahmedabad, Gujarat, India

Chandra S. Silori
RECOFTC-The Centre for People and
Forest,
Bangkok, Thailand

Yashwant S. Rawat
G.B. Pant Institute of Himalayan
Environment and Development,
Kosi-Katarmal, Almora, 263643,
Uttarakhand, India

Subhash C.R. Vishvakarma
G.B. Pant Institute of Himalayan
Environment and Development,
Kosi-Katarmal, Almora, 263643,
Uttarakhand, India

Jitendra S. Butola
G.B. Pant Institute of Himalayan
Environment and Development,
Kosi- Katarmal, Almora - 263643
Uttarakhand, India

S.S. Samant
G.B. Pant Institute of Himalayan
Environment and Development,
Mohal-Kullu-175126
Himachal Pradesh, India

Rajiv K. Vashistha
HAPPRC, Post Box No. - 14,
HNB Garhwal University
Srinagar Garhwal – 246174
Uttarakhand,
India

A.R. Malik
Division of Forestry,
SKUAST-K, Shalimar,
Srinagar - 191121
Jammu & Kashmir,India

Zubaida Yousaf
Department of Botany,
Lahore College for Women University,
Lahore, Pakistan
z4zubaida@yahoo.com

Uzma Hussain
Department of Botany,
Pir Mehr Ali Shah Arid Agriculture
University
Rawalpindi, Pakistan

Aisha Anjum
Department of Botany,
Pir Mehr Ali Shah Arid Agriculture
University, Rawalpindi
Pakistan

Daniel P. Kisangau
Department of Physical and Biological
Sciences,
South Eastern University College,
P.O. Box 170-90200, Kitui, Kenya

H. V.M. Lyaruu
Department of Physical and Biological
Sciences,
South Eastern University College,
P.O. Box 170-90200, Kitui, Kenya

K. M. Hosea
Department of Molecular Biology and
Biotechnology,
P.O. Box 35060,
University of Dar es Salaam,
Dar es Salaam, Tanzania

C. C. Joseph
Department of Chemistry,
University of Dar es Salaam,
P.O. Box 35061, Dar es Salaam,
Tanzania

L. N. Bruno
Department of Chemistry,
Organic and Bioorganic Chemistry,
Bielefeld University,
P.O Box 100131,
33501, Bielefeld, Germany

K. P. Devkota
Department of Chemistry,
Organic and Bioorganic Chemistry,
Bielefeld University,
P.O Box 100131,
33501, Bielefeld, Germany

T. Bogner
Department of Chemistry,
Organic and Bioorganic Chemistry,
Bielefeld University,
P.O Box 100131,
33501, Bielefeld, Germany

N. Sewald
Department of Chemistry,
Organic and Bioorganic Chemistry,
Bielefeld University,
P.O Box 100131,
33501, Bielefeld, Germany

Yudhvir K. Bhoon
Sri Venkateswara College,
University of Delhi, Dhaula Kuan,
New Delhi – 110021, India

Yamini Chaturvedi
Sugarcane Research Station,
Kunraghat, Gorakhpur
Uttar Pradesh, 273008, India

Madhupriya
Sugarcane Research Station,
Kunraghat, Gorakhpur
Uttar Pradesh, 273008, India

G.P. Rao
Sugarcane Research Station,
Kunraghat, Gorakhpur
Uttar Pradesh, 273008, India

Arvind Bhatt
School of Biological Sciences,
Universiti Sains Malaysia,
11800, Penang, Malaysia

A.K. Bisht
Department of Botany,
Govt. Degree College,
Narayan Nagar, Didihat
Pithoragarh, Uttarakhand, India

Bharat Babu Shrestha
Central Department of Botany,
Tribhuvan University,
Kathmandu, Nepal
bhabashre@yahoo.com

Stephano Dall'Acqua
Department of Pharmaceutical Sciences,
University of Padova, Padova, Italy

Jayanti Ray Mukherjee
Dept of Wildland Resources,
Utah State University,
Logan, Utah 84321, USA

V. Chelladurai
Survey of Medicinal Plant Unit,
Siddha, Palayamkottai,
Tamil Nadu, India

J. Ronald
Wildlife Institute of India,
P.B. # 18, Chandrabani,
Dehradun, Uttarakhand,
India

G. S. Rawat
Wildlife Institute of India,
P.B. # 18, Chandrabani,
Dehradun, Uttarakhand,
India

P. Mani
Survey of Medicinal Plant Unit,
Siddha, Palayamkottai,
Tamil Nadu, India

M. A. Huffman
Primate Research Institute,
Kyoto University,
Inuyama Aichi 484, Japan.

M. Ayyanar
Entomology Research Institute,
Loyola College,
Chennai – 600034,
Tamil Nadu, India

S. Ignacimuthu
Entomology Research Institute,
Loyola College,
Chennai – 600034,
Tamil Nadu, India

P.C. Phondani
G.B. Pant Institute of Himalayan
Environment & Development
P. Box 92, Garhwal Unit,
Srinagar Garhwal – 246174,
Uttarakhand, India

R.K. Maikhuri
G.B. Pant Institute of Himalayan
Environment & Development
P. Box 92, Garhwal Unit,
Srinagar Garhwal – 246174,
Uttarakhand, India

C.S. Negi
G.B. Pant Institute of Himalayan
Environment & Development
P. Box 92, Garhwal Unit,
Srinagar Garhwal – 246174,
Uttarakhand, India

Chandra Prakash Kala
Ecosystem & Environment Management,
Indian Institute of Forest Management,
Nehru Nagar, Bhopal– 462003,
Madhya Pradesh, India

M.S. Rawat
National Medicinal Plants Board,
Janpath, New Delhi, 110001, India

N.S. Bisht
H.N.B. Garhwal Central University,
B.G.R. Campus Pauri Garhwal
Uttarakhand – 246001, India

Maria Costanza Torri
University of Toronto Scarborough,

Department of Social Sciences,
Canada
mctorri@yahoo.it

Thora Martina Herrmann
Canada Research Chair in Etynoecology &
Biodiversity Conservation,
Université de Montréal,
Canada,
thora.martina.herrmann@umontreal.ca

Maria Luiza Schwarz
Department of Geography,
Université de Montréal,
Canada,
luizaschwarz@videotron.ca

L.S. Kandari
Research Centre for Plant Growth &
Development,
School of Biological & Conservation
Sciences,
Private Bag X01,
Scottsville 3209,
University of KwaZulu-Natal,
Pietermaritzburg, South Africa

K.S. Rao
Department of Botany,
University of Delhi,
Delhi-110007, India

Abhishek Chandra
Department of Environmental Science &
Engineering, Guru Jambheshwar University
of Science & Technology, Hisar 125001,
India

Index